Contemporary Treatment Techniques in Pediatric Dentistry

Meenakshi S. Kher • Ashwin Rao

Contemporary Treatment Techniques in Pediatric Dentistry

Springer

Meenakshi S. Kher
Happy Tooth Clinic for Kids
Mumbai
India

Ashwin Rao
MCODS Mangalore, Manipal Academy
of Higher Education
Manipal
India

ISBN 978-3-030-11859-4 ISBN 978-3-030-11860-0 (eBook)
https://doi.org/10.1007/978-3-030-11860-0

Library of Congress Control Number: 2019934822

This Springer imprint is published by the registered company Springer Nature Switzerland AG
The registered company address is: Gewerbestrasse 11, 6330 Cham, Switzerland

Preface

In clinical practice, to continually apply scientific evidence when planning treatment requires vigilant review of literature, recommendations, and guidelines. Very often, it is hard for a busy clinician to keep abreast of latest developments, and it becomes easy to get comfortable in one's old ways. As a young enthusiastic graduate, I first started practicing pediatric dentistry exclusively in 1995. Focused on the principles of pediatric dentistry I had learnt back then, I managed behavior with passion, treated lesions with dedication, and sincerely carried out preventive protocols. In the meantime, researchers were working hard at further understanding the disease dental caries. But as a practicing clinician, O. Fejerskov's landmark article of 1997 was lost on me, and nothing changed in the way I practiced pediatric dentistry. I continued treating lesions mechanically. Thankfully, I documented my clinical work and meticulously followed up on long-term treatment outcomes. And as more than a decade went by, I noticed dental caries affecting sections of society in India that had until then been unaffected. Families that could ill afford dentistry were succumbing to dental caries with the improving economy and rise in sugar consumption. Our treatment interventions did not seem to have any effect on the disease.

New evidence frequently requires us to unlearn and relearn, forcing us to conceptualize disease in entirely new ways. When I finally started looking at dental caries anew, the changes it brought to the way we practiced were immense! We stopped being "Lesion Obsessed" and worked harder at managing the "Disease." Predictably, our management of lesions became less aggressive and more minimally invasive with our change in perspective. The paradigm shift this brought to our practice and the immense benefits I saw it bring to the families and children we treated encouraged me to share my experiences.

This book discusses two crucial aspects of clinical pediatric dentistry—contemporary management of dental caries and strategies to manage the pulp in immature permanent teeth. When studying contemporary "Carious Lesion Management" techniques, a clinician reading this work must remember that dental caries being a disease of the plaque biofilm, the lesion is but a consequence of the disease. All efforts to treat a symptomatic tooth, stop the progression of an active lesion or improve aesthetics and function must be made keeping in mind that simultaneous disease management strategies are paramount. The last chapter discusses pulp therapy in immature permanent teeth. Our renewed understanding of the regenerative potential of the immature permanent tooth has brought about revolutionary changes in treatment approaches that enhance outcomes greatly.

The merits of visual learning cannot be overstated, and I believe we learn and reproduce procedures best when we see them. With the unflinching support of my team at the "Happy Tooth Clinic for Kids," I have painstakingly documented and followed up on each treatment technique, and the pictures explain every procedure step-by-step. My coauthor Dr. Ashwin Rao being a well-regarded teacher and academic has brought the wealth of his expertise to this book. Together we hope that this work encourages the practice of evidence-based pediatric dentistry in the best interests of the child because the child's well-being is ultimately of primary concern to us all!

Mumbai, India
November 2018

Meenakshi Sivasankar Kher

Acknowledgments

To realize a dream requires the help and support of many.

A visual essay, the value of this book lies in its photographic documentation. Thank you Udatta Kher for teaching me, more than two decades ago, how to hold an SLR camera and how to focus and shoot intraoral pictures. Even today, you help technologically challenged me with my camera, lens, and flash settings. I am grateful for your sharp clinical acumen that helps me ideate and makes me seek your advice from time to time. Thank you for being there!

This book is the product of teamwork and would have been impossible without the relentless hard work and support of my team at the "Happy Tooth Clinic for Kids." Thank you Dr. Priyanka Desai for helping me with the clinical documentation and organization each step of the way. Your dedication to my cause and your support have been invaluable. Dr. Mitali Kochar, thank you for your enthusiastic participation on this journey, for relentlessly following up on patient recalls and always staying positive. I could not have done this without the two of you and our team, Movin Lewis, Priya Kulkarni, Suvarna Chavan, Nirmala Waghmare, and Sunanda Bodke.

I appreciate Springer Nature for their faith in this project, Josie Quehl for expanding the scope of this book with her erudite suggestions, and Markus Bartels for being a supportive editor. Thank you Smitha Diveshan for your efficient coordination with the Production Team.

The young pediatric dental community in India has a fervent desire to keep up with contemporary dental science that is infectious! I thank them all for the constant interactions and impassioned discussions!

Dr. Ashwin Rao, I remember my first call to invite you to join this project. You have been an able and reassuring collaborator, and your vast experience, as a teacher and academic, has been invaluable to this work. I could not have asked for a better person to partner me. Thank you!

To my child Saatvik, "I am grateful for your presence and thankful to you for reminding me everyday that I must do for my patients exactly what I would have done for you!"

November 2018, Mumbai Meenakshi Sivasankar Kher

Contents

Lesion Management: No Removal of Carious Tissue

1

1.1 Overview

Treatment modalities for managing a carious lesion in primary teeth have been wide-ranging. At one end of the spectrum is the traditional now obsolete technique where carious tissue is removed completely and, on the other hand, is the contemporary approach where carious tissue is not removed at all or removed selectively [1]. Managing a carious lesion without removing carious tissue may sound extreme but is based on current evidence-based understanding, which expounds that the disease dental caries occurs at the level of the plaque biofilm. The pathogenicity of the plaque biofilm located on the tooth and lesion surface is dependent on the microbial environment in the biofilm. Hence controlling the activity of the biofilm on the tooth and lesion surface should be the aim of treatment [1].

Carious lesions can be described as cleansable, potentially cleansable, or non-cleansable depending on how accessible the biofilm on the surface of the lesion is. Cleansable lesions are non-cavitated lesions easily amenable to plaque disruption. Potentially cleansable lesions are cavitated dentinal lesions that permit evaluation of lesion activity and visual and tactile inspection by the operator and are judged by the operator to be cleansable by the caretaker/child. In non-cleansable carious lesions, the plaque biofilm is sheltered under the undercuts in the carious lesion and is inaccessible to a toothbrush or adjunctive cleaning devices. Cleansable and potentially cleansable lesions can be inactivated and managed conservatively without removing any carious tissue using the "non-restorative cavity control" method [2]. Non-cleansable lesions can be conservatively managed by transforming them to cleansable lesions by widening them and making them accessible to plaque disruption. They can then be treated in the same way as cleansable lesions. Other strategies include sealing in the carious lesion, which involves "fissure sealing" occlusal cleansable lesions and the "Hall technique" [1]. Early non-cavitated proximal lesions can be treated in a minimally invasive way using "resin infiltration" [3].

M. S. Kher, A. Rao, *Contemporary Treatment Techniques in Pediatric Dentistry*,
https://doi.org/10.1007/978-3-030-11860-0_1

These treatment modalities are of special value in children whose cooperation is limited by age, behavior, and disabilities. In the absence of these minimally invasive techniques, clinical intervention would require the use of pharmacological behavior management techniques. The lesion management techniques described here help the clinician arrest the progress of active carious lesions in these children and in some situations allow the operator to buy time for more definitive treatment alternatives until the child is older. This conservative method of managing carious lesions without removing carious tissue helps the anxious child cope with dental treatment and positively influences both treatment outcomes and children's attitudes toward dentistry. The following subchapters describe in detail the various treatment modalities under this novel approach of managing carious lesions in children.

1.2 Non-restorative Cavity Control Using 5% Sodium Fluoride Varnish

1.2.1 Introduction

Non-restorative cavity control (NRCC) using 5% sodium fluoride varnish is a progressive approach to carious lesion management, which seeks to inactivate and arrest carious lesions rather than removing carious tissue and restoring a lesion. This is a treatment modality for primary teeth where cleansable and potentially cleansable lesions can be managed in a manner that is minimally invasive. NRCC (also referred to as non-operative caries treatment) views the carious lesion as a localized symptom of the disease caused by the undisturbed accumulation of plaque. Certain areas of the teeth are subjected to limited mechanical forces of mastication and toothbrushing and to greater accumulation of plaque. These areas called the plaque stagnation areas (PSA) demonstrate increased propensity to developing a carious lesion [4]. NRCC using fluoride varnish aims at arresting the progression of the carious lesion by mechanical disturbance of plaque through toothbrushing, professional plaque removal, and fluoride delivery. In addition, narrow cavitated lesions with limited access to plaque removal can be transformed to cleansable lesions by opening up the cavity, thus making them amenable to mechanical plaque disruption and removal [2]. Caregivers play a decisive role in disrupting plaque through daily meticulous toothbrushing. Fluoride is delivered on the tooth and lesion surface through the use of dentifrices that contain fluoride in a high concentration ideally 1450 ppm [4, 5]. This is in conjunction with professional oral prophylaxis and fluoride varnish application regimens using 5% sodium fluoride varnish [4]. Due to the restricted remineralizing ability of fluoride varnish, the success of this technique is limited by the compliance of the parent [4] to stop inappropriate feeding habits, control sugar exposure, follow diligent oral hygiene methods, and maintain the affected areas free of plaque.

1.2.2 Indications and Contraindications

- Primary tooth surfaces that exhibit active enamel demineralization, white spot lesions, and non-cavitated cleansable lesions [2].
- In potentially cleansable lesions [2], when the caregiver does not consent to the use of silver diamine fluoride (Sect. 1.3) because of the black discoloration that it causes. It should be noted here that NRCC using 5% sodium fluoride varnish is most effective on enamel lesions.
- In children in whom cooperation is limited by age or disabilities and performing conventional operative dentistry becomes a challenge.
- A motivated caregiver being a prerequisite for the success of NRCC using sodium fluoride varnish [5], a positive outcome of the procedure is caregiver driven rather than operator driven.

1.2.3 Rationale

The carious lesion is currently viewed as a localized symptom of the disease—dental caries. When plaque accumulates and remains undisturbed on the tooth and lesion surface, it causes initiation and progression of the lesion. Non-restorative cavity control is founded on the rationale that mechanical disruption of plaque accompanied by controlling consumption of refined sugars will play a primary role in halting initiation and progression of the lesion. Simultaneously, exposure of the tooth and lesion surface to fluoride delivered by the caregiver and operator will contribute to lesion arrest. NRCC is an optimum combination of home and professional disruption of plaque along with the use of fluoridated dentifrices and professionally applied fluoride varnishes to comprehensively inactivate the carious lesions.

1.2.4 Case Study 1: NRCC with 5% Sodium Fluoride Varnish

1.2.4.1 Case Selection

Why Was This Case Selected for NRCC with 5% Sodium Fluoride Varnish?

- This 10-month-old child presented with extensive enamel demineralization and plaque stagnation on the entire labial and palatal surfaces of the partially erupted upper incisors.
- Carious lesions extending to the dentine were apparent on the incisal surfaces of teeth 52, 61, and 62. Tooth 51 had a small labial lesion extending to the dentine. The lesions were judged to be potentially cleansable.
- The child did not show any signs of discomfort or pain.
- Due to aesthetic concerns, the parents did not consent to the use of silver diamine fluoride to arrest the dentinal lesions on the incisal surfaces of teeth 52, 61, and 62 and the lesion on the labial surface of tooth 51.
- Parents appeared motivated and enthused to participate actively in the management of dental caries in their child.

Case Selection: Preoperative Labial View

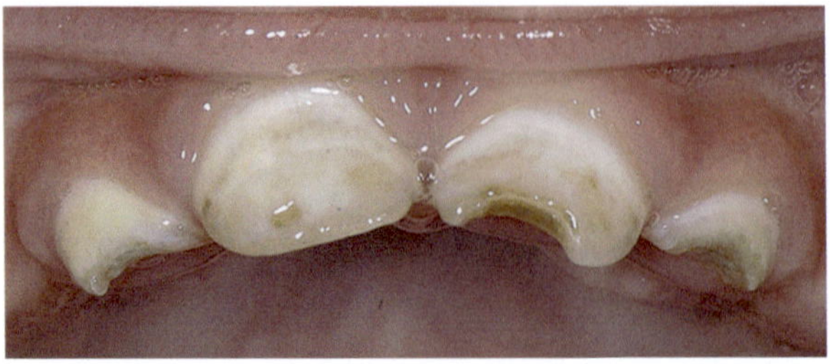

Teeth 51, 52, 61, and 62 showed extensive plaque stagnation and demineralization on the entire labial surface. Tooth 51 had a small labial lesion extending to dentine. Teeth 52, 61, and 62 showed carious lesions on the incisal surface

Case Selection: Preoperative Palatal View

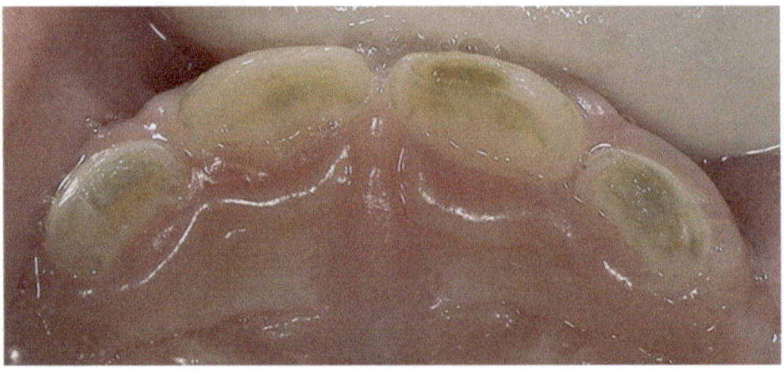

Preoperative palatal view showed carious lesions on the incisal surfaces of teeth 52, 61, and 62 extending to the dentine

1.2.4.2 Step-by-Step Guide

Step 1: Toothbrushing

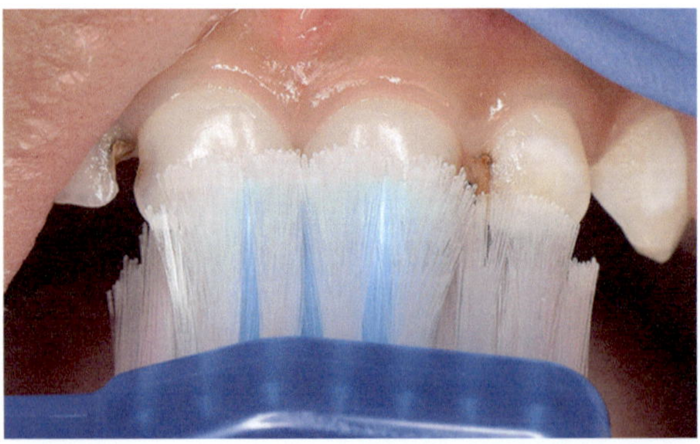

As an integral part of NRCC, the caregiver was motivated to perform meticulous toothbrushing twice a day with a fluoridated dentifrice. For the purpose of demonstration, illustration of a different case is presented here

Clinical Notes

Plaque must be accessed and mechanically disturbed/removed from all tooth surfaces, and the caregiver is advised on the correct toothbrushing technique. Brushing with a "pea-sized" amount of fluoridated dentifrice twice daily for over a minute is advised in a child who is less than 6 years of age. A 1–2 cm amount of fluoridated toothpaste is recommended in children older than 6 years [6]. Fluoridated toothpaste with at least 1000-ppm fluoride is recommended in a child with active carious lesions [7]. 1450-ppm toothpaste is considered ideal for NRCC, as the effects of fluoride are dose related [4]. It is beneficial to reduce rinsing to the minimum after brushing [8]. The caregiver is simultaneously educated to correct any faulty feeding habits and regulate intake of refined sugar.

Step 2: Oral Prophylaxis

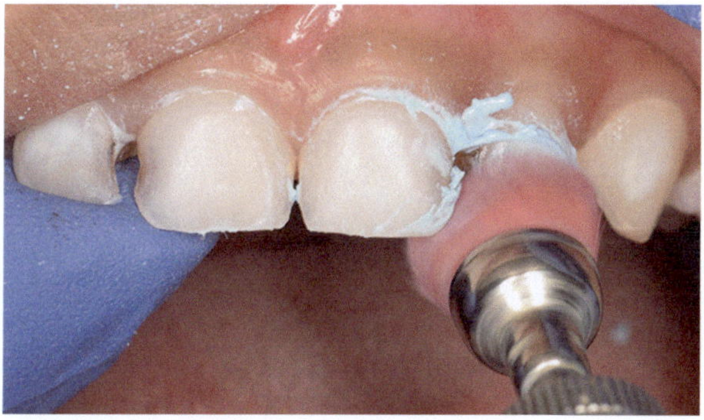

In-office oral prophylaxis is recommended when possible. For the purpose of demonstration, illustration of a different case is presented here

Clinical Notes

Mechanical disruption of plaque through toothbrushing in conjunction with professional oral prophylaxis forms the basis of NRCC. Professional oral prophylaxis will remove mature, stubborn plaque and suppress the activity of bacteria. It can be done with a rotating rubber cup or a rotating tuft along with a light abrasive paste [4].

Step 3: Application of Sodium Fluoride Varnish

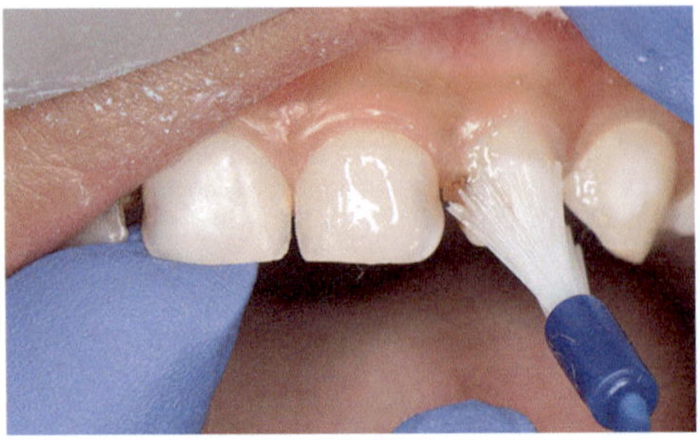

Following air-drying, 5% sodium fluoride varnish (NaF) was applied once per week for 3 weeks [9] followed by a three monthly application of NaF for 1 year. For the purpose of demonstration, illustration of a different case is presented here

Clinical Notes

Though some recent evidence suggests that an application of 5% NaF once per week for 3 weeks is favored for young children who are available regularly for treatment to arrest lesions [9], new guidelines [10] recommend application of 5% NaF varnish on non-cavitated carious lesions every 3–6 months and application of 38% SDF on cavitated lesions biannually.

Professional oral prophylaxis should precede the application of 5% sodium fluoride varnish. Application of high concentrations of topical fluoride leads to formation of a calcium fluoride reservoir in the active lesion. Calcium fluoride release serves to slow down the progression of lesion activity [11].

1.2.4.3 Long-Term Follow-Up

Twenty-Month Follow-Up: Labial View

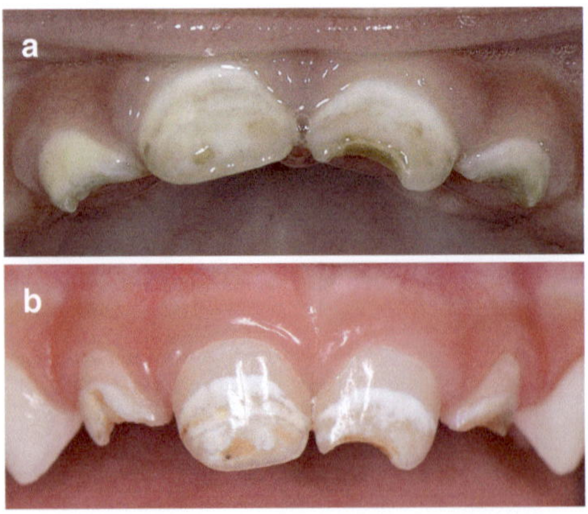

(**a**) Preoperative labial view, (**b**) 20-month follow-up, showed teeth 51, 52, 61, and 62 had erupted fully. Note the healthy enamel cervical to the demineralized zone on all four teeth. There were no signs of plaque stagnation or demineralization on the newly erupted tooth surfaces and the lesion on the labial surface of tooth 51 was contained, looked hard, and arrested. Enamel breakdown was noted but limited to the demineralized zone on tooth 52 and looked hard and arrested. Healthy plaque-free enamel on the newly erupted surfaces demonstrated that the disease process has been reversed

Twenty-Month Follow-Up: Palatal View

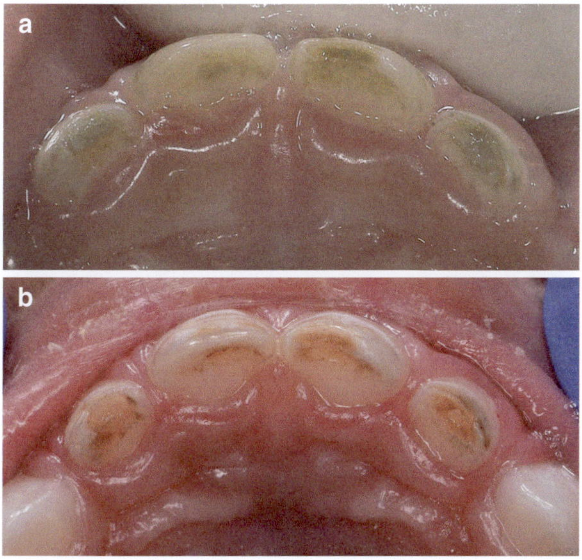

(**a**) Preoperative palatal view, (**b**) 20-month follow-up, showed that teeth 51, 52, 61, and 62 had reached full eruptive height. The carious lesions on the incisal surfaces of teeth 52, 61, and 62 remained contained and looked hard and shiny compared to the active lesions. The entire palatal surface was plaque-free, and the newly erupted enamel appeared healthy demonstrating that dental caries the disease has been treated

1.2.5 Case Study 2: Transforming Non-cleansable Lesions into Cleansable Lesions

1.2.5.1 Five-Year-Old Child with Multisurface Lesions in the Primary Lower Anterior Teeth

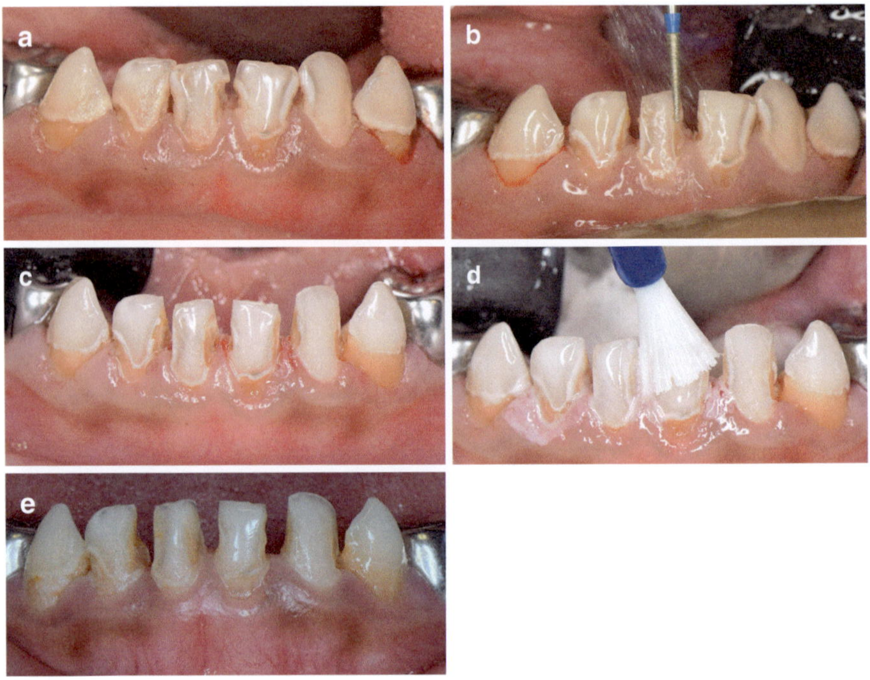

(**a**) Multisurface carious lesions were seen in the primary lower anterior teeth. Note that the proximal lesions were inaccessible to plaque disruption. They were also difficult to reach for the operator to perform prophylaxis or for fluoride delivery. (**b**) Overhanging tooth structure that sheltered the carious lesions was removed. (**c**) Carious lesions were made cleansable and accessible. (**d**) In-office application of 5% sodium fluoride varnish following oral prophylaxis. (**e**) Six-month follow-up demonstrates no further progress of the lesions. The lesions look darker and less active. The gingiva looks healthy and stippled compared to the preoperative image. Five percent NaF varnish was applied and the caregiver encouraged to take greater efforts at disrupting plaque in the lower right quadrant

Clinical Notes

Restoring lower anterior teeth for a long-term stable and durable outcome is a challenge. Arresting these lesions is often the most viable alternative. Once the lesions are made accessible, disruption of plaque by the caregiver and professional delivery of fluoride are made efficient and effective. In this case immediate arrest of the carious lesions in dentine would have been assured with the use of silver diamine fluoride (Sect. 1.3), but the caregivers chose to defer the use of SDF until NRCC using 5% sodium fluoride varnish proved ineffective.

1.3 Non-restorative Cavity Control Using Silver Diamine Fluoride

1.3.1 Introduction

Thirty-eight percent silver diamine fluoride (SDF) (approximately 44,800 ppm) [12] is a colorless fluoride delivery solution with the ability to arrest active dentinal carious lesions (frank lesions in dentine) [13]. In carious lesions treated with SDF, the remnant ionic silver inhibits further biofilm formation and makes the treated dentin more resistant to cariogenic bacteria thereby preventing further cavity formation [14]. While the silver in SDF solution plays the role of an antimicrobial, remineralization of the lesion is stimulated by fluoride. The solution is stabilized by ammonia [15]. SDF is an economical and a noninvasive mode of carious lesion management. The successful outcome of non-restorative cavity control (NRCC) with 5% sodium fluoride varnish discussed in Sect. 1.2 depends largely on the motivation and persistence of the parent to dislodge plaque mechanically through meticulous toothbrushing. SDF application on the other hand predictably arrests active dentinal caries soon after application [13]. As a corollary, it discolors the arrested carious tissue black. SDF is an invaluable tool in the management of carious lesions in precooperative children and in children where delivery of operative care is limited by disabilities. It is also a beneficial alternative when restorative options are not affordable or accessible [16].

1.3.2 Indications and Contraindications

- Primary tooth surfaces that exhibit areas of active cavitated dentinal lesions (frank soft carious lesions in dentin) with no signs or symptoms of pulp involvement. These are children where cooperation is limited by age or disabilities and performing conventional operative dentistry becomes a challenge [16].
- Deep active carious lesion where the clinician may want to scrub the lesion with SDF to arrest lesion progress predictably prior to restoring it with an intracoronal or an extra-coronal restoration.
- To arrest inaccessible proximal lesions where placing a restoration would involve extensive tooth preparation.
- In multisurface dentinal lesions or difficult to treat cavitated carious lesions [16], e.g., lower anterior primary teeth where longevity of the restoration is questionable.
- In children with limited access to dental care [16], SDF is the preferred choice of treatment given the evidence-based outcomes of predictable carious lesion arrest.

1.3.3 Rationale

The fundamentals of NRCC with SDF are similar to NRCC with 5% sodium fluoride varnish. However application of silver diamine fluoride as part of the NRCC protocol is very predictable in terms of caries arrest. Multiple mechanisms leading to this clinical outcome include [17]:

- Increased resistance to acid dissolution and enzymatic digestions through formation of silver protein conjugates.
- Increase in mineral density and hardness through hydroxyapatite and fluorapatite formation.
- Antiprotease activity preventing the breakdown of the dentinal organic matrix.
- A direct antibacterial action killing cariogenic bacteria.
- Lesions treated with SDF are also resistant to biofilm formation.

1.3.4 Case Study 1: SDF Application in Posterior Carious Lesions

1.3.4.1 Case Selection

Why Was This Case Selected for NRCC with SDF? [10]

- Tooth 64 presented with an active non-cleansable deep carious lesion in dentine.
- The child had no signs or symptoms of pulp pathology.
- The child was 28 months old and would have been unable to cooperate for operative procedures.

Case Selection: Preoperative Clinical View

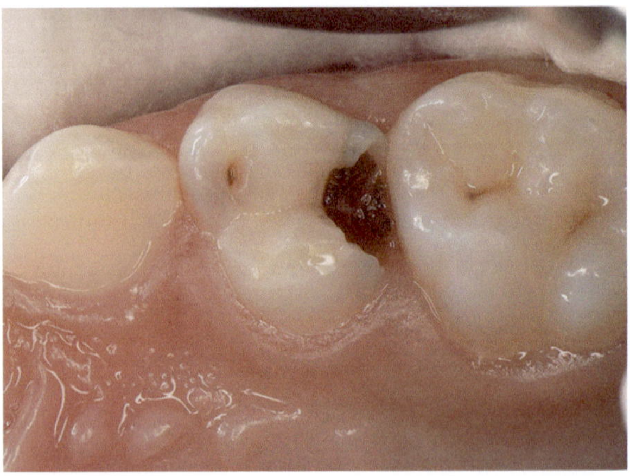

A deep carious lesion was seen in dentine on the disto-occlusal surface of tooth 64. A small stained pit was visible mesially. The occlusal grooves on tooth 65 appeared stained

Case Selection: Preoperative Radiograph

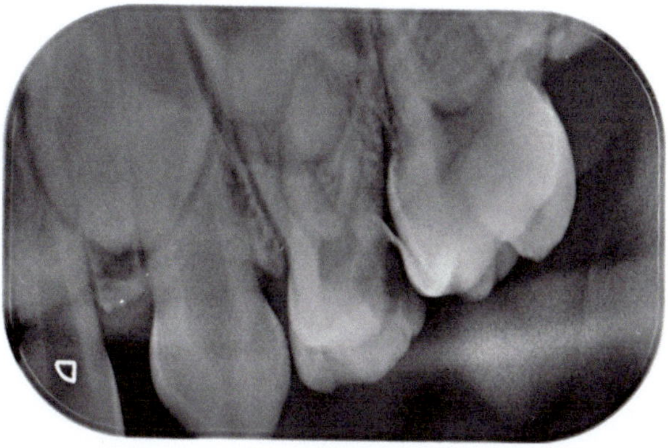

Radiograph showed the carious lesion in tooth 64 involving the inner third of dentin. A thin layer of dentine separated the carious lesion from the distal pulp horn

1.3.4.2 Step-by-Step Guide

Step 1: Application of Petroleum Jelly

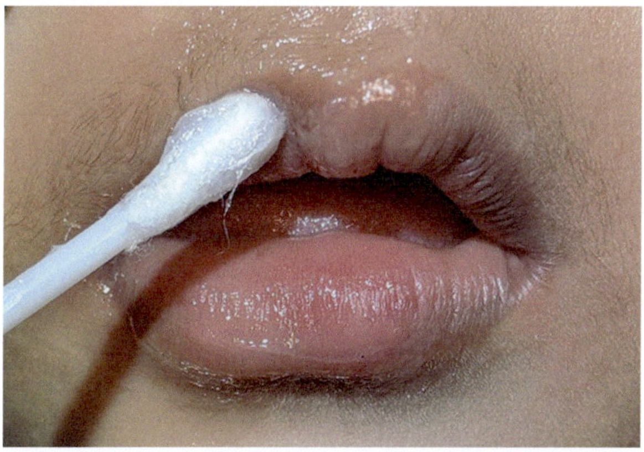

Petroleum jelly was applied to the perioral areas to prevent accidental staining

Clinical Notes

A temporary staining or silver tattoo occurs if SDF comes into accidental contact with the skin or mucosa. SDF will permanently stain clothing [18]. Equipment and all operating surfaces can also get stained, and hence adequate precaution must be taken to protect all such surfaces.

Step 2: SDF Application

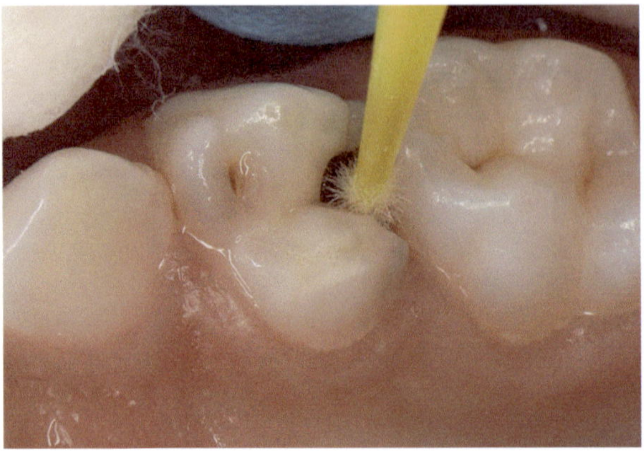

After air-drying the lesion, SDF was scrubbed into the lesion with a micro-brush

Clinical Notes
One drop of SDF dispensed in a plastic dish is sufficient to treat roughly 6 teeth [13]. Isolation with cotton rolls is adequate. When required, superficial loose debris can be removed to enable better contact of the SDF with carious dentin [18]. The lesion is air-dried, SDF scrubbed on for a minute, and gently dried [16]. The site of application should be isolated for up to 3 min when possible post application [18]. Fluoride varnish can be applied on the lesion post SDF application to keep the SDF in contact with the lesion and to mask the taste of SDF [19]. Patients are advised against eating or drinking for 30 min [16].

Step 3: Visualizing Lesion Arrest

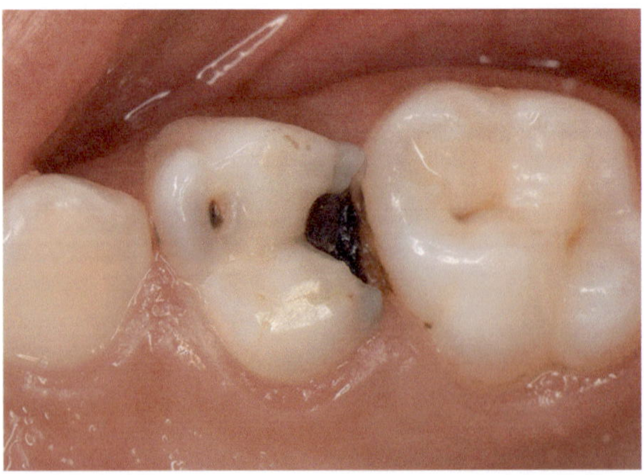

A well-arrested shiny dark lesion was visible

Clinical Notes

It should be noted that the hard tooth surface on probing and not the black color of the lesion indicates arrest of the lesion [10]. In large carious lesions in posterior teeth where the operator is uncertain of complete arrest after one application, reapplication after a week can be considered. Compared to posterior teeth, anterior teeth have higher rates of carious activity arrest. This can be due to their higher cleansability or more exposure to natural light, which results in higher precipitation of silver [13].

Step 4: Restoration with Glass Ionomer Cement: SMART

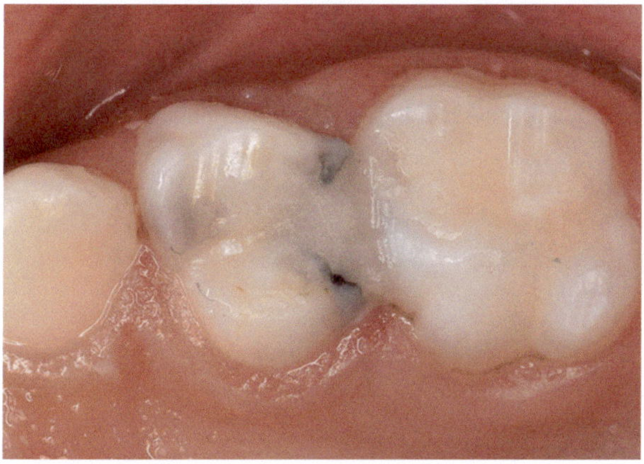

Tooth 64 was restored with high-viscosity glass ionomer cement—SMART. In tooth 65, the carious fissures were "sealed in" (Sect. 1.4)

Clinical Notes

Silver diamine fluoride Modified Atraumatic Restorative Technique, is a concept where the caries-arresting ability of SDF is combined with the ability of glass ionomer cement to seal the carious lesion. SMART is especially useful in cavitated non-cleansable carious lesions in posterior teeth [19]. In this case ideal proximal contacts could not be established, as child cooperation was limited and the priority was to achieve lesion arrest and sealing of the lesion.

Step 5: Postoperative Radiograph

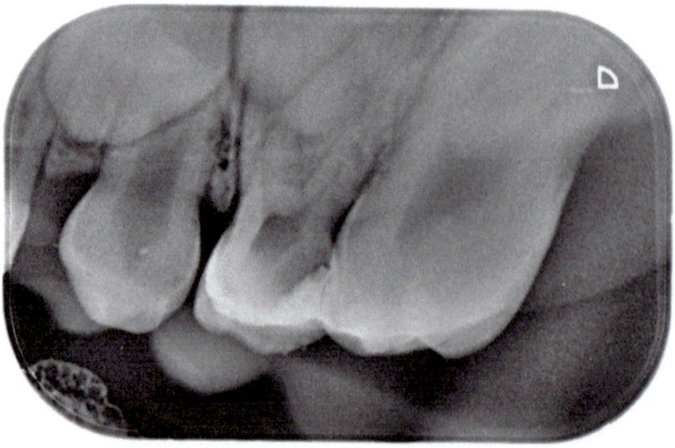

Postoperative radiograph was recorded to compare with a future radiograph

> **Clinical Notes**
> A postoperative radiograph serves to make a comparison with future radiographs to monitor remineralization of the carious lesion and lesion arrest.

1.3.4.3 Long-Term Follow-Up

Eighteen-Month Follow-Up

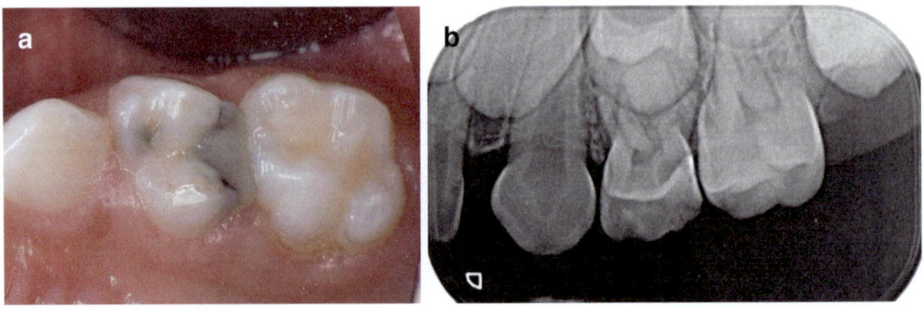

(**a**) Eighteen-month follow-up shows a stable restoration, and the soft tissue appears healthy. The dark hue of the arrested lesion underneath is showing through the restoration. (**b**) Note at the end of eighteen months that the restoration is stable, and periradicular tissue is healthy. There is an increase in the zone of mineralization between the lesion floor and the pulp indicating lesion arrest and mineralization

1.3.4.4 Follow-Up of a Lower Primary Molar Treated With SMART

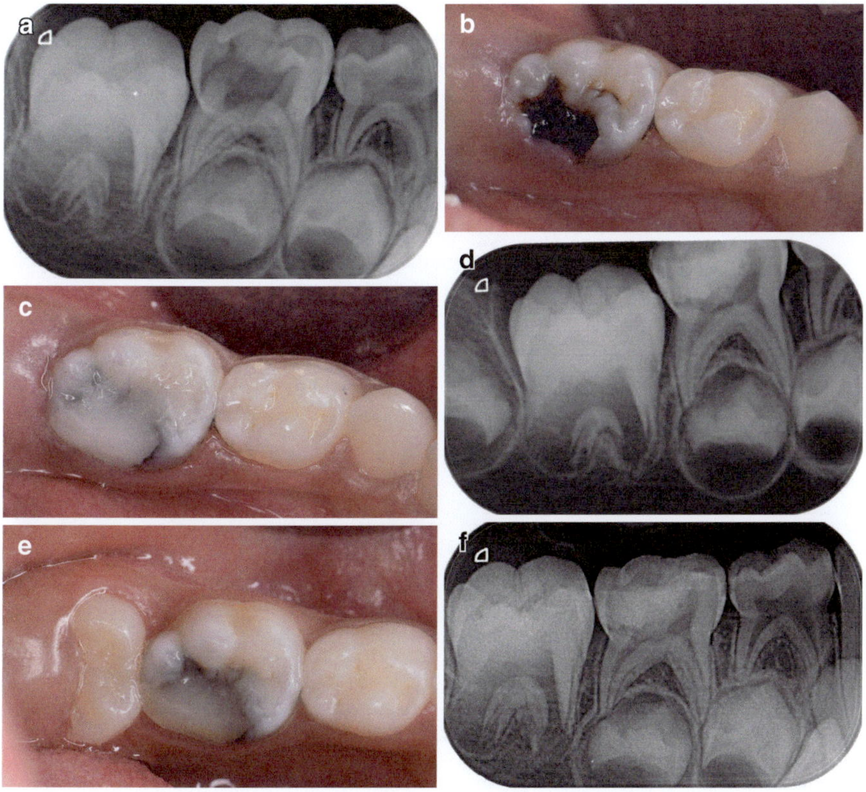

Four and a half-year-old girl presented with a deep carious lesion in tooth 85 involving part of the occlusal and lingual tooth structure. There were no signs or symptoms of irreversible pulp pathology (Chap. 3). (**a**) Radiograph showed a deep carious lesion approximating the pulp; however the lingual carious lesion could have superimposed on the pulp. (**b**) One week after application of SDF, the lesion looked discolored and was hard to touch, and the child was free of all discomfort while eating. (**c**) Glass ionomer cement placed in the lesion. (**d**) Postoperative radiograph after SMART. (**e**) One-year follow-up occlusal view showing stable restoration in tooth 85 and healthy gingival tissue. Note that tooth 46 is erupting. (**f**) One-year follow-up radiograph showing a stable restoration and healthy periradicular tissue. Note that tooth 46 has matured further and reached eruptive height

1.3.5 Case Study 2: Arrest of Interproximal Lesions Using SDF [19]

Though there are no randomized control trials to date examining the efficacy of SDF in non-cavitated proximal lesions, this clinical technique has generated a lot of interest [10].

1.3.5.1 Case Selection

Why Was This Case Selected for NRCC with SDF?

- Proximal lesions were noted in teeth 84 and 85 on bitewing radiograph extending to the inner half of enamel.
- There were no complaints of food impaction, pain, or discomfort.
- Arresting these lesions with SDF would be ultraconservative compared to placing a conventional restoration.
- Resin infiltration (Sect. 1.5) which was another conservative treatment alternative was disregarded for this child because it was the more expensive treatment alternative.

Case Selection: Preoperative Bitewing Radiograph

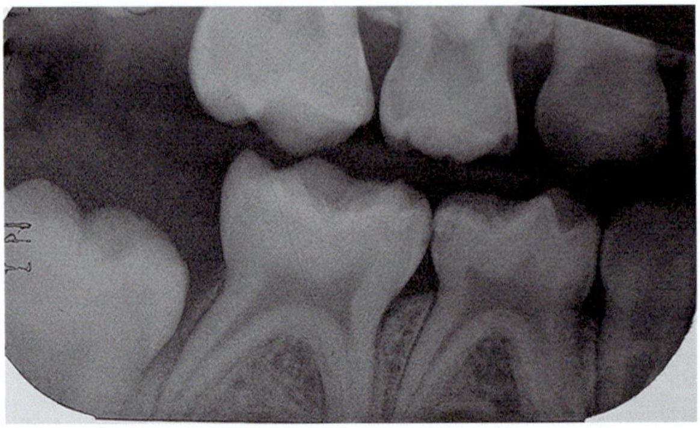

Bitewing radiograph showed teeth 84 and 85 demonstrating interproximal lesions

1.3.5.2 Step-by-Step Guide

Step 1: Patient Preparation

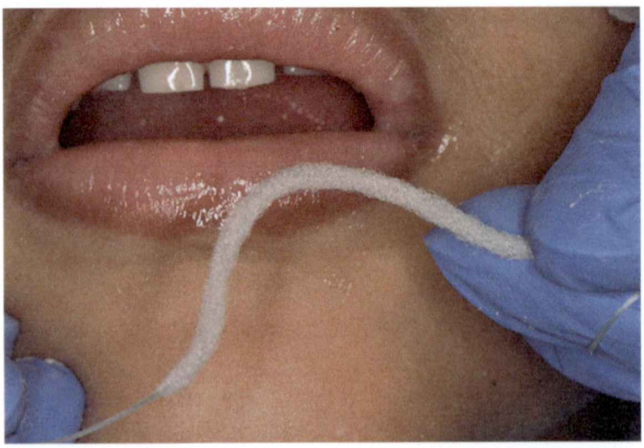

Petroleum jelly was applied, and a spongy dental floss was readied for application of SDF interproximally

Step 2: Insertion of Floss

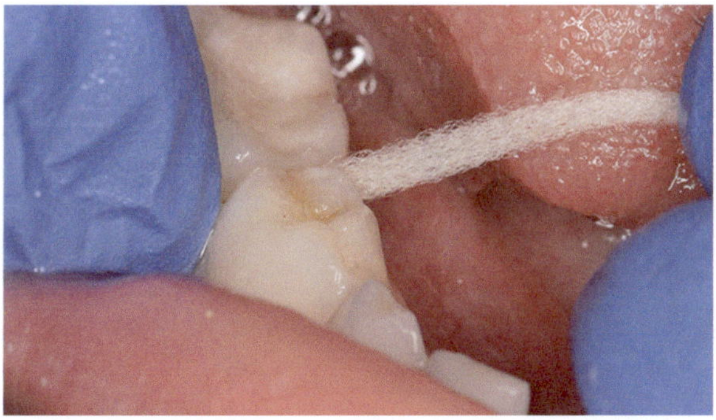

The interproximal area was air-dried gently and the floss was inserted interdentally

Step 3: Application of SDF

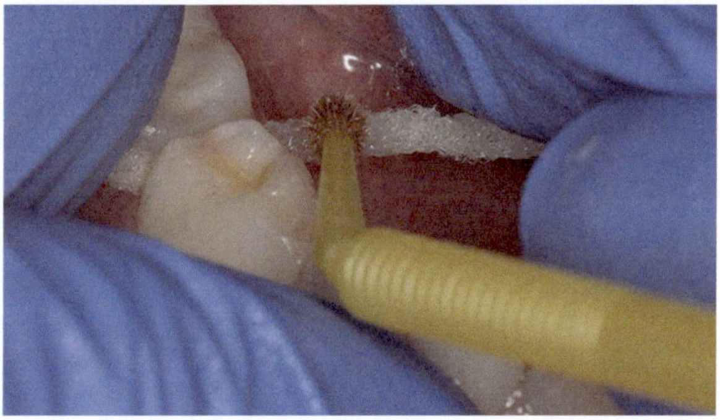

Floss was saturated with SDF solution via an applicator tip. The floss was pulled across and kept in place for a minute so as to allow the solution to be absorbed onto the lesion surface. The floss was soaked again and moved interproximally to assure thorough application of the SDF interproximally

1.3.5.3 Long-Term Follow-Up

One-Year Follow-Up: Bitewing Radiograph

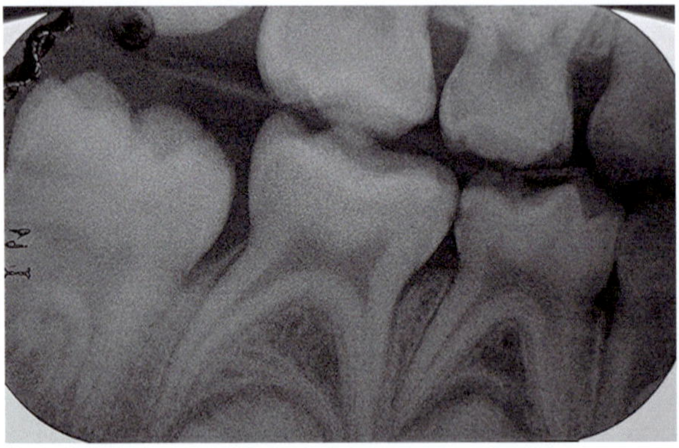

Note that the interproximal lesions in teeth 84 and 85 have not grown in size at the end of 1 year. This indicates arrest of the lesions and success of NRCC using SDF. Application of SDF was repeated after 6 months. Tooth 46 is seen close to eruption when compared to the preoperative radiograph

1.3.6 Case Study 3: Arrest of Anterior Lesions Using SDF

1.3.6.1 Case Selection

Why Was This Case Selected for NRCC with SDF? [10]

- Child was an 8-month-old baby.
- All surfaces of teeth 51 and 61 showed active deep carious lesions in dentine.
- Parents reported no signs or symptoms of pulp pathology.

Case Selection: Preoperative Clinical View

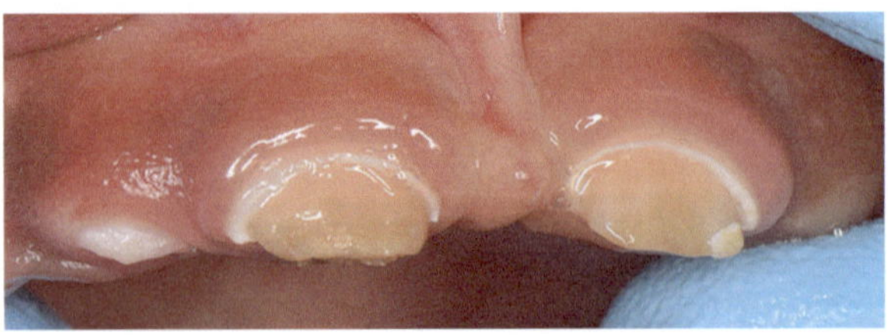

Teeth 51 and 61 were partially erupted and showed soft dentinal caries affecting all surfaces

Immediate Postoperative Clinical View

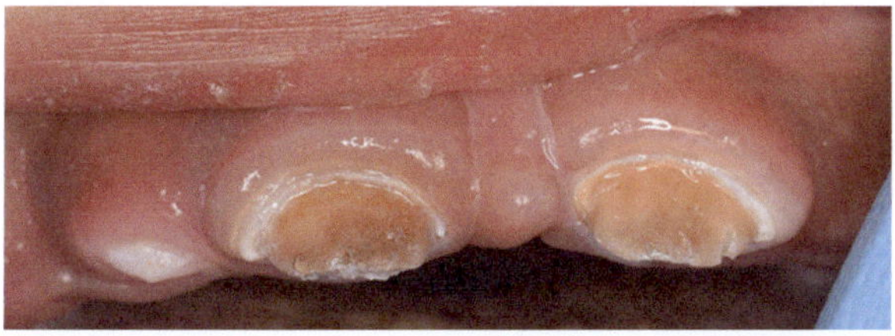

Teeth 51 and 61 after SDF application. Note the darkening of the dentine immediately post SDF application

Two-Week Follow-Up

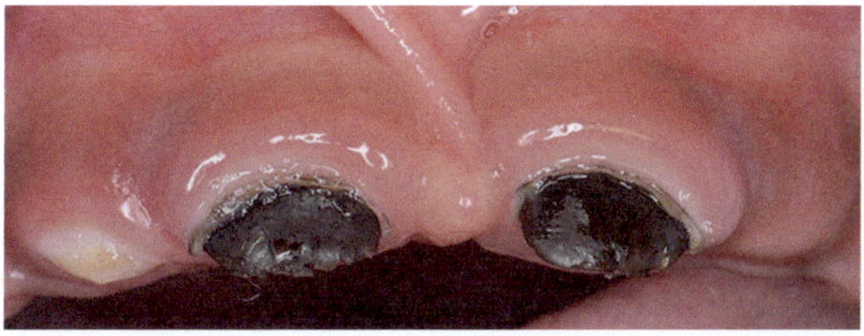

Carious tissue in teeth 51 and 61 turned completely dark on 2-week follow-up post SDF application

Clinical Notes

Lesion activity is monitored at 2–4 weeks following SDF application. The lesions should look dark and shiny and feel hard to pressure. SDF can be reapplied if necessary [16]. A popular protocol is to monitor on follow-up at 3 months and apply SDF biannually for 2 years thereafter [17]. A recent systematic review showed that the biannual application of SDF has a much greater chance of arresting cavitated lesions in primary teeth compared to an annual application [10].

Three-Month Follow-Up

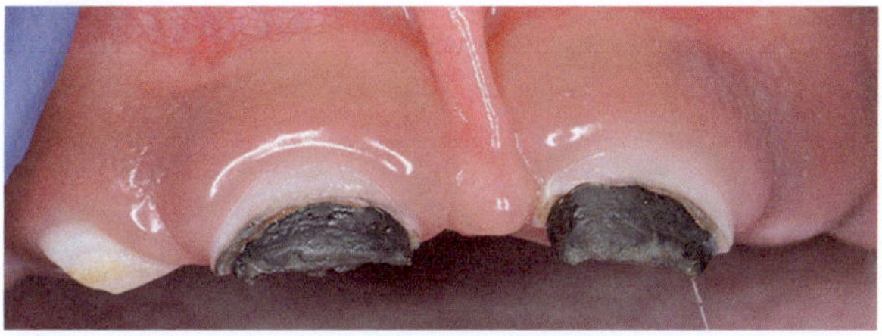

Note the stable arrested carious lesions on teeth 51 and 61. Teeth 51, 52, and 61 had erupted further. Healthy tooth structure was seen free of plaque, demineralization, or carious lesions on the freshly erupted teeth indicating that the disease "dental caries" has been treated

Clinical Notes

Children with a high plaque index show lower arrest rates [16]. Consequently, the motivation of the caregiver to manage plaque and correct faulty feeding habits and sugar intake becomes critical. Follow-ups are scheduled based on the child's disease activity at 3–6 months. Fluoride varnish application along with necessary intervention to reduce risk factors at the individual level can comprehensively tackle the disease dental caries [16].

1.3.6.2 Long-Term Follow-Up

One-Year Follow-Up: Labial View

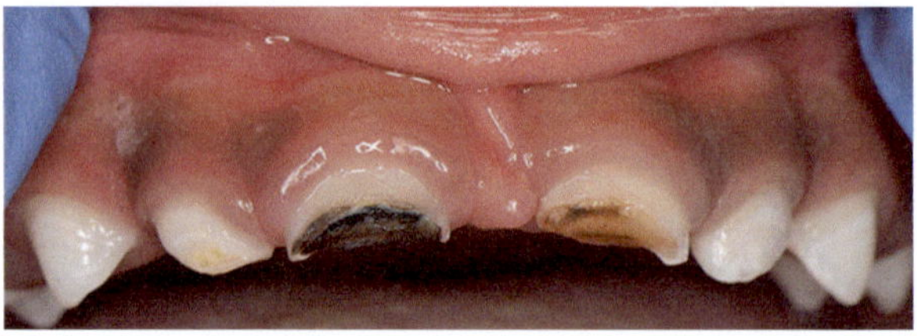

Teeth 51 and 61 have erupted further at the end of 1 year. No new areas of plaque stagnation or demineralization are seen indicating that NRCC has been successful. Parts of the arrested dentinal tissue in teeth 51 and 61 have chipped away, but the dentinal tissue is hard to touch indicating no new caries activity

One-Year Follow-Up: Palatal View

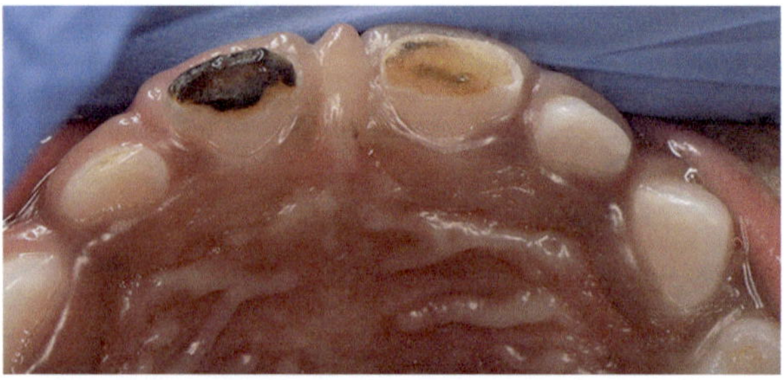

Palatal view clearly shows the arrested dentinal lesions on teeth 51 and 61 at the end of 1 year. Though some SDF treated arrested tissue has sheared away from the incisal edges of both teeth, the discolored dentine left behind is hard and arrested proving a successful outcome of NRCC with SDF

1.4 Resin Infiltration in Interproximal Lesions

1.4.1 Introduction

Non-cavitated proximal lesions are most commonly detected on bitewing radiographs. The correlation between the extent of a proximal lesion on the radiograph and the possibility of the lesion being cavitated is not well established [20]. A common classification of lesion severity on the radiographs is as follows: E0, no lesion; E1, lesion restricted to the outer half of enamel; E2, lesion extending into the inner half of enamel; D1, lesion restricted to the outer third of dentin; D2, lesion extending into the middle third of dentin; D3, lesion in the inner third of dentin [21]. Clinical studies have shown that a lesion extending into the mid (D2) or inner third (D3) of dentin will most likely be cavitated and are unsuitable for treatment with resin infiltration [22]. Lesions extending on the radiograph to enamel or the outer third of dentin are most likely non-cavitated and should be treated by non-restorative interventions [10]. Resin infiltration is an effective and contemporary method of arresting non-cavitated carious lesions in E1, E2, and D1 [23].

1.4.2 Indications and Contraindications

- For interproximal carious lesions, resin infiltration is indicated in lesions extending radiographically from E2 (inner half of enamel) to D1 (outer third of dentin) with no visible signs of clinical cavitation [22].
- The procedure being technique sensitive is difficult in children where behavior is challenged by age or special needs.

1.4.3 Rationale

Non-cavitated proximal lesions are characterized by a porous lesion body covered by intact surface layer. The porous lesion body presents a pathway for diffusion of acids into the dentin. Resin infiltration is a technique where a low-viscosity light-cured resin called “Infiltrant” is allowed to penetrate these porosities. The diffusion pathway of the proximal lesion is blocked thereby arresting the progress of the carious lesion [24]. The resin also coats the enamel crystals within the lesion body and prevents them from further dissolution [22].

1.4.4 Case Study

1.4.4.1 Case Selection

Why Was This Case Selected for Resin Infiltration?

- The bitewing radiograph showed that tooth 74 had an interproximal lesion on the distal surface that was extending to the outer third of dentine (D1).
- It was judged that the child would cooperate for this technique-sensitive procedure.

Case Selection: Preoperative Clinical View

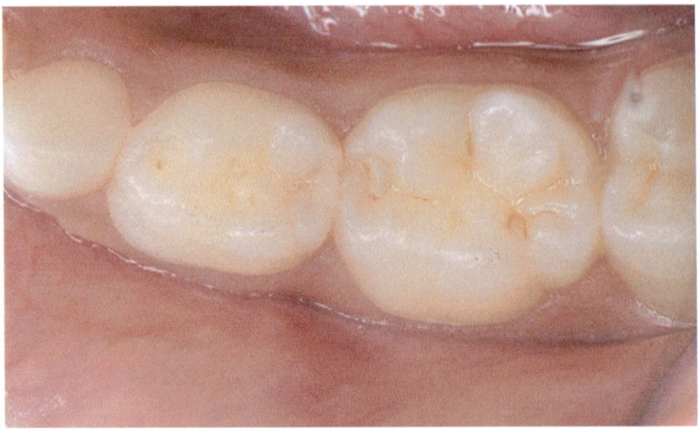

Clinical view showed slightly stained occlusal grooves in teeth 74, 75, and 36. There were interproximal lesions in teeth 54 and 55. Hence a bitewing radiograph was recommended

Case Selection: Bitewing Radiograph

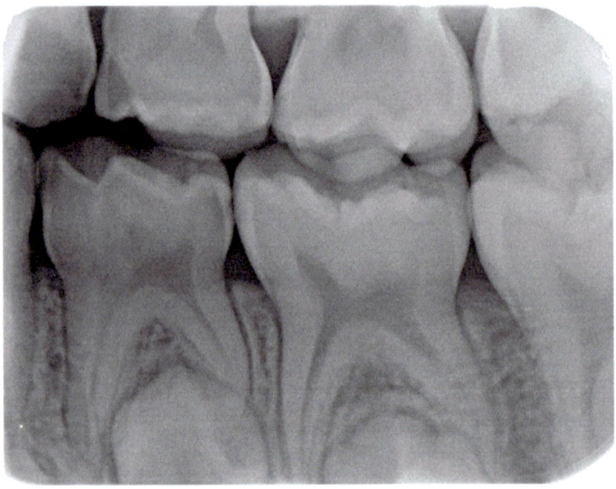

Note the interproximal lesion on the distal surface of tooth 74 extending into the outer third of dentine (D1)

Clinical Notes

Carious lesions in the interproximal area allow limited and often no visual access. Proximal lesions should be suspected in the primary molars in children who are at high risk or demonstrate an interproximal lesion in any primary molar. When bitewing radiographs are added as an adjunct to visual inspection of primary molars, there is a 45% increase in the detection of proximal lesions [25].

1.4.4.2 Step-by-Step Guide

Step 1: Isolation and Tooth Separation

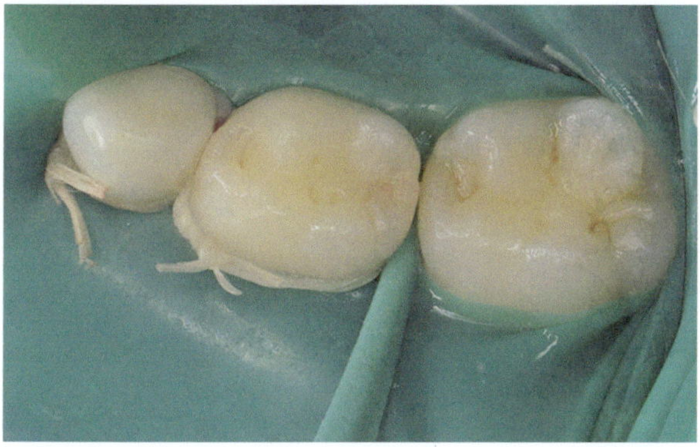

Meticulous rubber dam isolation is an integral part of the resin infiltration procedure. A special wedge available in the kit (Icon, DMG Hamburg, Germany) was inserted in the interproximal area in order to achieve tooth separation. This allowed access to the interproximal lesion

Clinical Notes
The resin infiltration kit consists of plastic flattened wedges, special foil applicators, 15% hydrochloric acid gel in a syringe, ethanol, and infiltrant resin in a syringe [22].

Foil Applicator

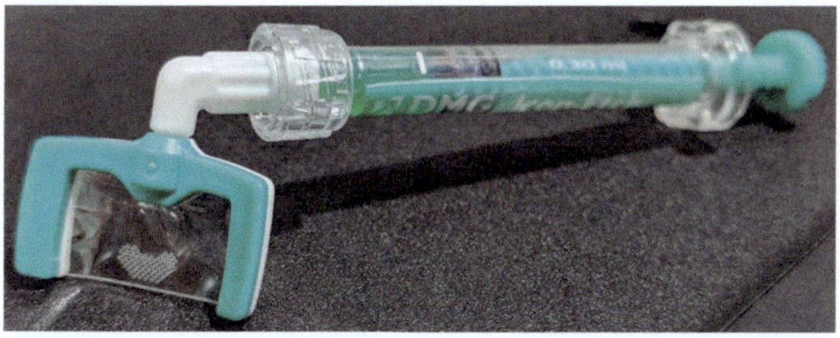

Foil applicator was attached to the syringe with 15% hydrochloric acid gel (Icon-etch, Icon, DMG Hamburg, Germany)

Clinical Notes
The foil applicator has two thin foil films welded to create a pocket into which the 15% hydrochloric acid is injected through an attached syringe. When inserted interproximally, one foil protects the adjacent tooth from the acid. The other foil has a small kidney-shaped area of perforations through which the acid discharges onto the lesion [22].

Step 2: Application of Hydrochloric Acid Gel

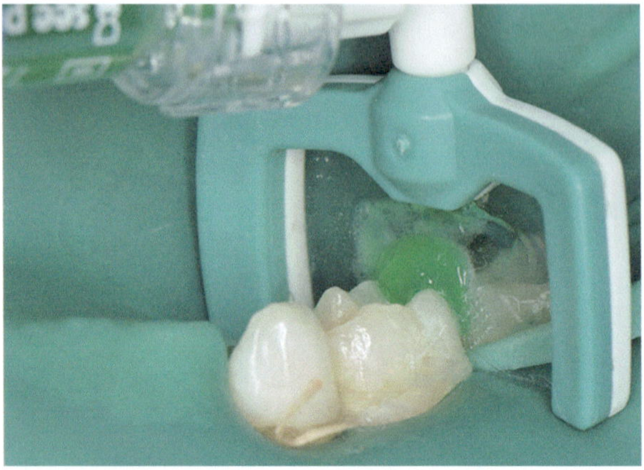

The foil applicator attached to the hydrochloric acid syringe was inserted interdentally after air-drying. The plunger was pushed gently so that 15% hydrochloric acid gel (Icon-etch®) deposited into the foil pocket and discharged onto the interproximal lesion. The gel has to wet the lesion for 120 s

Clinical Notes

In non-cavitated lesions, the porous lesion body is covered with an apparently intact surface layer. Fifteen percent hydrochloric acid gel is used to perforate or remove this surface layer so the resin can infiltrate the lesion [26].

Step 3: Rinsing the Gel

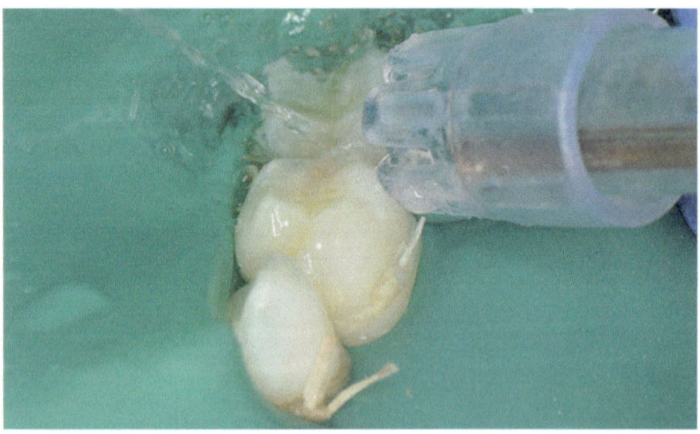

The gel was washed away with air water spray and dried with compressed air for 15 s

Step 4: Desiccation of the Lesion

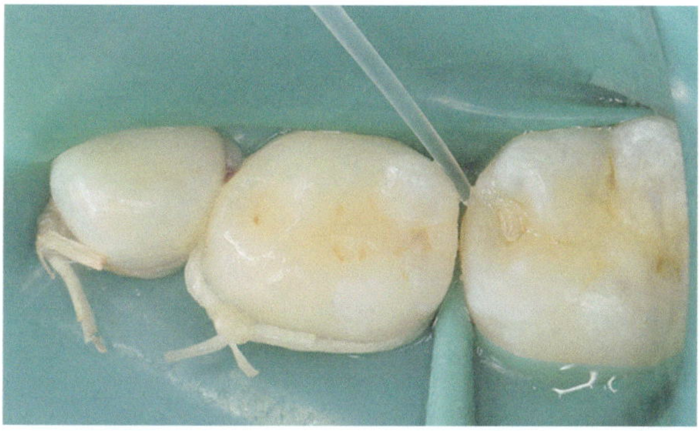

Ethanol provided in the kit (Icon-dry, Icon, DMG Hamburg, Germany) was applied for 15 s interproximally with the help of a syringe and fine delivery tip. This allowed complete desiccation of the proximal surface. This was followed by air-drying for 15 s

Clinical Notes

Resin infiltration is a process where the "infiltrate" is soaked up into the porous lesion body by capillary action. Any moisture within the lesion body will impede this capillary action. Therefore the lesion has to be thoroughly desiccated [22].

Step 5: "Infiltrate" Application

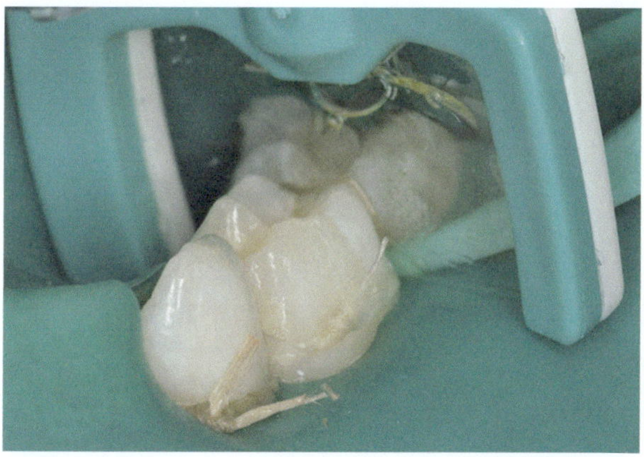

A fresh foil applicator was placed interdentally attached to the resin infiltrate syringe. The resin infiltrant (Icon-infiltrant) was injected onto the applicator and kept in place for 3 min

Clinical Notes
The light-cured, unfilled resin infiltrate (99% triethylene glycol dimethacrylate and camphorquinone) [27] is a resin of very low viscosity developed to easily soak up into the lesion body via capillary action.

Step 6: Contact Areas Cleaned

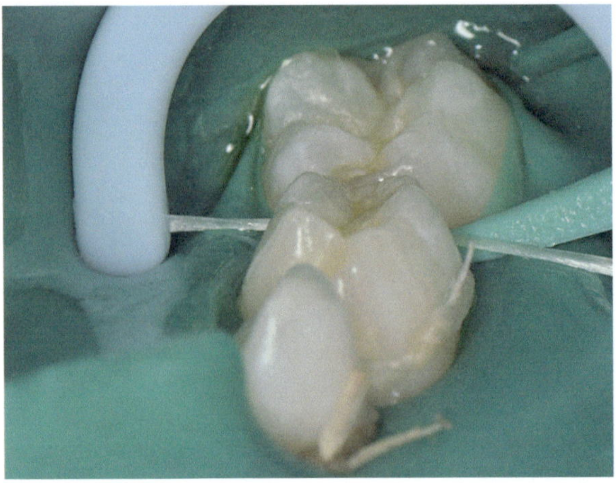

After 3 min, the excess material was air blown and the foil applicator removed. Dental floss was used to clean the contact areas

Clinical notes
A 3-min application is mandatory because the process of capillary penetration into the porous enamel lesion is slow and time dependent [28].

Step 7: Light Curing

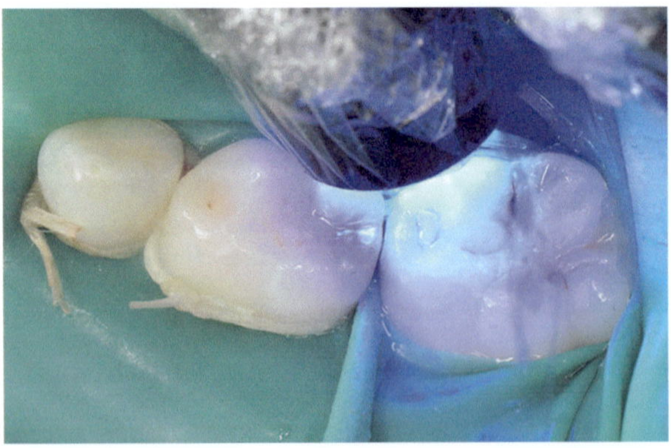

The resin infiltrant was light cured for a total of 40 s from the occlusal, buccal, and lingual aspects

Clinical Notes
A second 1-min application of the resin infiltrant improves the impermeability of the lesion [22].

Postoperative View

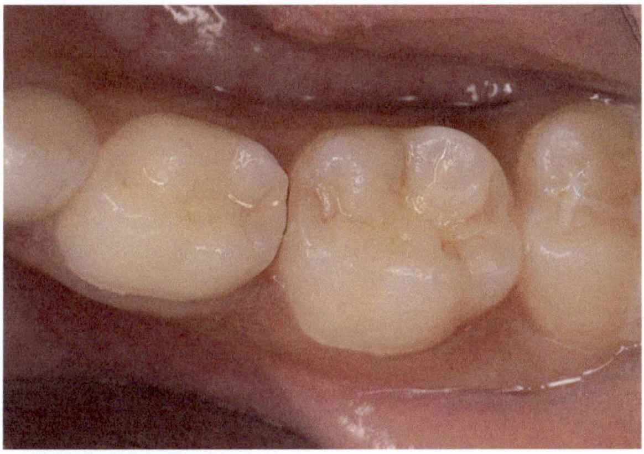

The infiltrant is not visible clinically

Clinical Notes
The "infiltrant" is radiolucent and will not show on the radiograph. The infiltrated carious lesions should be monitored radiographically on a regular basis to check for lesion progress [22].

1.5 Sealing Carious Tissue

1.5.1 Introduction

Sealing carious tissue is an approach to carious lesion management where the carious lesion is sealed in without removing any carious tissue [1]. It is a highly recommended mode of treatment in literature to arrest or reverse non-cavitated occlusal carious lesions in primary and permanent teeth [10]. It is especially useful in the young child anxious of traditional operative dentistry [29]. It helps the clinician defer conventional operative treatment until the child is old enough to cooperate for operative care. Resin-based sealants, polyacid-modified resin sealants, glass ionomer sealants, and resin-modified glass ionomer sealants are commonly used sealant materials [28]. Although resin-based sealants are popularly used to seal carious lesions [29], glass ionomer cements have several advantages over resin-based sealants. The fluoride release, chemical bond, hydrophilic nature, and ease of application of glass ionomer restorative cements make them an ideal choice for sealing carious tissue compared to the technique-sensitive placement of composite resin which requires multiple steps and meticulous isolation. Also no significant differences have been found in the caries-preventive effects of resin-based sealants and glass ionomer sealants [30]. Regular follow-ups to monitor the restoration for microleakage and integrity are recommended. Recent evidence recommends that non-cavitated occlusal lesions can be arrested or reversed with a combination of sealant and 5% NaF varnish [10]. More often than not, conventional operative dentistry can be obviated altogether in teeth where the sealants are intact on follow-up because sealing a carious lesion predictably arrests the lesion [29].

1.5.2 Indications and Contraindications

- Sealing carious tissue is best indicated in non-cavitated occlusal carious lesions in dentine and enamel [31] in children where obtaining cooperation for operative procedures is a challenge [29].
- In minimally cavitated potentially cleansable lesions in non-occlusal areas like buccal pits [1].

1.5.3 Rationale

The rationale for sealing carious tissue is that the disease "dental caries" is dependent on the environment of the plaque biofilm on the tooth. Altering the microenvironment within the carious lesion can challenge the pathogenicity of the cariogenic bacteria within the plaque biofilm. By hermetically sealing the biofilm under a restoration, the microorganisms are deprived of intraoral sugar substrates. This brings down their pathogenicity and diversity and thereby slows down progression of the carious lesion. The pulp-dentinal complex in turn is stimulated to promote reactionary dentin and tubular sclerosis further isolating the cariogenic bacteria leading to the arrest of the lesion [32].

1.5.4 Case Study

1.5.4.1 Case Selection

Why Was This Case Selected for Sealing In the Carious Lesion?

- Tooth 85 presented with a hypomineralized occlusal surface and a non-cavitated occlusal lesion.
- The child was 30 months old, and traditional operative dentistry would have been a challenge for both the child and the operator.

Case Selection: Preoperative Clinical View

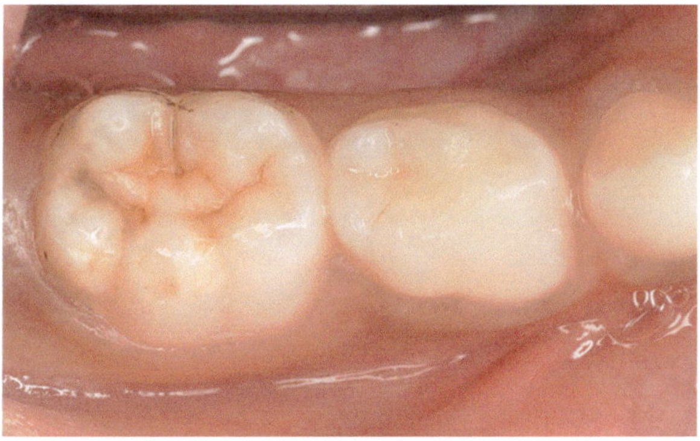

Tooth 85 showed hypomineralized occlusal surface and stained occlusal pits and fissures. The occlusal pits appeared carious with possible plaque stagnation and caries activity

1.5.4.2 Step-by-Step Guide

Step 1: Placing of Resin-Modified Glass Ionomer Cement Restoration

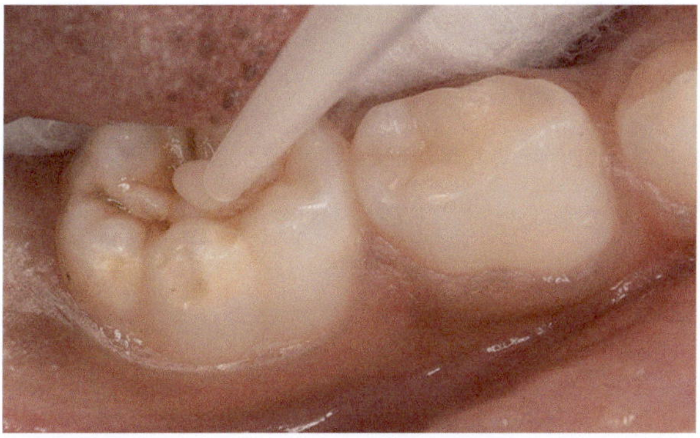

Following cotton roll isolation and air-drying, resin-modified glass ionomer cement RMGIC (Fuji II LC, GC Corporation, Tokyo, Japan) was squeezed onto the occlusal surface with a capsule

Clinical Notes

RMGIC is our preferred choice of restorative material because of its fluoride release, hydrophilic nature, resistance to microleakage, ease of application, command cure, and adequate wear resistance [33].

Step 2: Condensing the Material

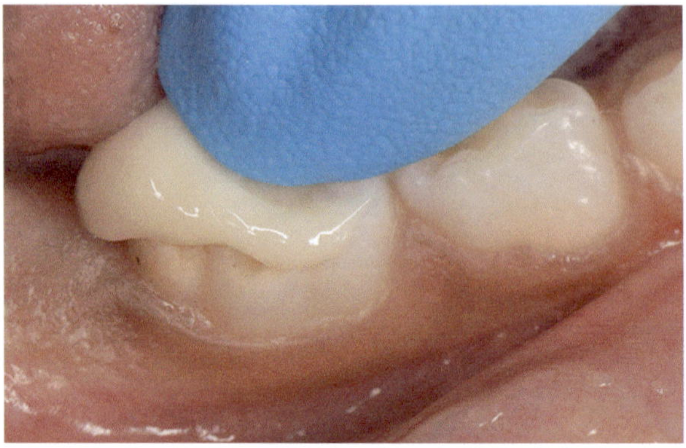

The material was placed in excess on the occlusal surface and pushed in with a gloved finger

> **Clinical Notes**
> The material should be condensed, ensuring it flows well into the deep pits and fissures on the surface of the tooth. The use of the capsule ensures the mix of an ideal restorative consistency. This allows the operator to manually condense the cement with the gloved finger. It also guarantees that no air bubbles are trapped in the restoration.

Step 3: Removing Cement Excess

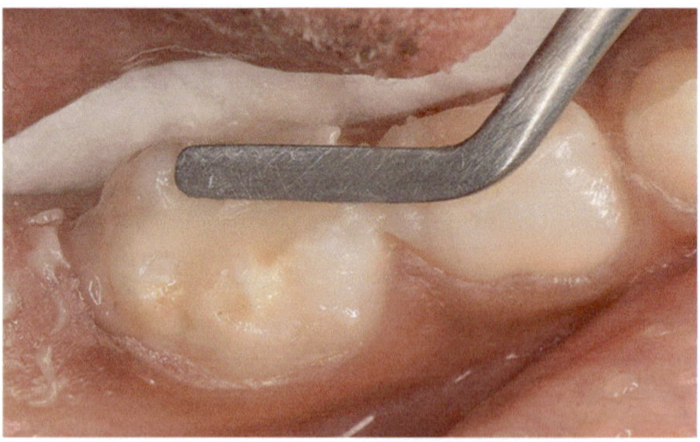

Excess cement was removed with an appropriate hand instrument

> **Clinical Notes**
> Cleanup post-cement placement depends on patient cooperation. In the event that cooperation does not permit a through cleanup, excess glass ionomer cement will eventually wear itself out. This is another advantage of using glass ionomer cement.

Step 4: Light Curing the Restoration

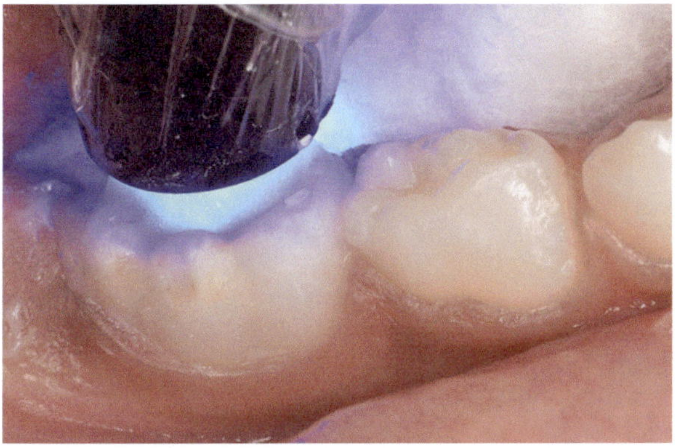

The restorative material was photo activated

> **Clinical Notes**
> Conventional autocure glass ionomer can also be used in place of RMGI restorative cement. However the command cure property of RMGI restorative cement in addition to the dual cure (tricure in some materials) ability makes it especially useful in children where time and patient cooperation may impede meticulous placement and bulk packing of the material in limited time may be necessary [33, 34].

Postoperative Occlusal View

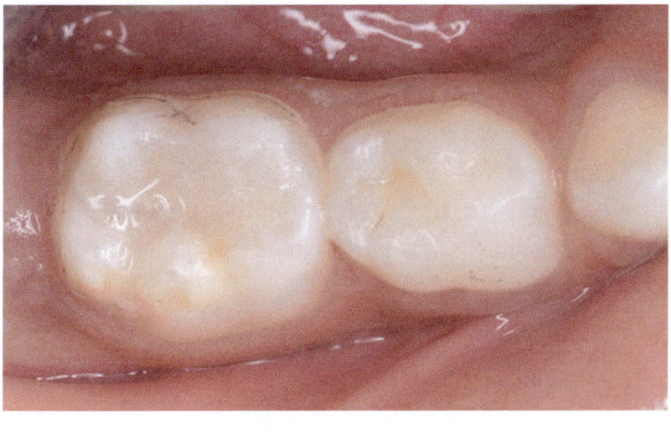

Note the well-sealed occlusal lesion in tooth 85. This not only arrests the initial occlusal lesion but also makes plaque disruption easy for the caregiver

Clinical Notes
Follow-up and monitoring to check the integrity of the sealant is critical when carious tissue is sealed. An additional advantage of glass ionomer sealants over resin sealants is that they have a cariostatic effect even if the sealant is lost clinically due to wear and tear. This is due to the remnants of the cement at the base of the fissure, and the fluoride release that takes place when the cement is still in place [35].

1.6 The Hall Technique

1.6.1 Introduction

The Hall technique is named after Dr. Norna Hall, a former general dental practitioner in Scotland [36]. The Hall technique is an extension of sealing carious tissue, by glass ionomer cementation of a preformed metal crown (PMC) over a carious primary molar—without any carious tissue removal, crown preparation, or the use of local anesthesia [37]. Once a clinical and radiographic assessment confirms that there is no irreversible involvement of the pulp, an appropriately sized PMC is selected and cemented over the tooth sealing in the carious lesion and coronal tooth structure under the crown [38]. Two recent studies concluded that when compared to conventional management of carious lesions involving complete removal of carious tissue followed by a pulpotomy or restoration, teeth that were treated with the Hall technique had equally successful outcomes at reduced treatment costs [39, 40]. The minimally invasive nature of the Hall technique positively influences treatment related anxiety in children [37].

1.6.2 Indications and Contraindications

For a tooth to be considered a candidate for the Hall technique, the diagnosis of irreversible pulpitis should be ruled out clinically and radiographically [38]. The radiograph should also confirm the presence of a definite dentinal layer over the pulp [36]. The Hall technique is indicated in:

- Small to moderate carious lesions, especially approximal lesions [37]
- Hypoplastic primary molars [37]
- In children whose cooperation during traditional operative dentistry poses a challenge

The contraindication is:

- Children with systemic problems like those at risk of bacterial endocarditis [36]

1.6.3 Rationale

The rationale behind this seemingly counterintuitive concept is scientifically based on the current understanding of the carious process. It relies on the fact that the pathogenicity of the plaque biofilm located on the surface of the carious lesion is dependent on its environment. If the biofilm is hermetically sealed with a restoration, the carious microorganisms are deprived of the micronutrients from the oral cavity. They then become less cariogenic, and the carious process slows down or gets arrested [41]. This leaves the pulp-dentinal complex with favorable conditions to deposit reactionary dentin over the pulp [37].

1.6.4 Case Study 1: Hall Crown in a Molar with Open Contacts

1.6.4.1 Case Selection

Why Was This Case Selected for Sealing the Carious Lesion with a Hall Crown?

- Tooth 74 had an old occlusal restoration and new carious lesions on the distal and buccal surfaces of tooth 74.
- The 4-year-old child was categorized at high risk for dental caries.
- The tooth showed no signs or symptoms of pulp pathology.

Case Selection: Preoperative Clinical View

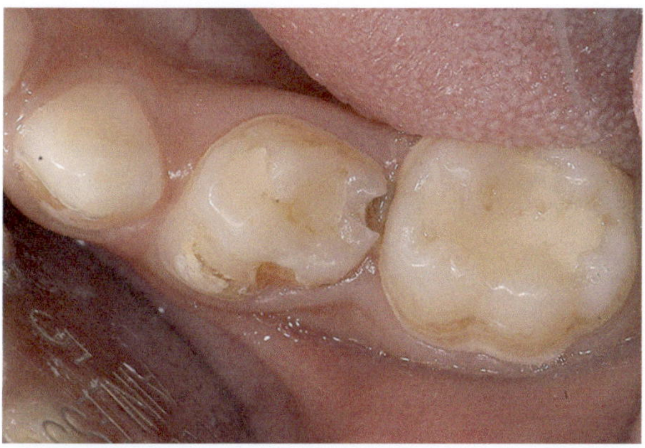

Teeth 74 and 75 had old stable restorations on the occlusal surface. New carious lesions were evident on the buccal and distal surfaces of tooth 74 and labial surface of tooth 73 indicating that the disease dental caries was still active

1.6.4.2 Step-by-Step Guide [36]

Step 1: Securing the Crown Before Trial

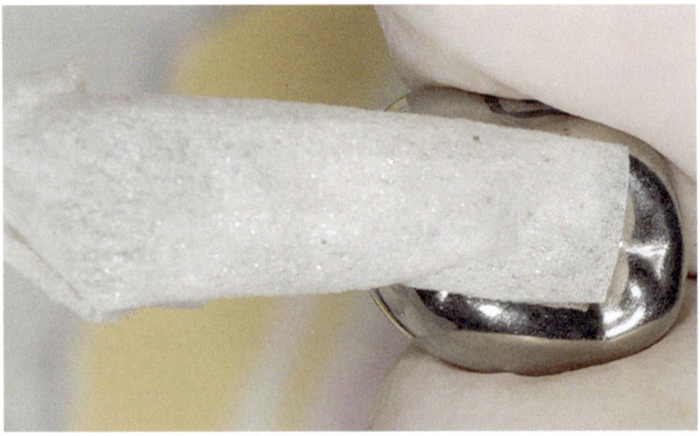

A medical grade tape was secured on the occlusal surface of the preformed metal crown (3M ESPE, St. Paul, MN, USA) before it was tried in the mouth for size selection

Clinical Notes

The steel crown being small can often feel slippery to a gloved finger. Securing it with a tape prevents it from slipping from the operator's fingers and accidental swallowing or aspiration of the crown. A gauze pack can also be placed in the oral cavity, distal to the teeth to be treated, to protect the airway.

Step 2: Selection of the Preformed Metal Crown

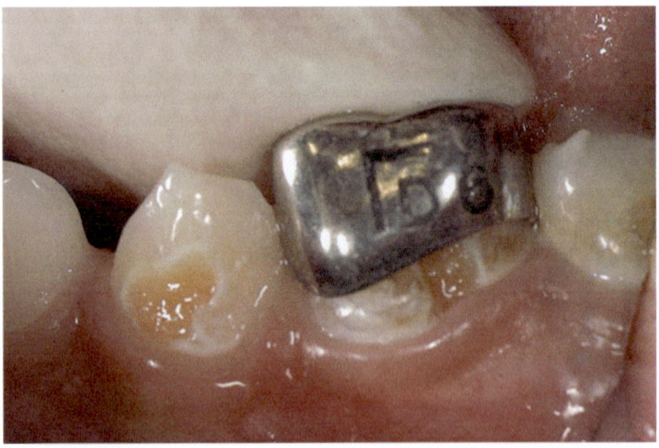

Note the selected crown pushed over three-fourths of tooth 74 by locking it lingual to the tooth and rolling it over the occlusal surface

Clinical Notes
The smallest crown that fits two-thirds of the tooth is selected by trial and error. The crown should exhibit a spring back at the contact areas. During trial the selected metal crown should not be pushed in completely as this can make crown removal difficult once the crown snaps in place.

Step 3: Loading the Hall Crown

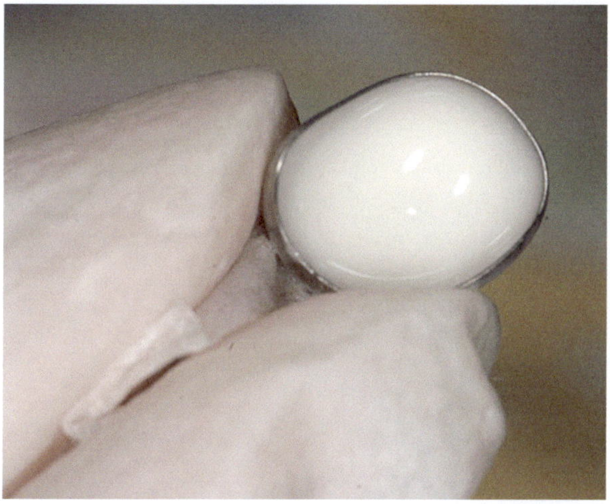

The selected crown was filled to the brim with glass ionomer luting cement without incorporating air bubbles

Clinical Notes
For any given tooth, the crown selected in the Hall technique is larger than a crown placed on the same tooth following conventional tooth preparation. When a Hall crown is placed on the second deciduous molar before eruption of the first permanent molar, special care to select the smallest crown possible is recommended to reduce chances of the erupting first permanent molar getting impacted under the margins of a larger steel crown. This is more likely in the maxillary arch [36]. We prefer tooth preparation to reduce crown size in these situations.

Step 4: Cementation of Crown

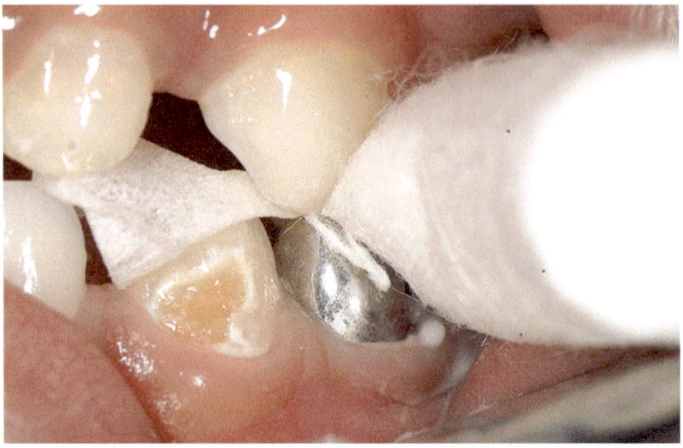

The loaded preformed metal crown was rolled over the tooth, and the child was encouraged to bite down on a cotton roll to aid in the seating of the crown

> **Clinical Notes**
> In case of an inadequate fit, the preformed metal crown is immediately removed with a suitable hooked hand instrument such as a sickle scaler before the luting cement sets.

Step 5: Interproximal Cleaning

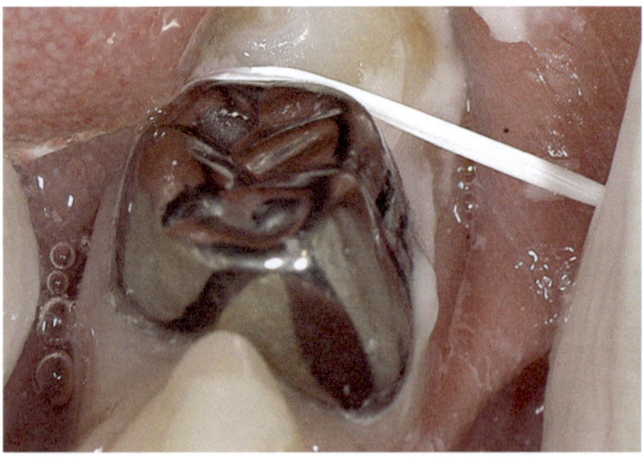

Luting cement in the interproximal areas was cleared with floss

Clinical Notes
The excess luting cement is wiped off and the adequacy of the fit is rechecked. The child should now continue to bite down on the PMC until the cement sets.

Postoperative Occlusal View

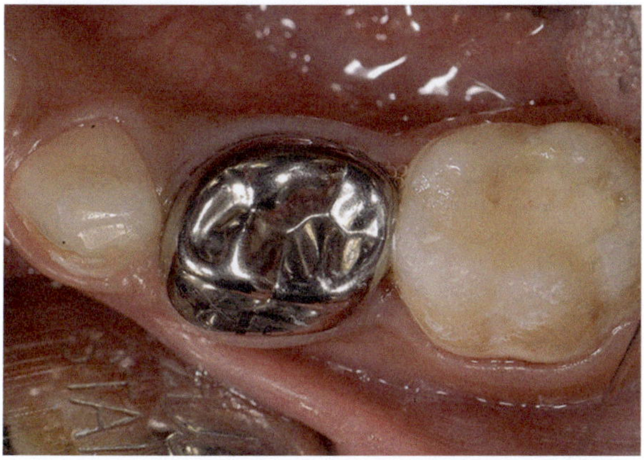

Note the well-seated Hall crown and proximal contacts post cementation

Clinical Notes
Gingival blanching is visible when the Hall crown is first cemented but is of no clinical significance in the primary dentition and resolves in a few days.

Postoperative Radiograph

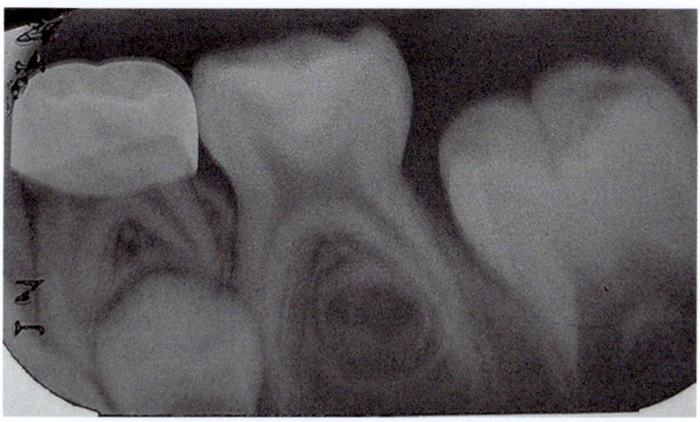

A postoperative radiograph was taken to compare with future radiographs and monitor the treated teeth

Postoperative View in Occlusion

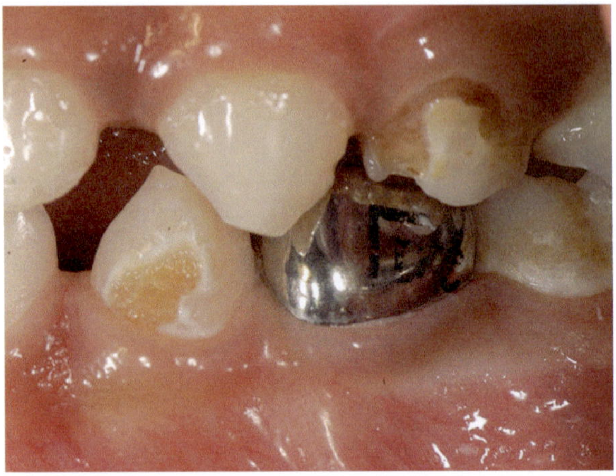

Note the Hall crown on tooth 74 in occlusion

> **Clinical Notes**
> Minor occlusal discrepancy may be seen post cementation because the tooth receiving the crown is not prepared operatively. This discrepancy will settle in a few days in the growing primary dentition [37].

1.6.4.3 Long-Term Follow-up

Two-Year Follow-Up Radiograph

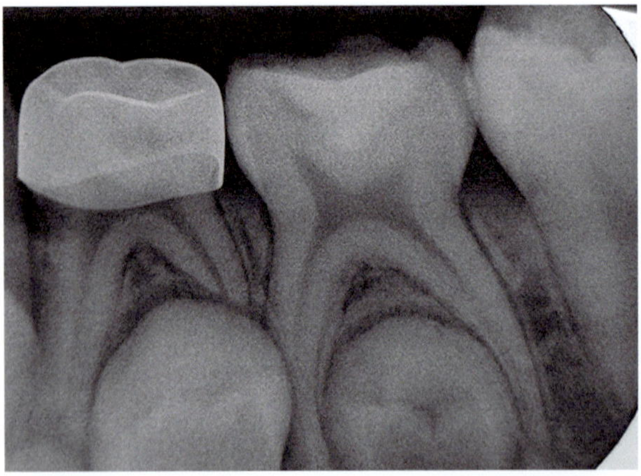

Note the stable restoration in tooth 74 and healthy radicular tissues at the end of 2 years indicating success of the Hall technique. Note that tooth 36 is now fully erupted

1.6.5 Case Study 2: Molar with Tight Contacts

1.6.5.1 Case Selection

Preoperative Clinical View of Tooth 54

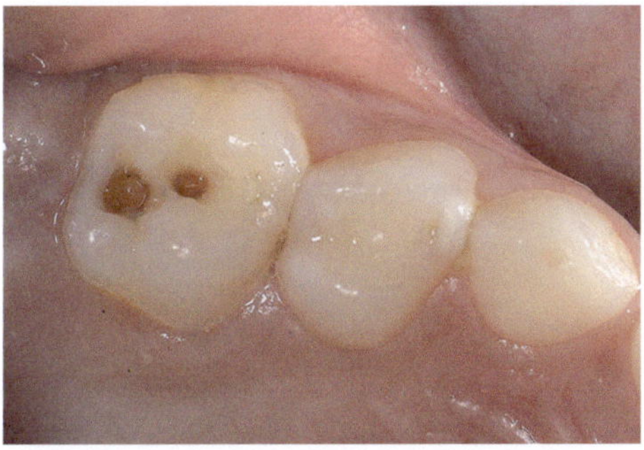

Note tooth 54 with tight proximal contacts indicated for a Hall crown. However no lesions were apparent clinically. An occlusal carious lesion was noted in tooth 55

Preoperative Bitewing Radiograph

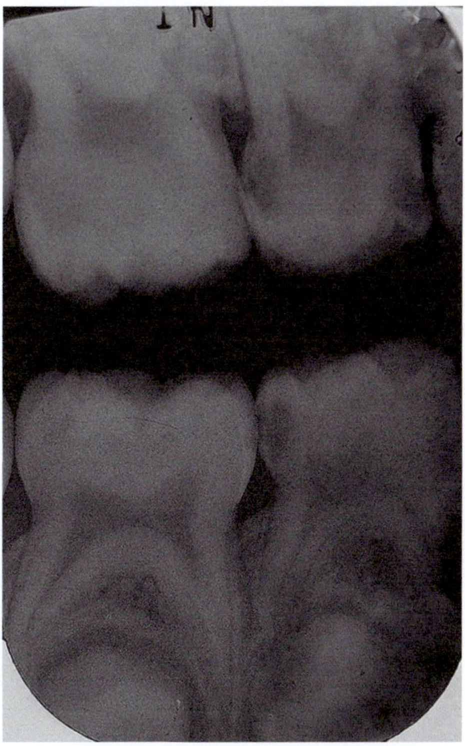

Upper first primary molar demonstrated mesial and distal proximal lesions. Note the distal proximal lesion in tooth 84

1.6.5.2 Step-by-Step Guide

Step 1: Orthodontic Separators Placed

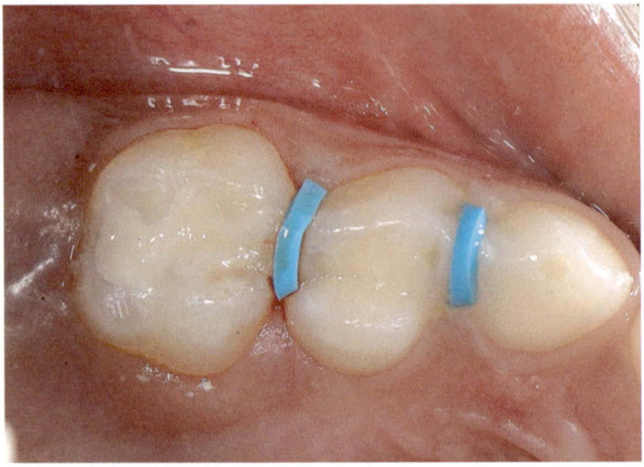

Orthodontic separators were passed through the tight contact areas mesial and distal to tooth 54. Tooth 55 was restored with resin-modified glass ionomer cement

Clinical Notes
Separators are placed in the proximal contact areas for 3 days to enable separation and opening of the contacts [36].

Step 2: Space Created After 3 Days

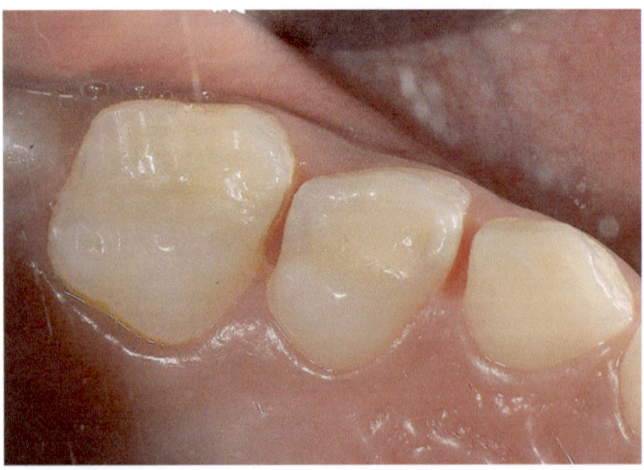

Note the proximal separation achieved 3 days later

Clinical Notes

Once separation is achieved, a Hall crown is selected to fit the tooth to seal in the proximal carious lesions. Reducing the mesiodistal dimension of the stainless steel crown (Chap. 4) makes seating the crown a smoother process.

Step 3: Cemented Hall Crown

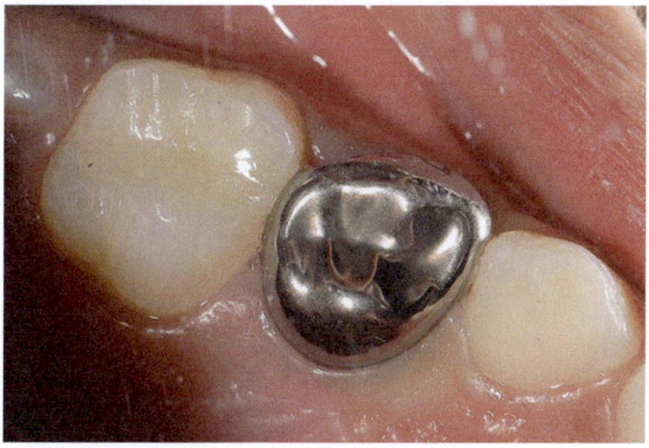

Note the tight proximal contacts and mild gingival blanching

Hall Crowns in Occlusion

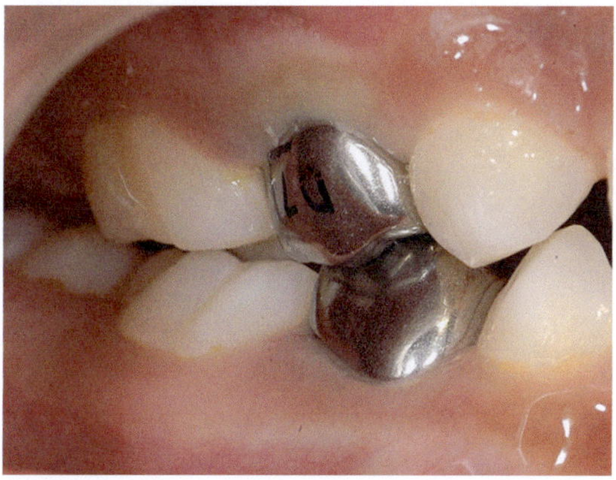

Hall crowns on teeth 54 and 84 seen in occlusion

Clinical Notes

Hall crowns placed on teeth in opposing arches should be placed a week to 10 days apart from each other. This will allow the occlusion in one arch to settle in before the crown is placed in the other arch [36].

Postoperative Radiograph

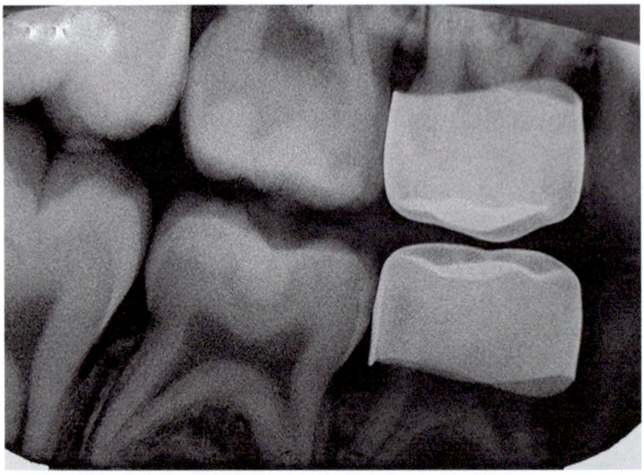

Teeth 54 and 84 showed well-placed Hall crowns

> **Clinical Notes**
> The radiograph was used to compare with follow-up radiographs to confirm success of treatment.

1.6.5.3 Long-Term Follow-Up

Four-Year Follow-Up Occlusal View

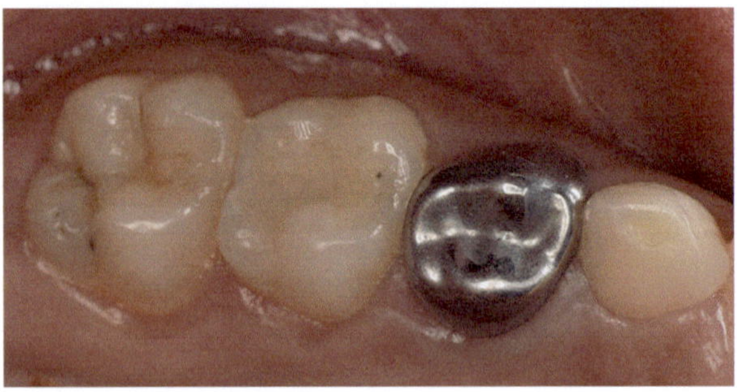

At the end of 4 years, tooth 54 shows a stable Hall crown and healthy soft tissue

Four-Year Follow-Up in Occlusion

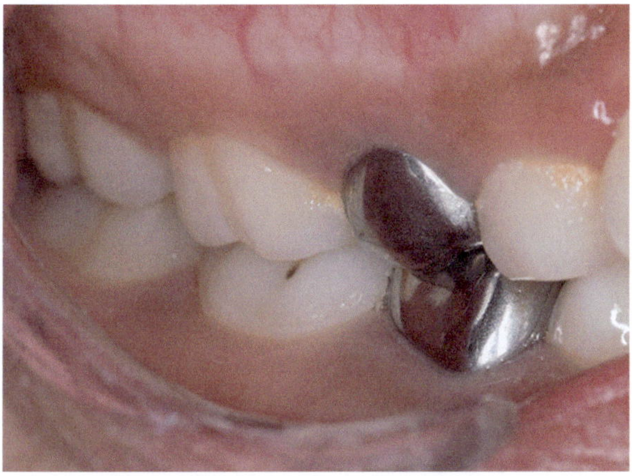

Teeth 54 and 84 show successful Hall crowns in occlusion 4 years post treatment

Four-Year Follow-Up Bitewing Radiograph

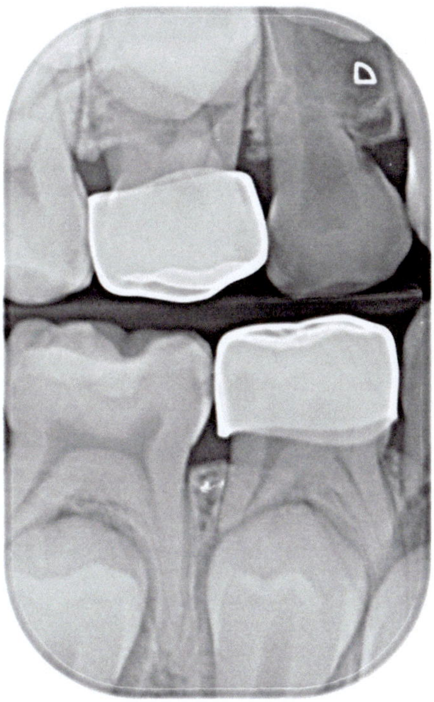

At the end of 4 years, teeth 54 and 84 show stable Hall crowns. Teeth 54 and 84 show healthy tooth structure, interradicular and periradicular tissue. This proves that carious lesion management by sealing the lesions with Hall crowns was a success. Also seen is a mesial proximal lesion developing in tooth 85 showing that the disease "dental caries" is still active requiring diligent caries management. The lesion in tooth 85 was treated with proximal application of silver diamine fluoride

1.7 Conclusion

Managing a carious lesion without removing carious tissue, though evidence based, is an absolute shift in treatment philosophy. It requires the clinician to unlearn past concepts and techniques in order to apply these lesion management strategies in clinical practice. An understanding and appreciation of the disease process and the role of the plaque biofilm will help implement these invaluable treatment protocols in the everyday practice of pediatric dentistry, making the dental experience less demanding on the operator and less stressful and more pleasant for the child.

References

1. Schwendicke F. Contemporary concepts in carious tissue removal: a review. J Esthet Restor Dent. 2017;29(6):403–8. https://doi.org/10.1111/jerd.12338.
2. Schwendicke F, Frencken JE, Bjørndal L, Maltz M, Manton DJ, Ricketts D, Van Landuyt K, Banerjee A, Campus G, Doméjean S, Fontana M, Leal S, Lo E, Machiulskiene V, Schulte A, Splieth C, Zandona AF, Innes NP. Managing carious lesions: consensus recommendations on carious tissue removal. Adv Dent Res. 2016;28(2):58–67. https://doi.org/10.1177/0022034516639271.
3. Dorri M, Dunne SM, Walsh T, Schwendicke F. Micro-invasive interventions for managing proximal dental decay in primary and permanent teeth. Cochrane Database Syst Rev. 2015;(11):CD010431. https://doi.org/10.1002/14651858.CD010431.
4. Christiansen J. Non-operative caries treatment. In: Splieth CH, editor. Revolutions in pediatric dentistry. Berlin: Quintessence; 2011. p. 21–35.
5. Hansen NV, Nyvad B. Non-operative control of cavitated approximal caries lesions in primary molars: a prospective evaluation of cases. J Oral Rehabil. 2017;44(7):537–44. https://doi.org/10.1111/joor.12508.
6. European Academy of Paediatric Dentistry. Guidelines on the use of fluoride in children: an EAPD policy document. Eur Arch Paediatr Dent. 2009;10(3):129–35.
7. Toumba J. Current guidelines for the use of fluorides for caries prevention. In: Splieth CH, editor. Revolutions in pediatric dentistry. Berlin: Quintessence; 2011. p. 37–48.
8. dos Santos AP, Nadanovsky P, de Oliveira BH. A systematic review and meta-analysis of the effects of fluoride toothpastes on the prevention of dentalcaries in the primary dentition of preschool children. Community Dent Oral Epidemiol. 2013;41(1):1–12. https://doi.org/10.1111/j.1600-0528.2012.00708.x.
9. Duangthip D, Wong MCM, Chu CH, Lo ECM. Caries arrest by topical fluorides in preschool children: 30-month results. J Dent. 2018;70:74–9.
10. Slayton RL, Urquhart O, Araujo MWB, Fontana M, Guzmán-Armstrong S, Nascimento MM, Nový BB, Tinanoff N, Weyant RJ, Wolff MS, Young DA, Zero DT, Tampi MP, Pilcher L, Banfield L, Carrasco-Labra A. Evidence-based clinical practice guideline on nonrestorative treatments for carious lesions: a report from the American Dental Association. J Am Dent Assoc. 2018;149(10):837–849.e19. https://doi.org/10.1016/j.adaj.2018.07.002.
11. Bruun C, Givskov H. Formation of CaF2 on sound enamel and in caries-like enamel lesions after different forms of fluoride applications in vitro. Caries Res. 1991;25(2):96–100.
12. Chu CH, Lo EC. Promoting caries arrest in children with silver diamine fluoride: a review. Oral Health Prev Dent. 2008;6(4):315–21.
13. Crystal YO, Niederman R. Silver diamine fluoride treatment considerations in children's caries management. Pediatr Dent. 2016;38(7):466–71.
14. Knight GM, McIntyre JM, Craig GG, Mulyani, Zilm PS, Gully NJ. Inability to form a biofilm of Streptococcus mutans on silver fluoride- and potassium iodide-treated demineralized dentin. Quintessence Int. 2009;40(2):155–61.

15. Rosenblatt A, Stamford TC, Niederman R. Silver diamine fluoride: a caries "silver-fluoride bullet". J Dent Res. 2009;88(2):116–25. https://doi.org/10.1177/0022034508329406.
16. Use of silver diamine fluoride for dental caries management in children and adolescents, including those with special health care needs. Pediatr Dent. 2017;39(6):146–55.
17. Horst JA, Ellenikiotis H, Milgrom PL. UCSF protocol for caries arrest using silver diamine fluoride: rationale, indications and consent. J Calif Dent Assoc. 2016;44(1):16–28.
18. Chairside guide: silver diamine fluoride in the management of dental caries lesions. Pediatr Dent. 2017;39(6):478–9.
19. Bendit J, Young D. Silver diamine fluoride: the newest tool in your caries management kit. In: Dental academy of continuing education. July 2017; 2017. https://www.dentalacademyofce.com/courses/3347/PDF/1707cei_Bendit_Young_web.pdf. Accessed 6 Sep 2018.
20. Ratledge DK, Kidd EA, Beighton D. A clinical and microbiological study of approximal carious lesions. Part 1: the relationship between cavitation, radiographic lesion depth, the site-specific gingival index and the level of infection of the dentine. Caries Res. 2001;35(1):3–7.
21. Anusavice KJ. Present and future approaches for the control of caries. J Dent Educ. 2005;69(5):538–54.
22. Paris S, Meyer-Lueckel H. Microinvasive caries treatment by resin infiltration. In: Splieth CH, editor. Revolutions in pediatric dentistry. Berlin: Quintessence; 2011. p. 103–17.
23. Paris S, Hopfenmuller W, Meyer-Lueckel H. Resin infiltration of caries lesions: an efficacy randomized trial. J Dent Res. 2010;89(8):823–6. https://doi.org/10.1177/0022034510369289.
24. Robinson C, Brookes SJ, Kirkham J, Wood SR, Shore RC. In vitro studies of the penetration of adhesive resins into artificial caries-like lesions. Caries Res. 2001;35(2):136–41.
25. Huysmans MC. New diagnostic approaches: promise or reality? In: Splieth CH, editor. Revolutions in pediatric dentistry. Berlin: Quintessence; 2011. p. 1–10.
26. Paris S, Meyer-Lueckel H, Kielbassa AM. Resin infiltration of natural caries lesions. J Dent Res. 2007;86(7):662–6.
27. Bagher SM, Hegazi FM, Finkelman M, Ramesh A, Gowharji N, Swee G, Felemban O, Loo CY. Radiographic effectiveness of resin infiltration in arresting incipient proximal enamel lesions in primary molars. Pediatr Dent. 2018;40(3):195–200.
28. Paris S, Meyer-Lueckel H, Cölfen H, Kielbassa AM. Resin infiltration of artificial enamel caries lesions with experimental light curing resins. Dent Mater J. 2007;26(4):582–8.
29. Hesse D, Bonifácio CC, Mendes FM, Braga MM, Imparato JC, Raggio DP. Sealing versus partial caries removal in primary molars: a randomized clinical trial. BMC Oral Health. 2014;14:58. https://doi.org/10.1186/1472-6831-14-58.
30. Evidence-based clinical practice guideline for the use of pit-and-fissure sealants. Pediatr Dent. 2016;38(6):263–79.
31. Borges BC, de Souza Borges J, Braz R, Montes MA, de Assunção Pinheiro IV. Arrest of non-cavitated dentinal occlusal caries by sealing pits and fissures: a 36-month, randomised controlled clinical trial. Int Dent J. 2012;62(5):251–5. https://doi.org/10.1111/j.1875-595X.2012.00117.
32. Ricketts DNJ, Innes NPT. To drill or not to drill? How much caries removal do we need? In: Splieth CH, editor. Revolutions in pediatric dentistry. Berlin: Quintessence; 2011. p. 119–34.
33. Hewlett ER, Mount GJ. Glass ionomers in contemporary restorative dentistry--a clinical update. J Calif Dent Assoc. 2003;31(6):483–92.
34. Berg JH. Glass ionomer cements. Pediatr Dent. 2002;24(5):430–8. Review.
35. Ovrebö RC, Raadal M. Microleakage in fissures sealed with resin or glass ionomer cement. Scand J Dent Res. 1990;98(1):66–9.
36. Evans D, Innes N. The hall technique. A minimal intervention, child centred approach to managing the carious primary molar: a users manual. November 11, 2010. 3rd ed. Dundee: University of Dundee; 2010. https://dentistry.dundee.ac.uk/files/3M_93C%20HallTechGuide2191110.pdf. Accessed 15 Sep 2018.
37. Innes NPT, Evans DJP. The Hall technique as a new method for managing caries in primary molars: is it really a revolution? In: Splieth CH, editor. Revolutions in pediatric dentistry. Berlin: Quintessence; 2011. p. 151–62.
38. Schwendicke F, Innes N. Removal strategies for carious tissues in deep lesions. In: Schwendicke F, editor. Management of deep carious lesions. New York, NY: Springer; 2018. p. 15–35.

39. BaniHani A, Toumba K, Duggal M, Deery CH. Outcomes of the conventional and biological treatment approaches for the management of caries in the primary dentition. Int J Paediatr Dent. 2018;28:12. https://doi.org/10.1111/ipd.12314.
40. BaniHani A, Deery C, Toumba K, Duggal M. Effectiveness, costs and patient acceptance of a conventional and a biological treatment approach for carious primary teeth in children. Caries Res. 2019;53:65–75. https://doi.org/10.1159/000487201.
41. Paddick JS, Brailsford SR, Kidd EA, Beighton D. Phenotypic and genotypic selection of microbiota surviving under dental restorations. Appl Environ Microbiol. 2005;71(5):2467–72.

Lesion Management: Selective Removal of Carious Tissue in Shallow, Moderately Deep, and Deep Carious Lesions

2

2.1 Overview

The traditional approach of "complete removal" of carious tissue, currently termed nonselective removal, advocated removal of all carious tissue in both the peripheral and pulpal areas of the carious lesion [1]. This implied removal of contaminated (infected) as well as demineralized (affected) dentine completely. Research subsequently showed that complete removal of carious tissue was unnecessary because demineralized dentine had the potential to remineralize when the lesion was sealed hermetically [2]. The practice of removing carious tissue completely posed a high risk of causing pulp exposures and complete removal was not required for a successful outcome as long as the restoration was sealed well [3, 4]. To prevent these unintentional pulp exposures, numerous alternatives were suggested under varying terminologies such as partial, incomplete, and ultraconservative carious tissue removal [5]. However, these terminologies were confusing for a clinician in terms of the actual extent and degree of carious tissue removal.

Hence the International Caries Consensus Collaboration (ICCC) [5] proposed newer standardized terminologies and definitions. "Selective" removal of carious tissue implies different degrees of carious tissue removal in the "peripheral" and "pulpal" areas depending on the depth of the lesion [5]. The goals of selective removal of carious tissue are:

1. To remove adequate carious tissue from the lesion so that there is sufficient depth to allow a stable restoration to be placed
2. To ensure that no pulp exposure occurs when carious tissue is removed

Since they can counter each other, it is essential for the clinician to carefully balance both these goals when performing operative care.

The ICCC recommendations divide the carious lesion into zones based on tactile sensation to hand instrumentation. Beginning from the outer surface of the carious lesion in the direction of the pulp, the three zones of carious tissue in a

M. S. Kher, A. Rao, *Contemporary Treatment Techniques in Pediatric Dentistry*,
https://doi.org/10.1007/978-3-030-11860-0_2

carious lesion suggested are soft, firm, and hard [5]. In selective carious tissue removal, carious tissue on the floor of the lesion is removed to a sufficient depth thereby leaving the lesion either in "firm dentine" (second zone) in moderately deep lesions or in "soft dentine" (first zone) in very deep lesions [5]. Though the terms soft, firm, and hard are subjective, they provide the operator with a more tangible guide. Removing "firm" or "soft" dentine is a tactile parameter as compared to previously used histological terminologies like infected and affected dentine [5]. Selective carious tissue removal is always followed by a hermetically sealed restoration [6]. To enable a good adhesive seal, carious tissue is removed to "hard" dentine and sound enamel along the periphery of the lesion [5]. In situations where the depth of the carious lesion does not permit an intracoronal restoration with a good seal, a full coronal coverage restoration is preferred in order to ensure a hermetic seal. The following sub-chapters explain these terminologies and treatment modalities in detail.

2.2 Selective Carious Tissue Removal to Firm Dentine

2.2.1 Introduction

Selective removal of carious tissue to firm dentine is the recommended technique for treating carious lesions that are shallow to moderately deep in teeth with no signs of irreversible pulp pathology [6].

In a moderately deep carious lesion, the first zone of soft carious tissue is relatively narrow (Fig. 2.1). Following the goal of removing carious tissue to an adequate depth allowing placement of a stable restoration, the soft zone of carious tissue is first removed followed by removal of carious tissue from the second zone, i.e., firm dentine (Fig. 2.2). The peripheral areas of the lesion are cleaned to hard enamel and dentine to enable a good restorative seal [1].

2.2.2 Indications and Contraindications

- Selective removal of carious tissue to "firm" dentine is indicated in the management of moderately deep carious lesions [6] in teeth that demonstrate no clinical symptoms of pulp inflammation such as severe, spontaneous, or persistent pain consistent with a diagnosis of irreversible pulpitis. (Distinguishing reversible from irreversible pulpitis is detailed in Chap. 3.)
- Radiographically, these lesions extend to less than the pulpal third of dentine [6] with no signs of bone loss or furcal pathology.

2.2.3 Rationale

When carious tissue is removed selectively to firm dentine, the aim is to remove tissue to a depth that provides for a restoration of adequate bulk and at the same time

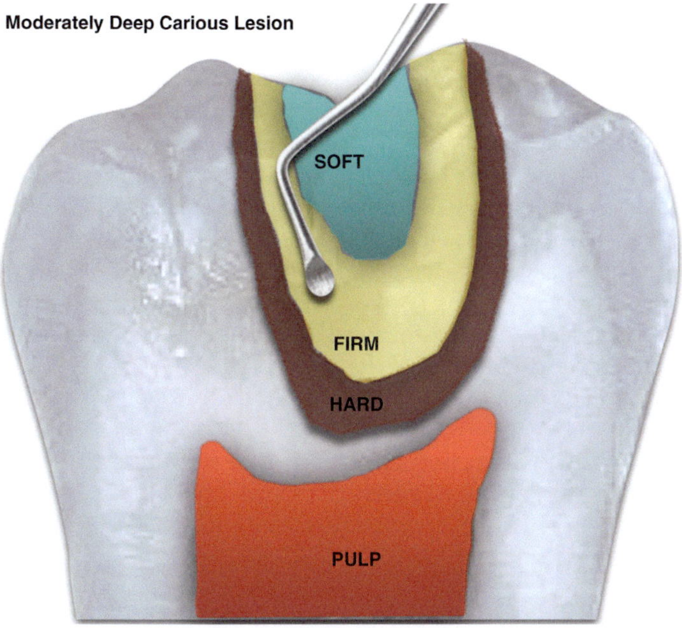

Fig. 2.1 Cross section of a moderately deep carious lesion: Note the three zones of carious tissue based on tactile sensation to hand instrumentation

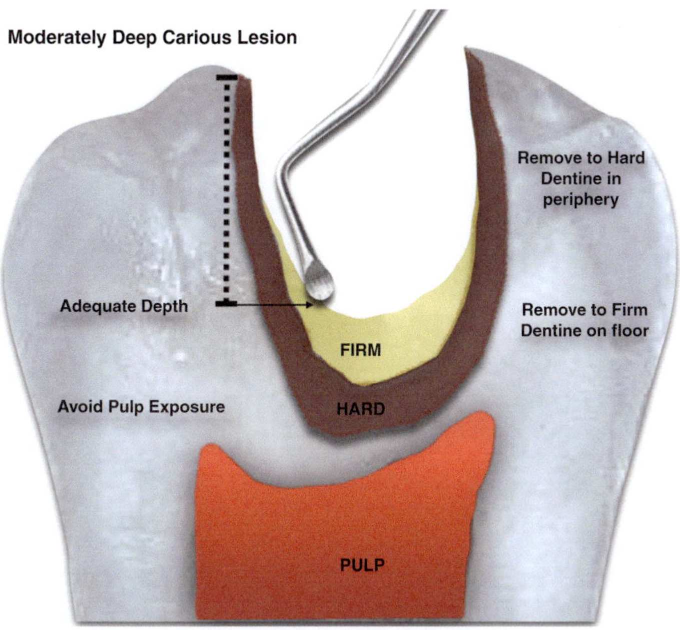

Fig. 2.2 Carious tissue removal in a moderately deep carious lesion: Note that carious tissue is removed to an adequate depth that leaves the base of the lesion in firm dentine. However carious tissue at the periphery of the lesion is removed to hard dentine

prevents pulpal irritation [5]. The microorganisms present in the carious tissue that is left behind are deprived of micronutrients from the oral cavity when the carious lesion is hermetically sealed [7, 8]. Their consequent reduction in potency inactivates the carious lesion. Subsequent deposition of reactionary dentin protects the pulp [7]. Managing a carious lesion in this minimally invasive manner has the advantage in children of reducing the likelihood of the more aggressive, anxiety- and pain-inducing treatment modalities. It allows for undisturbed root maturation in the sensitive immature permanent tooth.

The following is a step-by-step description of management of primary molars where moderately deep carious lesions were treated by removing carious tissue selectively to firm dentine. This is followed by the same restorative principle applied to an immature permanent molar.

2.2.4 Case Study: Selective Carious Tissue Removal to "Firm" Dentine in Primary Teeth

2.2.4.1 Case Selection

Why Were Teeth 74 and 75 Elected for Selective Carious Tissue Removal to "Firm" Dentine?

- Clinically tooth 74 demonstrated an active occlusal lesion. Tooth 75 had a moderately deep carious lesion.
- Teeth 74 and 75 did not have any signs or symptoms of irreversible pulp inflammation.
- Radiographically, the lesions in teeth 74 and 75 appeared moderately deep, but lesions in both teeth did not involve the pulpal third of dentine.
- There were no signs of furcal pathology on the radiograph.

Case Selection: Preoperative Clinical View

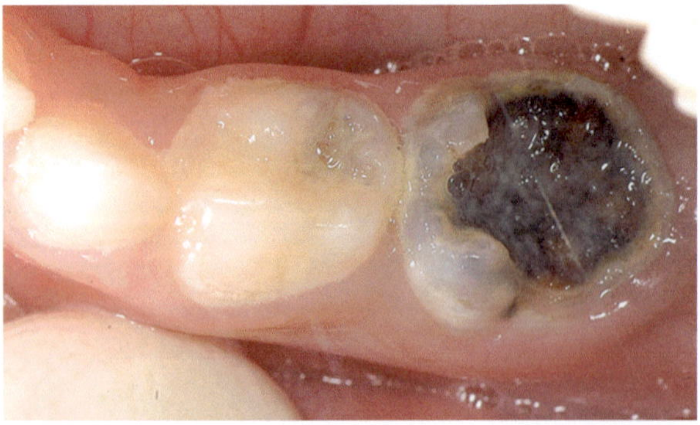

The child reported with carious lesions in teeth 74 and 75. Clinically tooth 74 demonstrated an active occlusal lesion. The carious lesion in tooth 75 appeared moderately deep clinically

Case Selection: Preoperative Radiograph

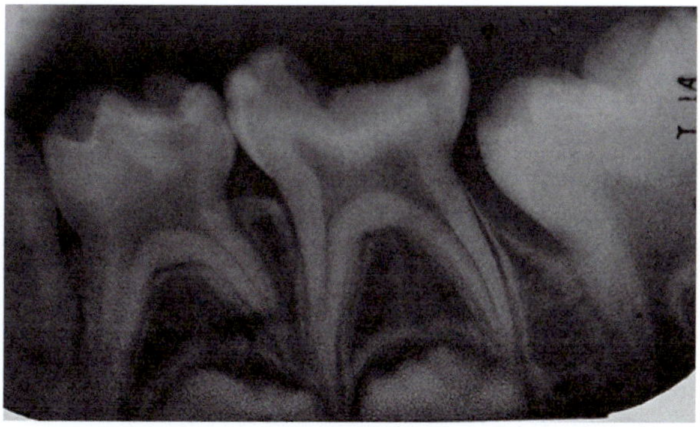

The radiograph showed the carious lesions involving the middle third of dentine with a visible layer of dentine over the pulp in both teeth 74 and 75

2.2.4.2 Step-by-Step Guide

Step 1: Teeth Isolated

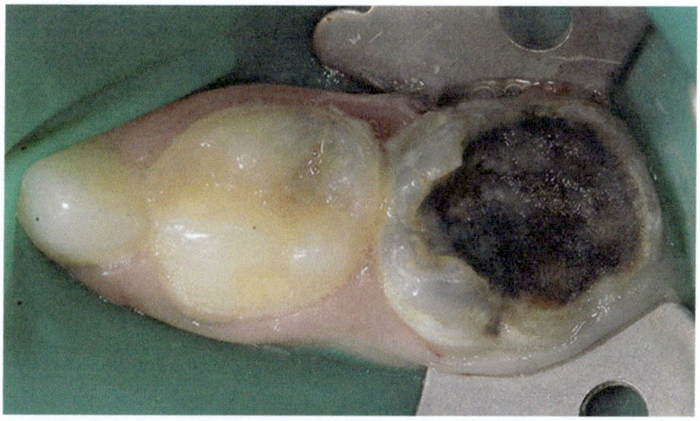

Teeth 74 and 75 were isolated and the carious lesions clearly visualized

Clinical Notes

An alternative treatment option for tooth 75 was to place a Hall crown (Chap. 1). We preferred to remove carious tissue selectively and prepare the second primary molar before placing a crown since the first permanent molar had not yet erupted. This reduces disturbances in eruption of the first permanent molar due to the potentially large Hall crown placed on the second primary molar.

Step 2: Carious Tissue Removal in 74

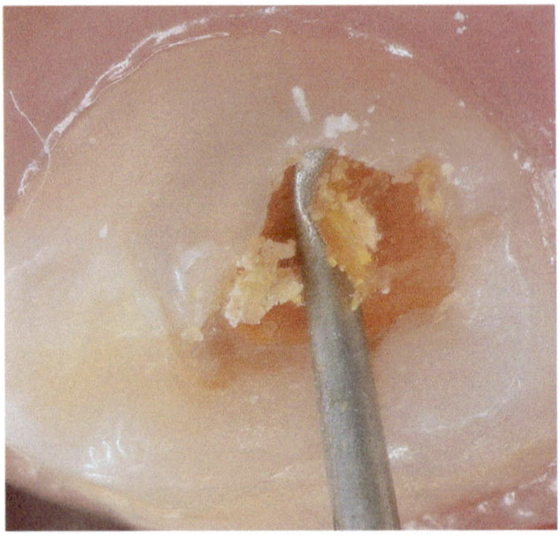

Carious tissue in the periphery of the lesion was removed to "hard" dentine, and tissue was removed to firm dentine in the depth of the lesion

> **Clinical Notes**
> "Hard" dentine is discolored but has tactile sensation similar to "sound" dentine. A "cry dentinaire" or a scratchy sound is heard when a spoon excavator runs through "hard" dentine [5]. "Firm" dentine resists hand excavation and some force is required to lift it [5].

Step 3: Restoration of Tooth 74 and Carious Tissue Removal in Tooth 75

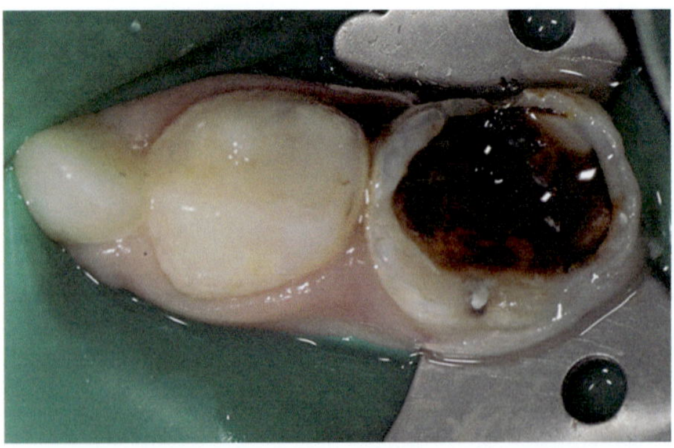

Tooth 74 received a resin-modified glass ionomer cement restoration. In tooth 75, peripheral carious tissue was removed to "hard" dentine. Carious tissue was then removed to firm dentine from the floor of the lesion

Clinical Notes
The depth of the cavity in tooth 75 after removal of carious tissue to firm dentine was insufficient to support an intracoronal restoration. However no further removal of carious tissue was performed in order to avert any possibility of pulp irritation or exposure. A full coronal coverage restoration was planned for tooth 75 with the aim of providing a stable restoration.

Step 4: Full Coronal Coverage Restoration in Tooth 75

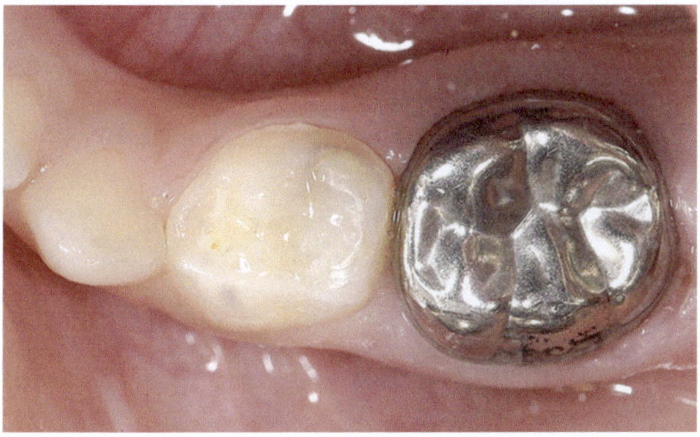

Tooth 75 was restored with a preformed metal crown in order to ensure a stable restoration

Clinical Notes
Long-term stability of the restoration and a hermetic seal is critical to the success of the restoration [6]. An appropriate restoration must be chosen with this in mind.

Step 5: Postoperative Radiograph

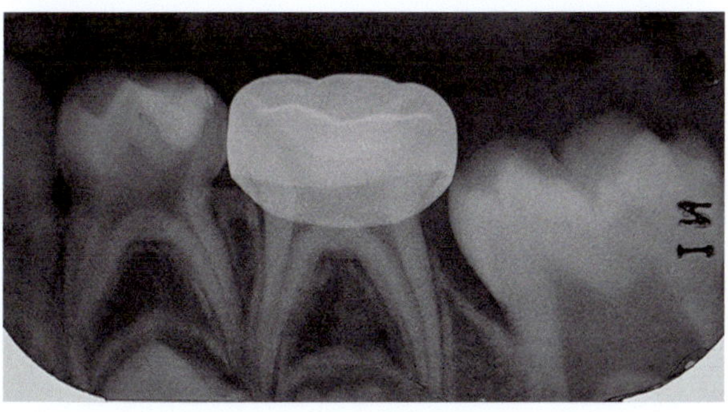

Posttreatment periapical radiograph demonstrates intracoronal restoration in tooth 74 and full coronal coverage restoration in tooth 75

Clinical Notes

Reinforced glass ionomer and resin-modified glass ionomer restorative cements make for good intracoronal restorations after selective removal of carious tissue in primary posterior teeth. However if there is a concern that marginal leakage or fracture of the restoration will compromise the hermetic seal and caries could progress unchecked below the restoration, the option of full coronal restoration must be explored. A postoperative radiograph serves as a baseline to compare with future radiographs to determine success of the treatment.

2.2.4.3 Long-Term Follow-Up

Two-Year Follow-Up Radiograph

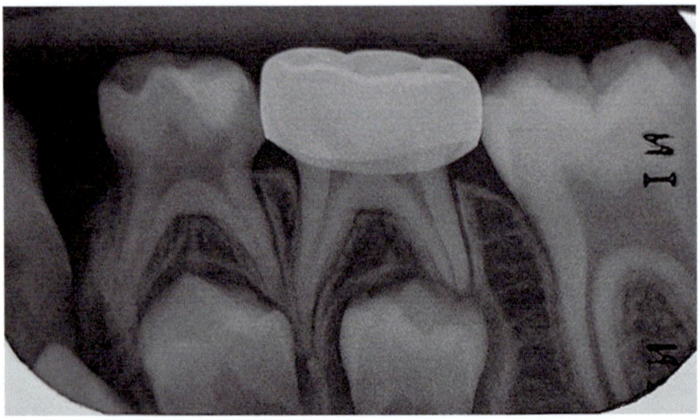

Radiograph on 2-year follow-up shows teeth 74 and 75 with stable restorations and healthy periapical tissue. Note the erupting first permanent molar

Three-Year Follow-Up

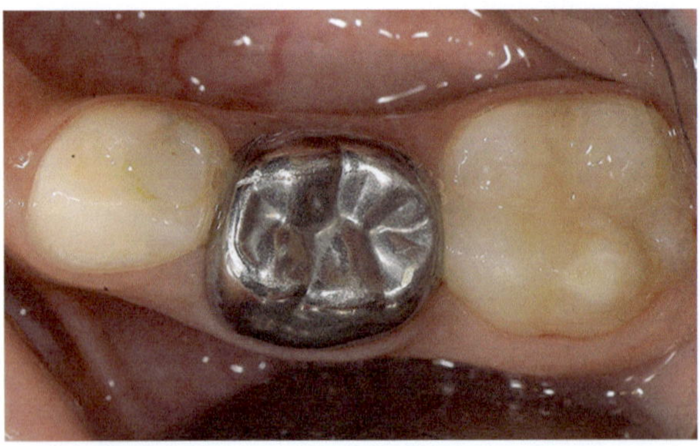

Three-year follow-up shows stable restorations in teeth 74 and 75. Note the well-erupted first permanent molar

Four-Year Follow-Up Radiograph

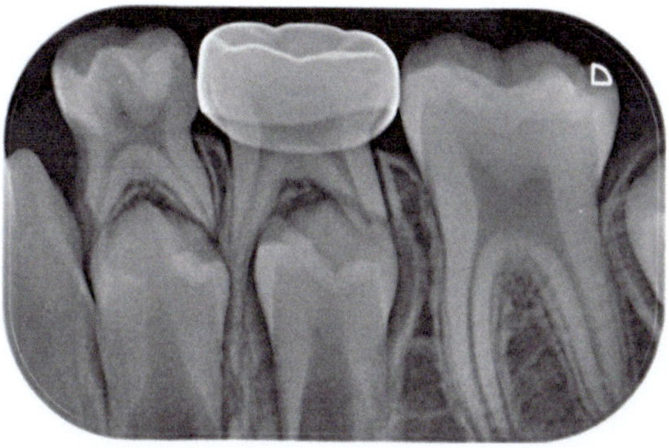

The radiograph shows that selective removal of carious tissue has ensured success of treatment in teeth 74 and 75. Stable restorations and healthy periapical tissue and physiologic root resorption are evident. Note the fully erupted first permanent molar and erupting permanent canine

2.2.5 Case Study: Selective Carious Tissue Removal to "Firm" Dentine in the Immature Permanent Tooth

2.2.5.1 Case Selection

Why Was Tooth 46 Selected for Selective Carious Tissue Removal to "Firm" Dentine?

- Clinically tooth 46 demonstrated a moderately deep carious lesion.
- There were no signs or symptoms of irreversible pulp inflammation.
- Radiographically, the lesion appeared moderately deep and did not involve the pulpal third of dentine.
- There were no signs of periapical pathology on the radiograph.

Case Selection: Preoperative Occlusal View

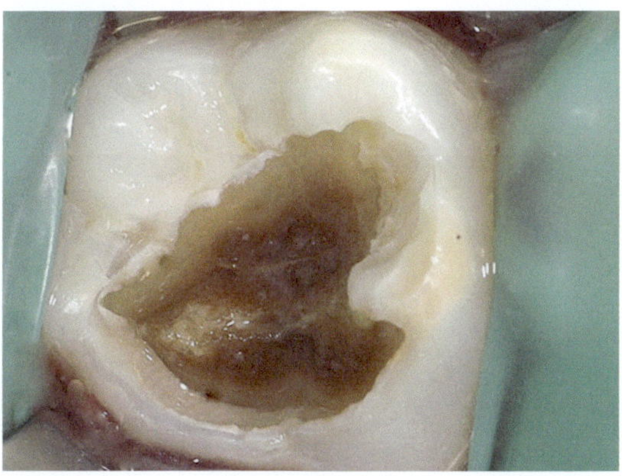

Tooth 46 demonstrated a moderately deep occlusal carious lesion. There was no history or clinical symptoms of pulp inflammation

Case Selection: Preoperative Radiograph

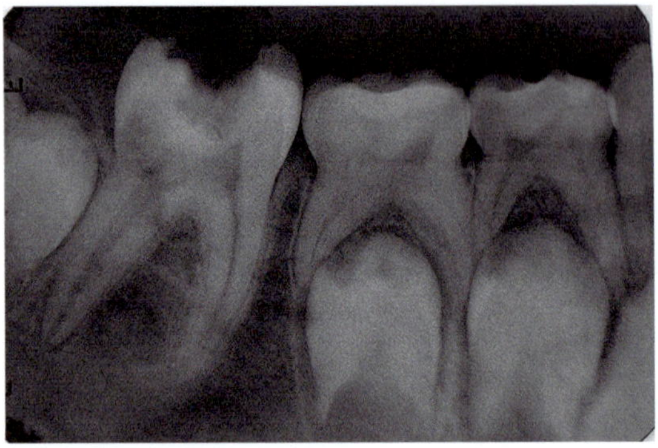

The radiograph showed a moderately deep carious lesion in tooth 46 with a definite layer of dentin over the pulp and no signs of periapical pathology

2.2.5.2 Step-by-Step Guide

Step 1: Selective Removal to "Firm" Dentine

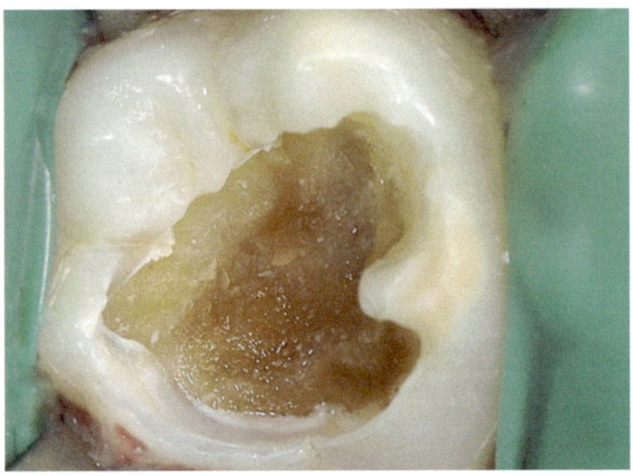

Carious tissue was removed so that the periphery or walls of the lesion are in sound (hard) enamel and dentine to allow the best seal for the restoration. Carious tissue was removed to firm dentine so that a durable restoration of sufficient bulk can be placed

Clinical Notes

An additional terminology, "Leathery" dentin, describes a phase of transition in dentine hardness between "soft" and "firm" dentin. In this lesion distinct "leathery" dentine was encountered and removed to reach firm dentine. Leathery dentine is dentine that does not deform when an excavator is pressed into it but can be removed without much force. "Firm" dentine resists hand excavation and some force is required to lift it [5].

Step 2: Layer of MTA Placed

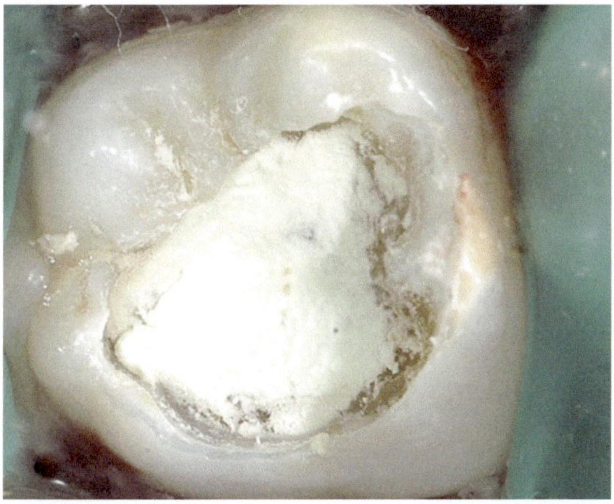

A thin layer of MTA was placed on the floor of the carious lesion [9]

Clinical Notes

In moderately deep lesions, a cavity liner is not a necessity but can be placed if there is sufficient depth in the lesion. Evidence shows that a well-sealed restoration is a prerequisite to success and the type of liner is less important [10].

Step 3: Placement of Final Restoration

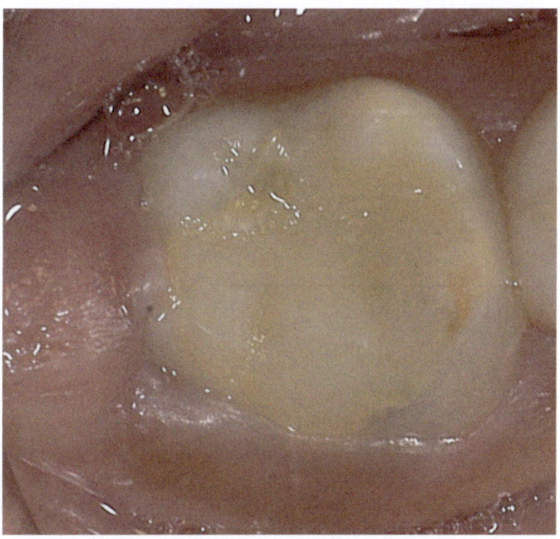

Resin-modified glass ionomer restorative cement was chosen as the final restoration since the tooth had not gained complete eruptive height

Clinical Notes

RMGI cements have the advantage of being less technique sensitive, bonding chemically, releasing fluoride with no marginal shrinkage. They can also be placed immediately over MTA allowing it to set underneath [10]. A composite resin restoration can be added when the tooth erupts completely and the restoration shows wear. In case of extensive lesions, a preformed metal crown can also be used.

Step 4: Postoperative Radiograph

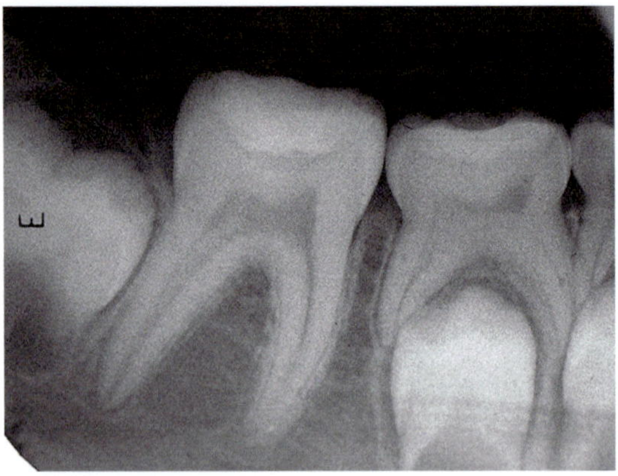

The postoperative radiograph serves as a baseline to compare with future radiographs to confirm lesion arrest and further root maturation

2.2.5.3 Long-Term Follow-Up

Four-Year Follow-Up

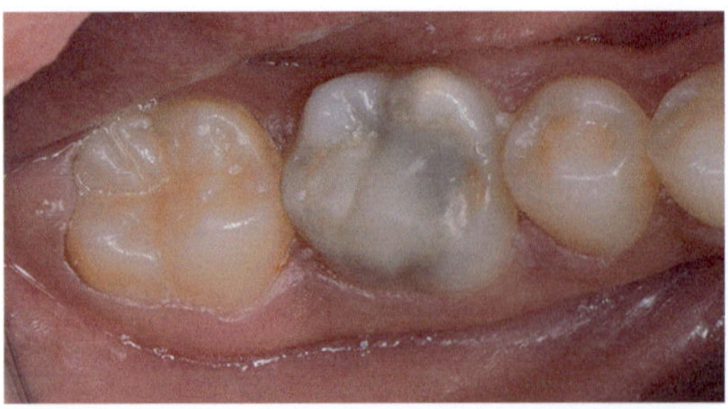

At the end of 4 years, note the stable restoration in tooth 46 and well-erupted teeth 44, 45, and 47. A composite resin restoration was placed over the resin-modified glass ionomer restoration 2 years after the initial treatment when the tooth had gained sufficient eruptive height. Healthy soft tissue and an asymptomatic tooth demonstrate success of the restorative technique. Note that the MTA lining has discolored the tooth and the gray hue is seen through the composite resin restoration

Four-Year Follow-Up Radiograph

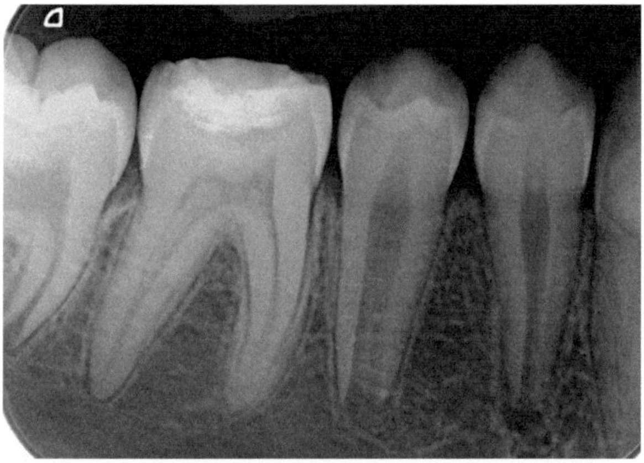

At 4-year follow-up, the demineralized tissue below the restoration looks less radiolucent and has not increased in size proving that the carious lesion has been arrested. Note apical maturation of the distal root, healthy periodontal tissue, and narrowing of pulp chamber and canals indicating further root maturation. This demonstrates success of the lesion management technique

2.3 Selective Carious Tissue Removal to Soft Dentine

2.3.1 Introduction

Complete removal of carious tissue in deep carious lesions, in primary and young permanent teeth, often results in pulp exposure [3, 4]. This is due to the large pulp chamber and high pulp horns in these teeth. When these teeth have no symptoms of irreversible pulp pathology, such an inadvertent carious exposure results in the need for unnecessary and invasive pulp therapy [11]. The anxiety, discomfort, and distress that these demanding procedures cause in children are best avoided. In the immature permanent tooth, circumventing pulp therapy has the added advantage of allowing the immature tooth to mature. It prevents endodontics in the young permanent tooth and the long-term burden of care for the patient.

The main aim of selective removal of carious tissue to soft dentine is to prevent this unnecessary pulp exposure. While achieving this primary objective, the clinician has to ensure that the carious tissue is removed to an adequate depth that allows placement of a restoration of sufficient volume. It is noteworthy that the zone of soft carious dentine increases with an increase in the depth of the carious lesion (Fig. 2.3). Hence in a deep carious lesion, adequate depth can be achieved in soft dentine (Fig. 2.4). Peripheral areas of the lesion are cleaned to hard enamel and dentine to enable a good restorative seal [1]. In the absence of sound peripheral tooth structure, a full coronal coverage restoration is cemented in case of extensive lesions to ensure a hermetic seal.

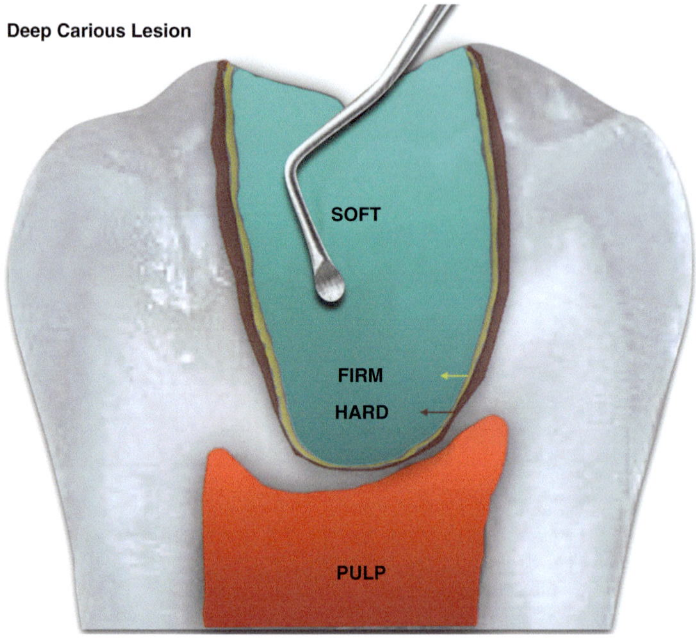

Fig. 2.3 Cross section of a deep carious lesion: Note that the zone of soft carious tissue increases in a deep carious lesion and can occupy almost all of the depth of the lesion

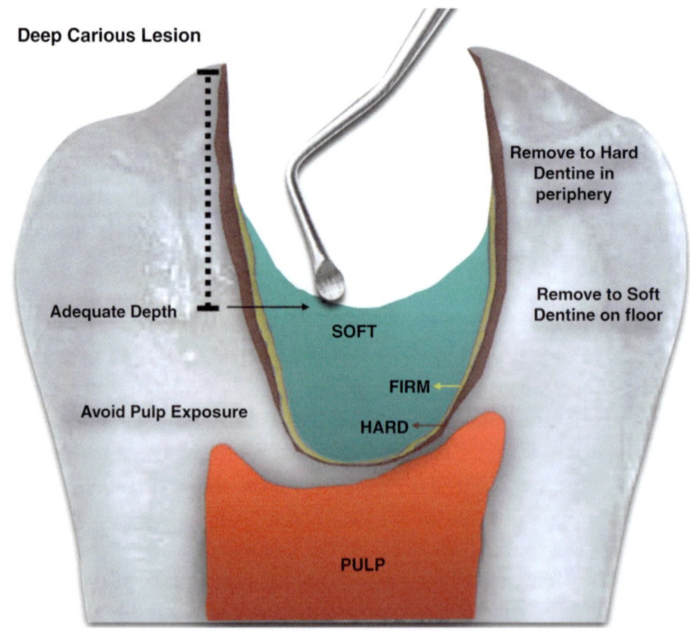

Fig. 2.4 Carious tissue removal in a deep carious lesion: Note that carious tissue is removed to an adequate depth that leaves the base of the lesion in soft dentine. However carious tissue at the periphery of the lesion is removed to hard dentine

2.3.2 Indications and Contraindications

- Selective removal of carious tissue to "soft" dentine is indicated in the management of deep carious lesions in teeth with no history or clinical symptoms and signs of pulp inflammation [1].
- Radiographically, the carious lesion is seen extending into the inner (pulpal) third of dentine with no signs of bone loss or furcal pathology [1].

2.3.3 Rationale

In a deep carious lesion, the outer zone of soft dentine comprises a greater part of the carious lesion. Hence adequate depth for a stable restoration can be achieved while still staying in soft dentine. However soft carious tissue can be scooped out easily and offers little resistance. Hence incessant excavation can lead to unintentional and needless pulp exposure. Discontinuing the removal of carious tissue at the appropriate level of soft dentine requires informed effort on the part of the operator. In a deep carious lesion, the removal of carious tissue to an adequate depth in soft dentin has to be balanced against the primary aim of avoiding pulp exposure [11].

The success of the technique relies on cautious removal of soft tissue over the pulpal areas and the presence of a hermetic seal provided by the peripheral sound enamel/hard dentin. The hermetic seal ensures that the remaining zones of carious tissue that are left behind get inactivated due to lack of substrate [12]. This averts the need for pulp therapy, making treatment less demanding and challenging and more comfortable for the child [13].

The following is a step-by-step guide to selective carious tissue removal to "soft" dentine in primary molars with deep carious lesions. Selective removal of carious tissue to soft dentine in the immature permanent tooth is also detailed.

2.3.4 Case Study: Selective Carious Tissue Removal to "Soft" Dentine in Primary Teeth

2.3.4.1 Case Selection

Why Was This Case Selected for Selective Carious Tissue Removal to "Soft" Dentine?

- Teeth 53, 54, and 55 presented with multisurface lesions.
- The carious lesion in tooth 54 is apparently deep.
- There were no signs or symptoms of irreversible pulp pathology in any tooth.

- The radiograph demonstrated deep carious lesions in teeth 54 and 55 involving the inner pulpal third of dentine.
- Radiographically there were no signs of calcifications in the pulp chamber and interradicular bone loss or signs of internal resorption.

Case Selection: Preoperative Clinical View

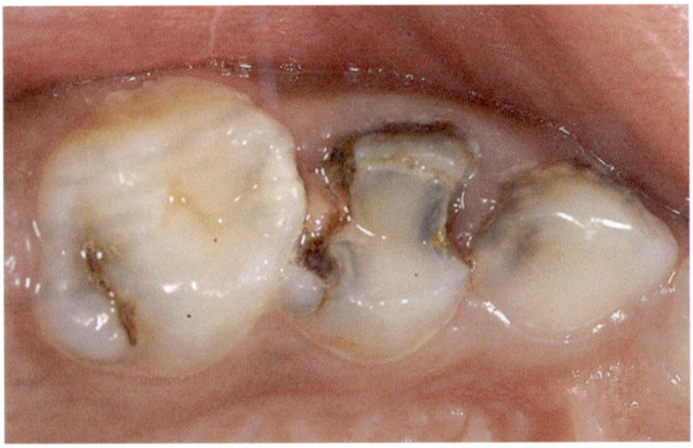

Multisurface carious lesions were seen in teeth 53, 54, and 55. The carious lesion in tooth 54 appeared deep. No clinical signs of pulp pathology were noted

Case Selection: Preoperative Radiograph

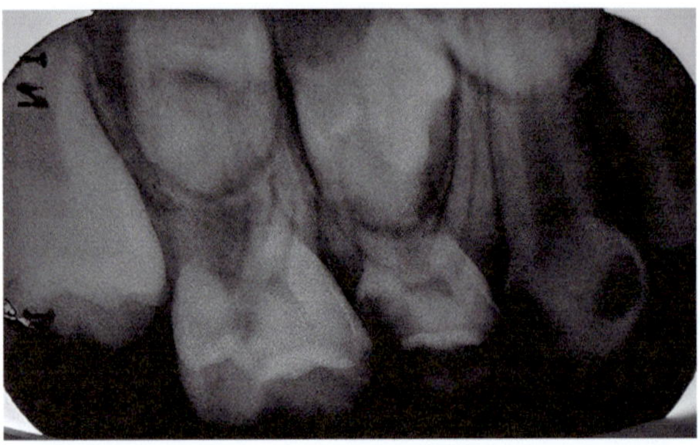

The radiograph showed a deep carious lesion in teeth 54 and 55 involving the inner third of dentine. A layer of dentin was visible over the pulp in tooth 54. No definitive layer of dentine was noticed over the pulp in the carious lesion in tooth 55. There were no signs of furcal or inter radicular pathology. The carious lesion in tooth 53 was moderately deep and did not extend into the inner third of dentine

Clinical Notes
No definitive layer of dentine was noticed over the pulp in the carious lesion in tooth 55. However in the absence of any signs or symptoms of irreversible pulp pathology, a judgment call was taken to restore the tooth after selective removal of carious tissue to soft dentine.

2.3.4.2 Step-by-Step Guide

Step 1: Teeth Isolated

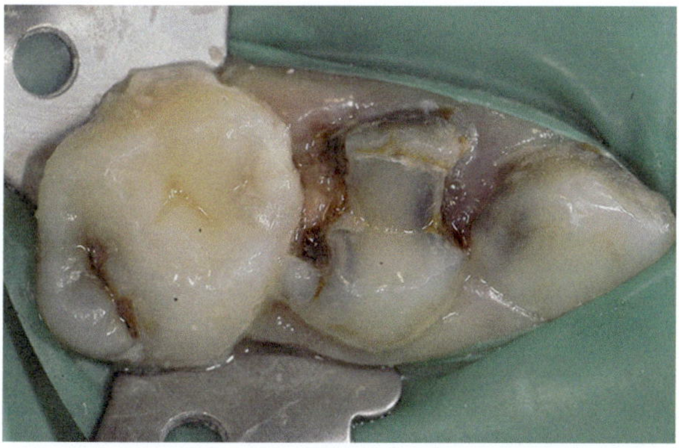

Careful examination after air-drying revealed proximal lesions in all three teeth. Distopalatal cusp of tooth 55 appeared to be undermined beneath the carious lesion

Clinical Notes
Though isolation under a rubber dam is ideal, it is not mandatory for this treatment protocol. A Hall crown was the alternate treatment modality for tooth 54. However, we preferred to selectively remove carious tissue to "soft" dentin to reduce the bacterial load and possibly influence a positive pulp outcome. It should be noted though that there is no strong evidence in literature suggesting that sealing large amounts of bacteria could harm the dental pulp [11].

Step 2: Carious Tissue Removal to "Soft" Dentine in Tooth 55

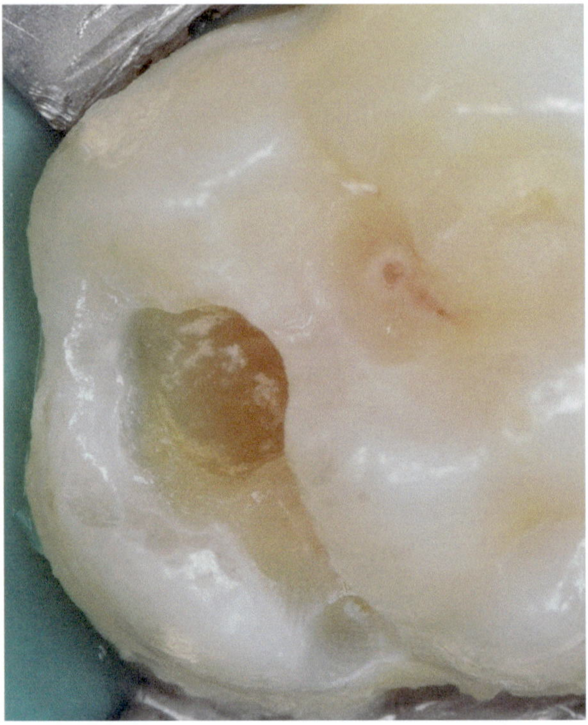

In tooth 55, carious tissue was removed to "hard" dentine along the periphery of the lesion. Carious tissue was then removed to soft dentine at the floor of the carious lesion making a conscious effort to avoid pulp exposure but also obtaining adequate depth for a stable intracoronal restoration

Step 3: Restoration of 53 and 55

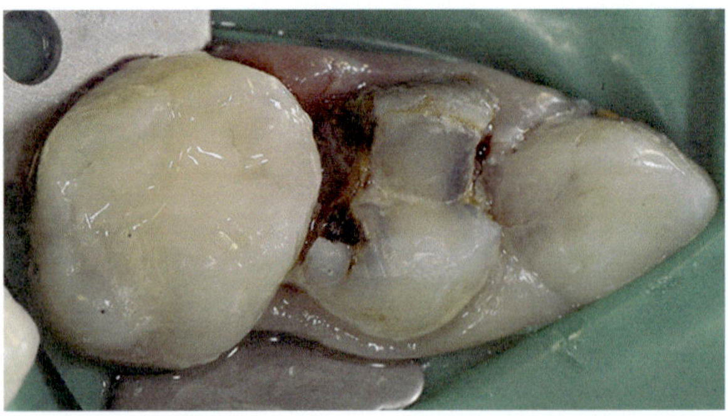

Teeth 53 and 55 were restored with resin-modified glass ionomer cement

Step 4: Carious Tissue Removal to "Soft" Dentine in Tooth 54

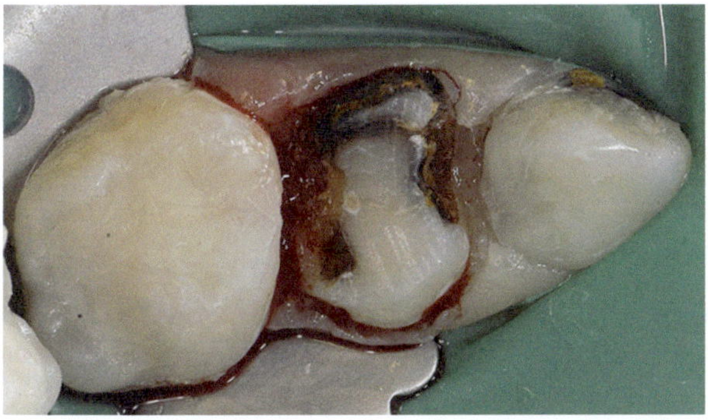

Carious tissue was removed cautiously and selectively to "soft" dentine in tooth 54 without exposing the pulp. Adequate depth could not be gained to place an intracoronal restoration. Hence the tooth was prepared to receive a preformed metal crown

Clinical Notes
The clinical guide to removing "soft" dentine is that pressing an excavator onto it can easily deform the carious tissue. Soft dentine can also be removed without much force.

Step 5: Full Coronal Coverage

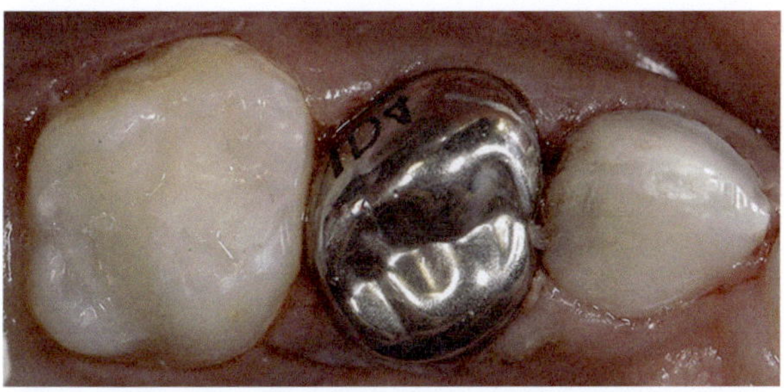

Tooth 54 received a full coronal coverage crown for the best hermetic seal

Clinical Notes
Further removal of carious tissue is terminated if it increases the risk of pulp exposure. When the depth of the resultant lesion is inadequate to support a stable intracoronal restoration, a full coronal coverage must be considered. Success of the treatment depends on achieving a good hermetic seal [6].

Step 6: Postoperative Radiograph

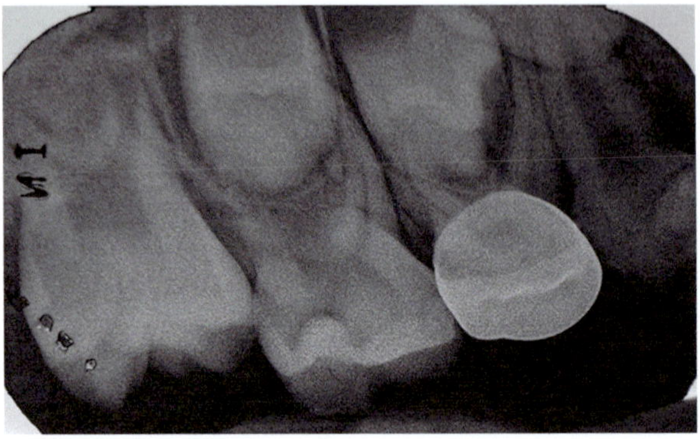

Note the intracoronal restorations in teeth 53 and 55 and the full coronal coverage on tooth 54

> **Clinical Notes**
> The radiograph serves as a record to be compared with follow-up radiographs to check for the stability and health of the restorations and periradicular area. In addition any remineralization of the carious tissue can be appreciated better when a comparison is made with earlier radiographs.

One-Week Postoperative View

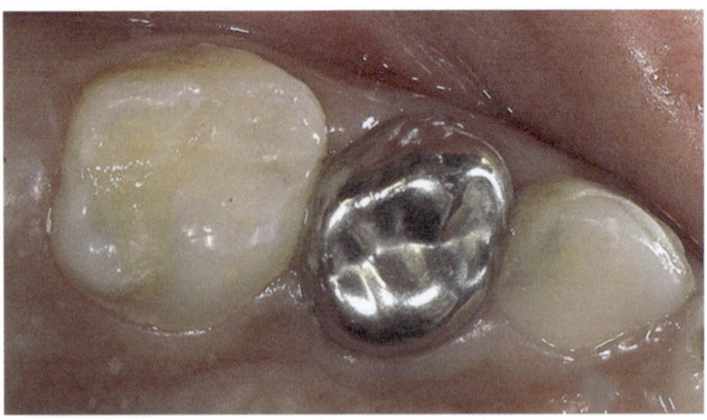

Follow-up at the end of a week showed excellent soft tissue healing and stable restorations

2.3.4.3 Long-Term Follow-Up

Two-Year Follow-Up Radiograph

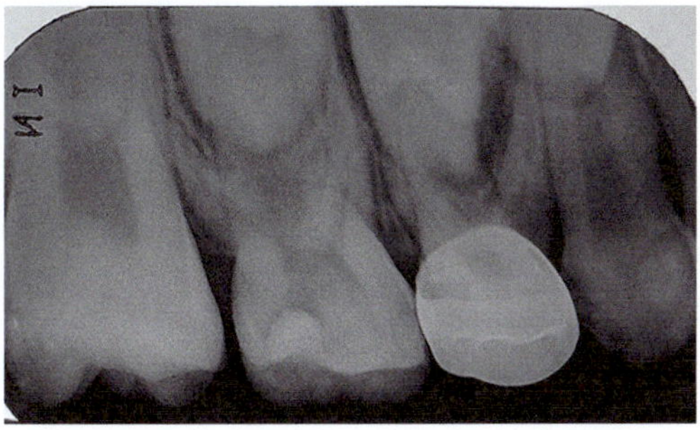

Follow-up at the end of 2 years shows stable restorations in teeth 54 and 55. Note the increase in the remineralization of dentine between the distal pulp horn and the base of the restoration in tooth 55, when compared to the immediate postoperative radiograph. The first permanent molar is seen erupting

Three-Year Follow-Up

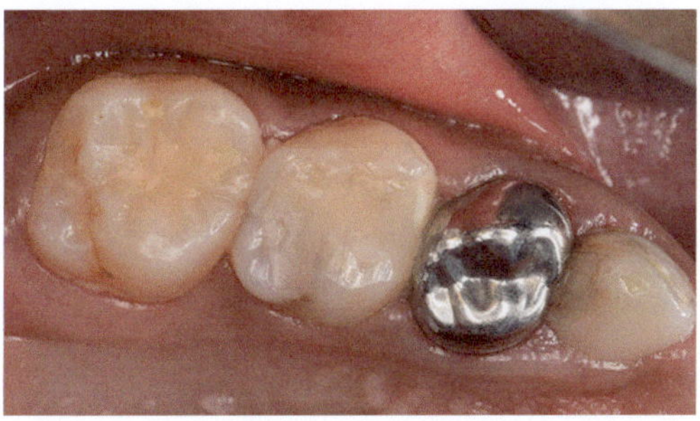

Three-Year follow-up shows stable restorations and healthy gingival tissue. Note the well-erupted first permanent molar

Three-Year Follow-Up Radiograph

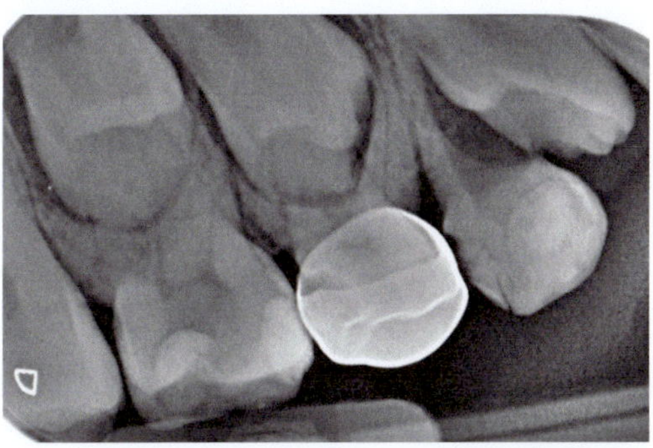

Three-year follow-up radiograph shows stable restorations and no periapical pathology. The first permanent molar is well erupted. Careful observation of the occlusal restoration in tooth 55 shows a substantial increase in the zone of remineralization between the base of the restoration and distal pulp horn. This demonstrates success of the treatment technique

2.3.5 Case Study: Selective Carious Tissue Removal to "Soft" Dentine in the Immature Permanent Tooth

2.3.5.1 Case Selection

Why Was This Case Selected for Selective Carious Tissue Removal to "Soft" Dentine?

- Tooth 36 presented with a deep carious lesion.
- There were no signs or symptoms of irreversible pulp pathology in the tooth.
- The radiograph demonstrated deep carious lesions involving the inner pulpal third of dentine.
- Radiographically there were no signs of calcifications in the pulp chamber, inter-radicular bone loss, or periapical pathology.

Case Selection: Preoperative View of Tooth 36

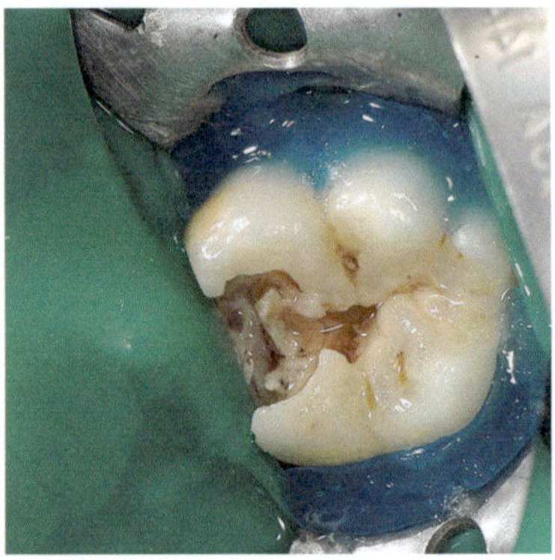

The tooth 36 demonstrated a deep carious lesion on the mesial and occlusal surfaces. There was no history or clinical symptoms and signs of pulp inflammation

Case Selection: Preoperative Radiograph

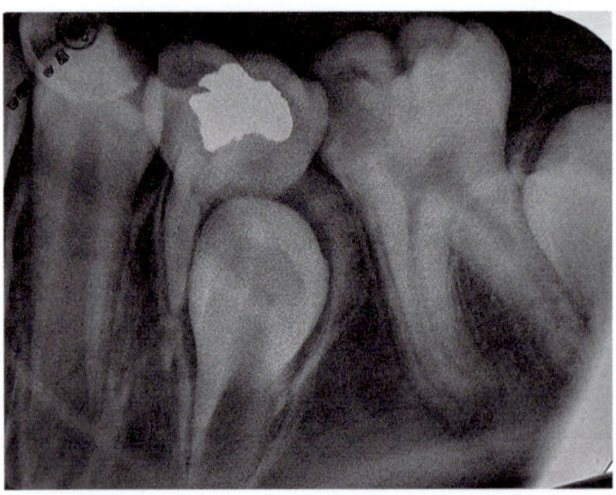

The radiograph showed tooth 36 with a deep carious lesion involving the pulpal third of dentine. The mesial roots showed immature apices, and there were no signs of periapical pathology

2.3.5.2 Step-by-Step Guide

Step 1: Carious Lesion Accessed

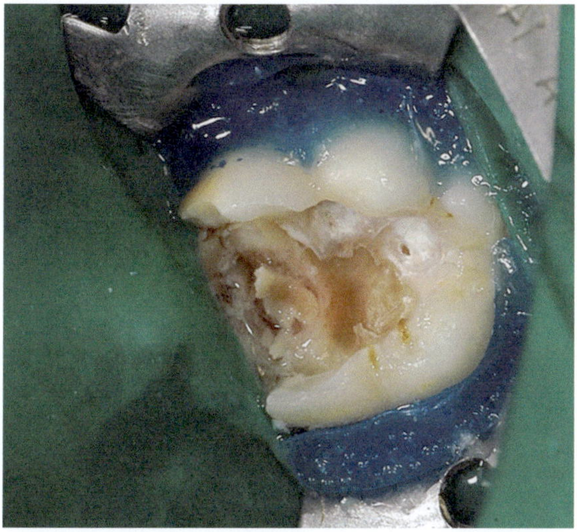

In order to gain access to and remove soft carious tissue, some of the undermined tooth structure was removed to visualize the lesion better

Step 2: Carious Tissue Removed to Soft Dentine

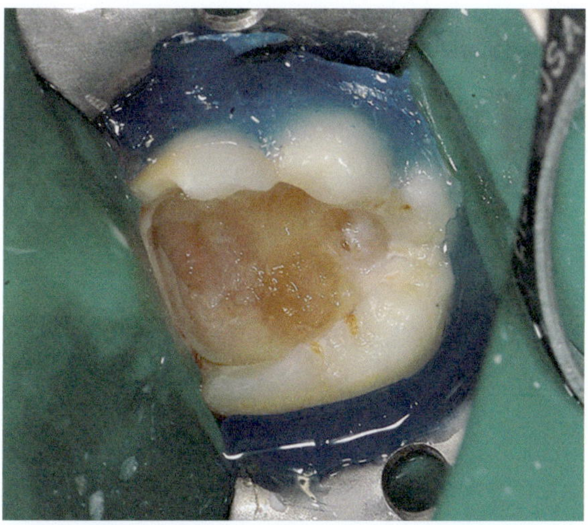

Carious tissue was removed from the walls to hard dentine and sound enamel and from the floor to soft dentine. Care was taken not to expose the pulp

Step 3: Placement of a Liner

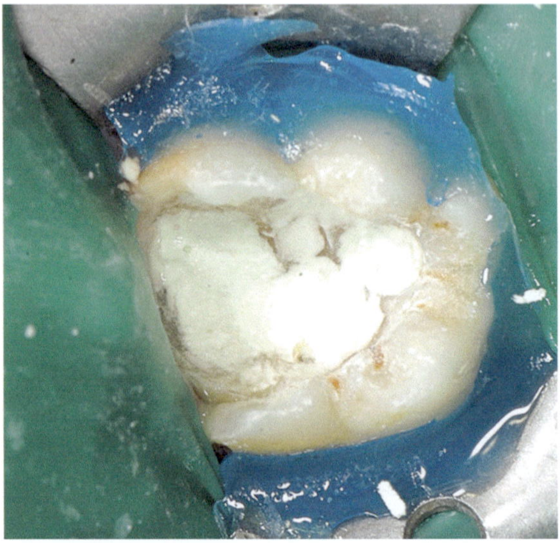

The carious dentin left behind was covered with MTA as a liner [9]

Clinical Notes

Calcium hydroxide or glass ionomer cement can also be used as a liner. Alternately the carious floor can be treated with silver diamine fluoride to arrest the remaining carious tissue. Evidence shows that a restoration with a good hermetic seal is a prerequisite for the success of this technique rather than the material used to line the cavity [10].

Step 4: Restoration of the Tooth

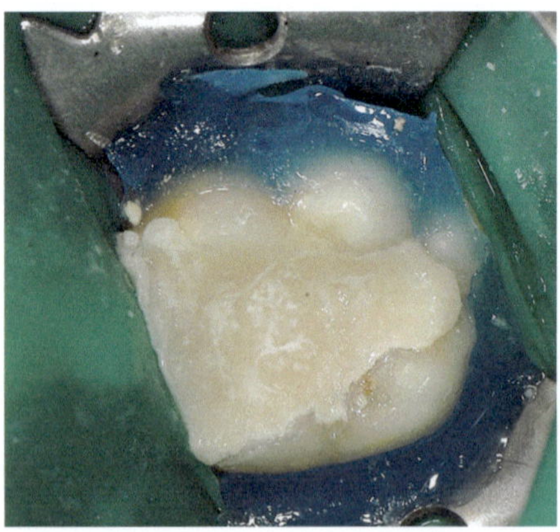

The tooth was restored with resin-modified glass ionomer cement

Clinical Notes

Since the setting time of MTA is prolonged, resin-modified glass ionomer (RMGI) restorative cement has to be placed over the MTA to protect it. This allows the final restoration to be placed in the same sitting and does not compromise the seal [10]. In the absence of RMGI, a temporary restoration would have to be placed until the MTA sets necessitating a second appointment and risking breakdown of the coronal seal [10].

Step 5: Restoration with a Preformed Metal Crown

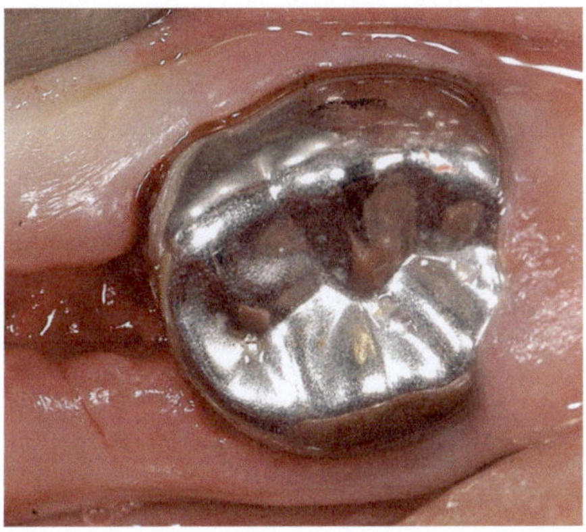

A preformed metal crown was cemented as a full coverage restoration in view of the extensive nature of the lesion. This provided a stable restoration with the best hermetic seal. Tooth 75 was extracted

Step 6: Postoperative Radiograph

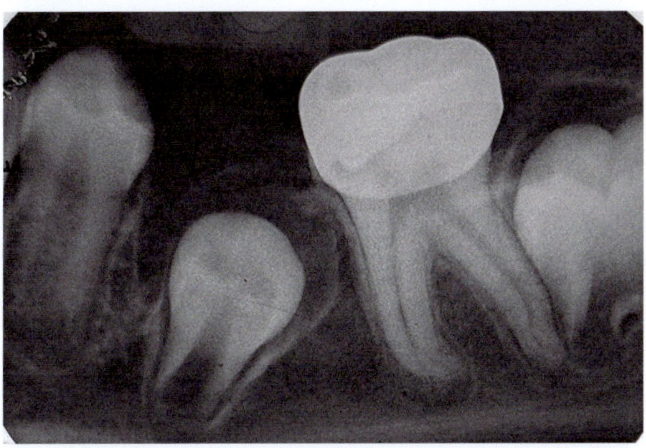

A postoperative radiograph was recorded to help make a comparison with future follow-up radiographs. Note that tooth 75 was extracted

2.3.5.3 Long-Term Follow-Up

Two-Year Follow-Up: Clinical View

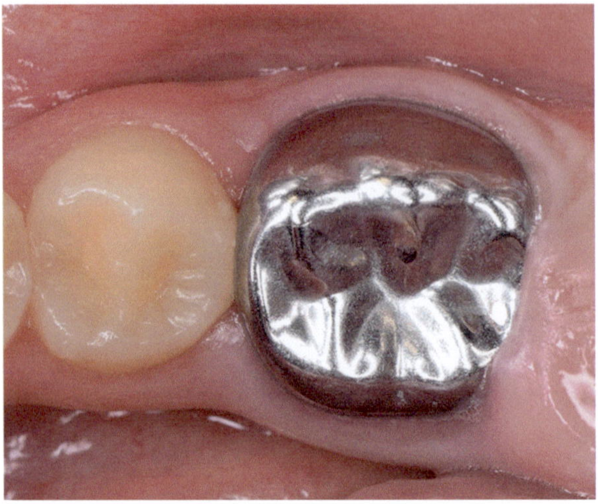

At the end of 2 years, note the healthy gingival tissue and stable restoration in tooth 36. Tooth 35 has erupted in the arch

Two-Year Follow-Up Radiograph

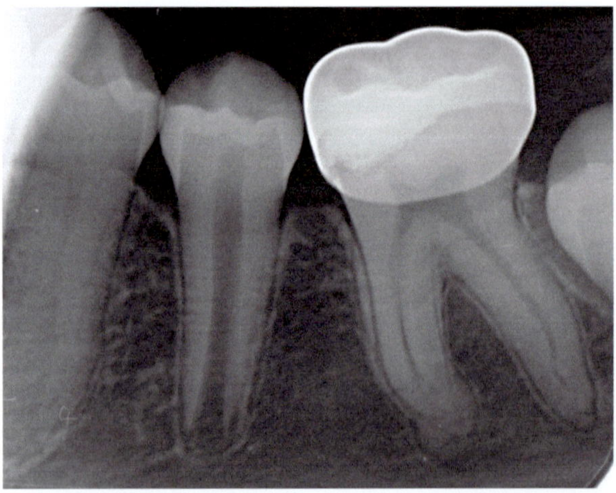

Two-year follow-up radiograph shows a stable restoration in 36, with healthy periradicular tissue. The roots of tooth 36 show further maturation. Tooth 35 has erupted in the arch

2.4 Conclusions

Our approach to the prevention and management of dental caries is determined by how we conceptualize the disease [14]. With this in mind, contemporary methods of managing the carious lesion advocate a minimally invasive approach that involves arresting the carious lesion, conserving tooth structure, and preserving pulp vitality. This approach maximizes long-term restorative success outcomes while ensuring that the more invasive and expensive treatment options are reduced to the minimum. The positive dental experience that this approach in lesion management gives our pediatric patients is invaluable.

References

1. Schwendicke F, Frencken JE, Bjørndal L, Maltz M, Manton DJ, Ricketts D, Van Landuyt K, Banerjee A, Campus G, Doméjean S, Fontana M, Leal S, Lo E, Machiulskiene V, Schulte A, Splieth C, Zandona AF, Innes NP. Managing carious lesions: consensus recommendations on carious tissue removal. Adv Dent Res. 2016;28(2):58–67. https://doi.org/10.1177/0022034516639271.
2. Ngo HC, Mount G, Mc Intyre J, Tuisuva J, Von Doussa RJ. Chemical exchange between glass-ionomer restorations and residual carious dentine in permanent molars: an in vivo study. J Dent. 2006;34(8):608–13.
3. Ricketts DN, Kidd EA, Innes N, Clarkson J. Complete or ultraconservative removal of decayed tissue in unfilled teeth. Cochrane Database Syst Rev. 2006;(3):CD003808.
4. Thompson V, Craig RG, Curro FA, Green WS, Ship JA. Treatment of deep carious lesions by complete excavation or partial removal: a critical review. J Am Dent Assoc. 2008;139(6):705–12.
5. Innes NP, Frencken JE, Bjørndal L, Maltz M, Manton DJ, Ricketts D, Van Landuyt K, Banerjee A, Campus G, Doméjean S, Fontana M, Leal S, Lo E, Machiulskiene V, Schulte A, Splieth C, Zandona A, Schwendicke F. Managing carious lesions: consensus recommendations on terminology. Adv Dent Res. 2016;28(2):49–57. https://doi.org/10.1177/0022034516639276.
6. Schwendicke F. Contemporary concepts in carious tissue removal: a review. J Esthet Restor Dent. 2017;29(6):403–8. https://doi.org/10.1111/jerd.12338.
7. Ricketts DNJ, Innes NPT. To drill or not to drill? How much caries removal do we need? In: Splieth CH, editor. Revolutions in pediatric dentistry. Berlin: Quintessence; 2011. p. 119–34.
8. Bjørndal L, Larsen T. Changes in the cultivable flora in deep carious lesions following a stepwise excavation procedure. Caries Res. 2000;34(6):502–8.
9. Petrou MA, Alhamoui FA, Welk A, Altarabulsi MB, Alkilzy M, Splieth CH. A randomized clinical trial on the use of medical Portland cement, MTA and calcium hydroxide in indirect pulp treatment. Clin Oral Investig. 2014;18(5):1383–9. https://doi.org/10.1007/s00784-013-1107-z.
10. Hilton TJ. Keys to clinical success with pulp capping: a review of the literature. Oper Dent. 2009;34(5):615–25.
11. Schwendicke F, Innes N. Removal strategies for carious tissues in deep lesions. In: Schwendicke F, editor. Management of deep carious lesions. New York, NY: Springer; 2018. p. 15–35.
12. Oong EM, Griffin SO, Kohn WG, Gooch BF, Caufield PW. The effect of dental sealants on bacteria levels in caries lesions: a review of the evidence. J Am Dent Assoc. 2008;139(3):271–8.
13. Schwendicke F, Stolpe M, Meyer-Lueckel H, Paris S, Dörfer CE. Cost-effectiveness of one- and two-step incomplete and complete excavations. J Dent Res. 2013;92(10):880–7. https://doi.org/10.1177/0022034513500792.
14. Fejerskov O. Concepts of dental caries and their consequences for understanding the disease. Community Dent Oral Epidemiol. 1997;25:5–12.

Pulp Therapy in Primary Teeth

3

3.1 Overview

The objectives of pulp therapy for primary teeth differ largely from permanent teeth. The premature loss of primary teeth leads to loss of arch length and decreased masticatory efficiency among other esthetic and functional needs. The rationale for performing primary tooth pulpotomy and pulpectomy is to maintain arch length and integrity by preserving the pulpally involved tooth as a natural space maintainer. Accurate case selection, use of contemporary materials, meticulous attention to clinical protocol, and efforts to achieve a good coronal seal determine the long-term success of pulp therapy in primary teeth. The following subchapters delve in detail into these treatment aspects.

3.2 MTA Pulpotomy

3.2.1 Introduction

Pulpotomy is the removal of the entire coronal portion of the pulp followed by the placement of a suitable medicament to preserve the remaining vital radicular pulp within the root canals.

A pulpotomy has traditionally been considered a classic pulp therapy protocol for all primary teeth exhibiting signs of reversible pulpits. Therefore for the tooth to be considered a pulpotomy candidate, the infection or inflammation should be confined to the coronal portion of the pulp [1]. However with the current understanding of the disease dental caries and of carious tissue removal, the need to do a pulpotomy in a primary tooth has concurrently reduced. Evidence suggests greater success rates of indirect pulp therapy when compared to pulpotomies using formocresol and ferric sulfate in primary teeth with deep carious lesions [2]. Recent studies comparing the complete removal of carious tissue (followed by a pulpotomy or restoration) to the biological approach (Hall technique or selective removal) when treating deep

M. S. Kher, A. Rao, *Contemporary Treatment Techniques in Pediatric Dentistry*,
https://doi.org/10.1007/978-3-030-11860-0_3

carious lesions found that both techniques showed equally successful final outcomes [3]. Selective removal of carious tissue to soft dentine in deep carious lesions (Chap. 2) hence decreases the need for a pulpotomy procedure in teeth with a diagnosis of reversible pulpits. Nevertheless, the pulpotomy procedure has an important place in pediatric endodontics provided the clinician understands its case selection, indications, and contraindications.

3.2.2 Indications and Contraindications

Pulpotomy is indicated in a tooth diagnosed with reversible pulpits in the following situations:

1. When a reliable pain history is compromised by the age of the child and the presence of multiple deep carious lesions in the same side of the mouth. This situation can leave the clinician uncertain of the actual nature and area of pain leading the clinician to play safe and perform a pulpotomy over the more conservative selective removal of carious tissue approach.
2. When the radiograph does not show a layer of mineralized dentine separating the carious lesion from the pulp.
3. When an inadvertent pulp exposure occurs in the process of removal of carious tissue.

Pulpotomy is recommended in a tooth with a diagnosis of *reversible pulpitis*. A tooth with a diagnosis of *irreversible pulpits* is contraindicated for a pulpotomy procedure. A differentiation should be made between provoked pain indicative of reversible pulpitis and spontaneous pain indicative of irreversible pulpitis [1]. The following is a simple guide to arriving at a diagnosis of either reversible or irreversible pulpitis.

3.2.2.1 Reversible Pulpitis

- The tooth may be sensitive to cold or sweet foods. The child may complain of discomfort while chewing.
- The pain, sensitivity, or discomfort is temporary in nature and disappears when the stimulus is removed.
- Clinically there is no sign of mobility, tenderness to percussion, or presence of a gingival draining sinus.
- Radiographically there should be no signs of calcifications in the pulp chamber, interradicular bone loss, signs of internal resorption or periapical pathology.

3.2.2.2 Irreversible Pulpitis

- There is a history of spontaneous, persistent pain, severe shooting pain or a dull throbbing ache. Pain continues even after the stimulus is withdrawn.
- Pain, if persistent, should be differentiated from pain that occurs due to food impaction interdentally and resultant papillitis, which is common in children [4].
- There may be a history of an extra oral swelling.

- There could be increased sensitivity to hot food.
- Clinical examination may reveal an intra oral abscess, draining sinus, pathologic mobility, or pain on percussion.
- Radiograph may show signs of bone loss or furcal pathology.

3.2.3 Rationale for MTA Pulpotomy

Historically, the pharmacotherapeutic medicament used in primary teeth pulpotomy was one-fifth dilution formocresol. Formocresol devitalizes the pulp tissue and does not fulfil the objective of maintaining the vitality of the radicular pulp tissue. It also has cytotoxic and carcinogenic concerns [5].

Currently, 15% ferric sulfate, mineral trioxide aggregate (MTA), and calcium silicate-based cements [6] are popular, while non-pharmacologic techniques include the use of an electrocautery and carbon dioxide laser.

Ferric sulfate being a potent hemostat may arrest hyperemic bleeding from the canal orifices [7]. This could mask a diagnosis of irreversible pulpitis. In addition, ferric sulfate only creates a metal protein clot at the orifices and does not seal the floor of the pulp chamber, thus leaving open accessory channels of communication between the pulp chamber and the surrounding tissue. This is also true when an electrocautery or a laser is used.

More recently, a rich body of evidence has favored pulpotomies with MTA [8–10]. When used as a pulpotomy agent, MTA maintains healthy radicular pulp vascularity by sealing the root canal orifices. It also offers good resistance to bacterial microleakage by plugging the accessory canals on the pulpal floor [7]. An alternative to the use of MTA is Biodentine. A recent systematic review concluded that neither material showed superior outcomes [11]. For pulpotomies in posterior teeth, we prefer the evidence-based use of MTA. The following is a step-by-step guide to performing an MTA pulpotomy in a primary molar.

3.2.4 Case Study: MTA Pulpotomy in a Primary Molar

3.2.4.1 Case Selection

Why Was This Case Selected for a Pulpotomy?

- From the pain history, a diagnosis of reversible pulpitis was made in tooth 75.
- There was no history of spontaneous or persistent pain indicating irreversible pulpitis.
- Clinically there were no signs of mobility, tenderness to percussion, presence of a gingival abscess, or draining sinus that are signs of irreversible pulpitis.
- The radiograph demonstrated a deep carious lesion approximating the distal pulp horn with no visible layer of dentine separating the lesion from the pulp.
- Radiographically there were no signs of calcifications in the pulp chamber, inter-radicular bone loss, or signs of internal resorption

Case Selection: Preoperative Clinical View

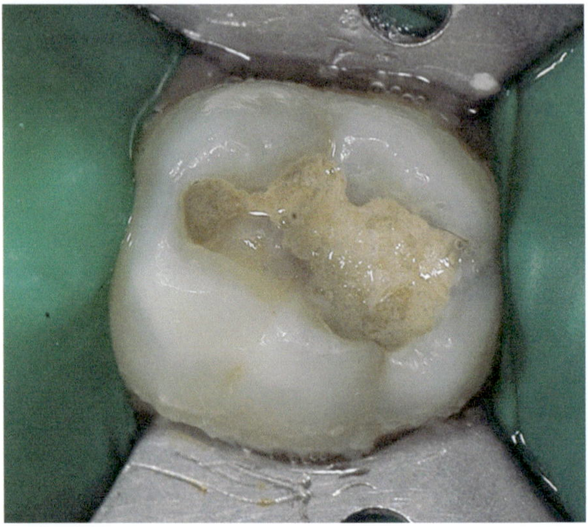

The child reported with a temporary restoration in tooth 75

Case Selection: Preoperative Radiograph

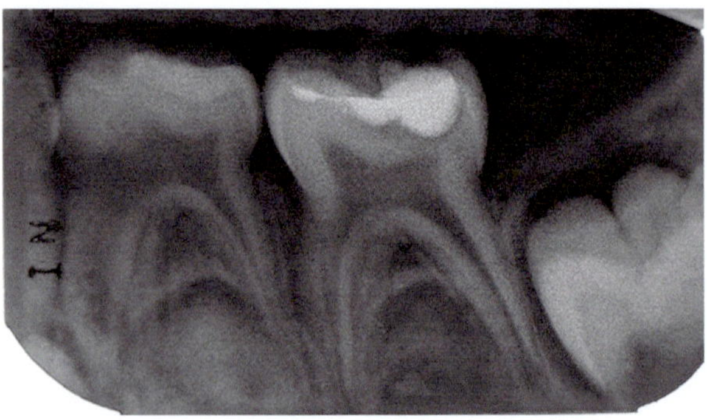

The radiograph demonstrated a deep carious lesion approximating the distal pulp horn with no visible layer of dentine separating the two. Radiographically there were no signs of calcifications in the pulp chamber, interradicular bone loss, or signs of internal resorption

3.2.4.2 Step-by-Step Guide

Step 1: Occlusal View of Carious Lesion

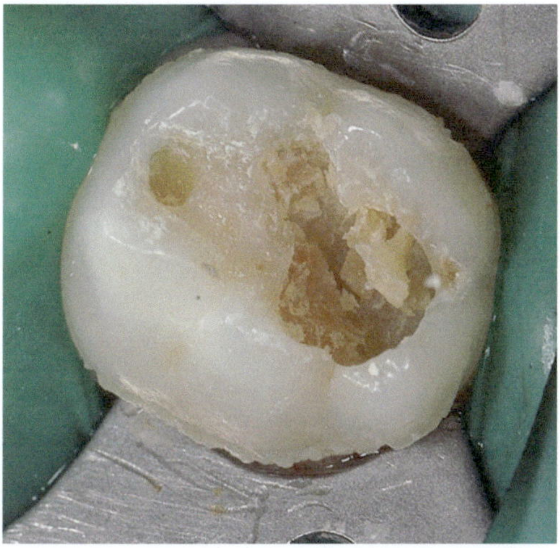

Temporary restorative cement was removed to reveal a deep carious lesion with soft carious tissue debris

> **Clinical Notes**
> Adequate local anesthesia is obtained. Before exposing the pulp, complete removal of carious tissue is important, to prevent inadvertent infection of the pulp tissue.

Step 2: Access Cavity Preparation

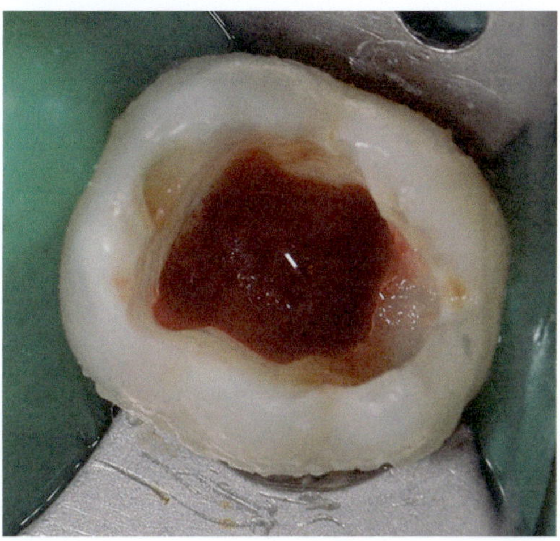

Complete unroofing of the pulp chamber was achieved with a sterile bur after complete removal of carious tissue

Clinical Notes
Unroofing of the pulp chamber should not leave undercuts. Undercuts make complete removal of pulp tissue difficult which results in continued hemorrhage.

Step 3: Coronal Pulp Amputation

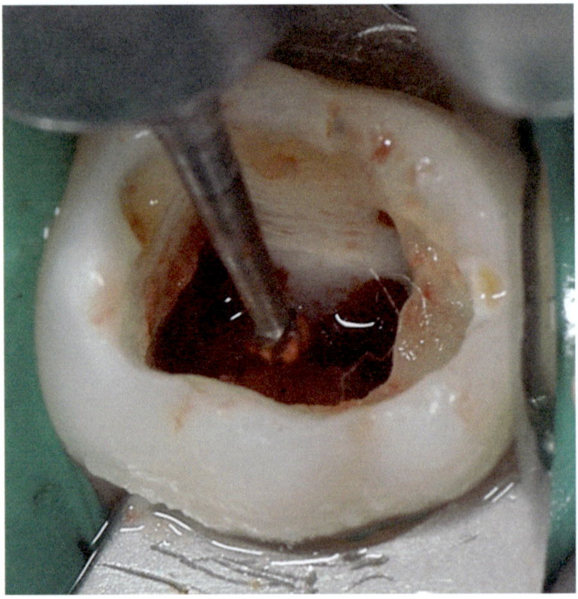

The coronal pulp amputation was completed with a sterile slow speed round bur

Clinical Notes
A conscious effort should be made to remove all pulpal filaments. Any remaining pulp tissue will result in continued hemorrhage. The pulp chamber is thoroughly debrided with saline to remove debris.

Step 4: Hemorrhage Control

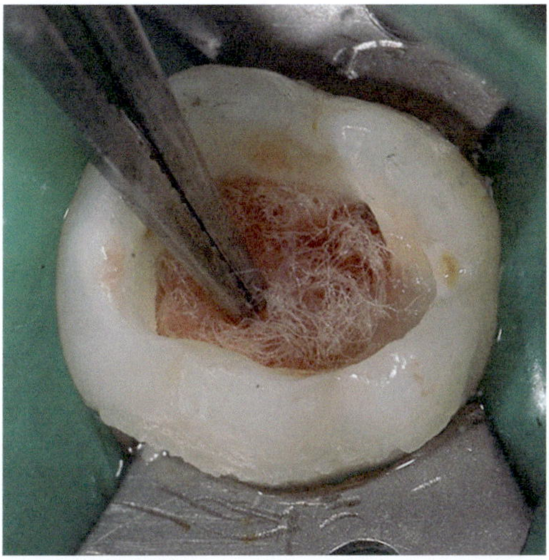

Cotton pellets soaked in saline and blot dried were placed over the orifices of the root canals under moderate pressure to control hemorrhage

Clinical Notes
Dry cotton pellets are not used as the fibers can engage the clot and induce bleeding [1].

Step 5: Hemostasis Obtained

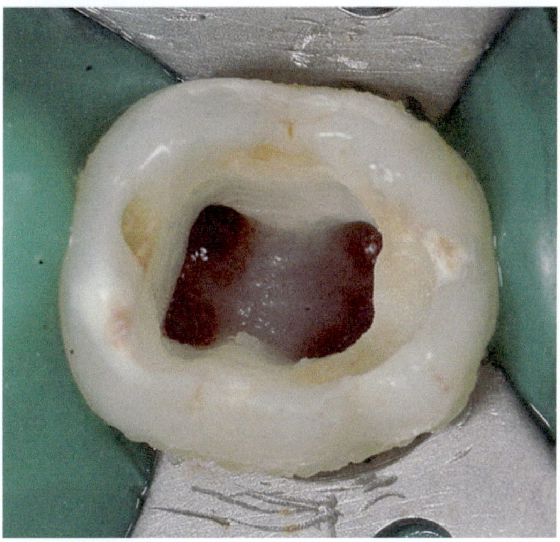

Note the hemostasis achieved in all four canal orifices

Clinical Notes
Hemostasis should be obtained in no more than 5 min [12]. Intrapulpal anesthesia or use of any hemostatic agent should be avoided as continued bleeding is a clinical sign of radicular pulp inflammation. In case of continued bleeding, the operator should proceed to perform a pulpectomy [8]. However recent evidence shows that acheiving hemostasis may not have a direct corelation to whether the radicular pulp is inflamed [13]. Hence all the parameters of case selection should be taken into consideration.

Step 6: Sodium Hypochlorite Sweep

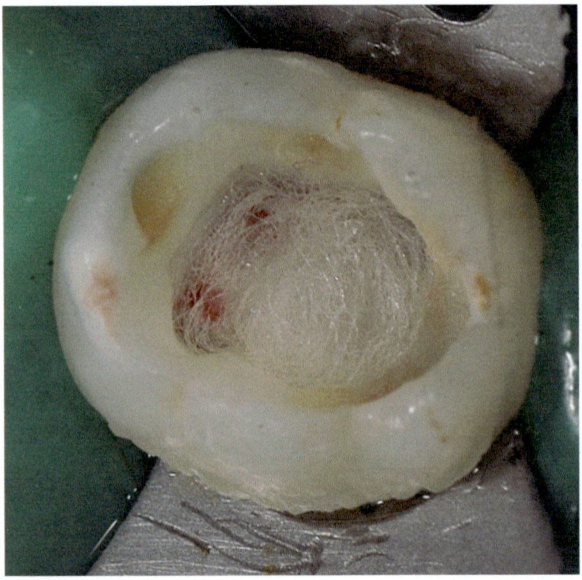

The chamber was swept with a pellet soaked in 1% sodium hypochlorite for an antibacterial effect [7]

Clinical Notes
Regardless of the medicament used, the technique of pulpotomy is constant up to this step.

Step 7: Application of MTA

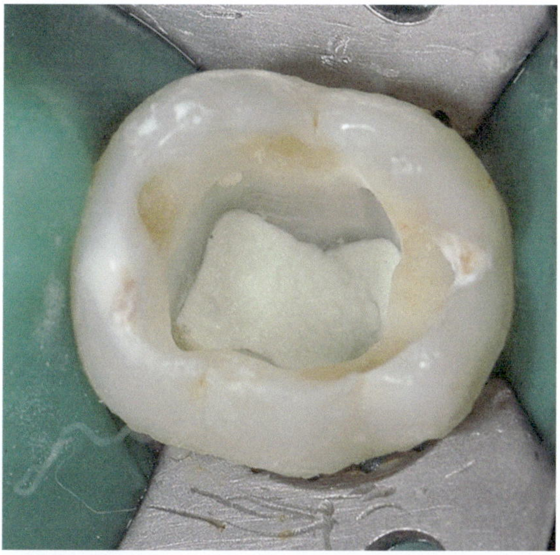

An adherent mix of MTA was placed on the root canal orifices and the pulpal floor and gently condensed with moist dry cotton pellets to a uniform thickness. The MTA is placed evenly on the entire pulpal floor and condensed in order to cover all accessory canals

Step 8: Core Buildup

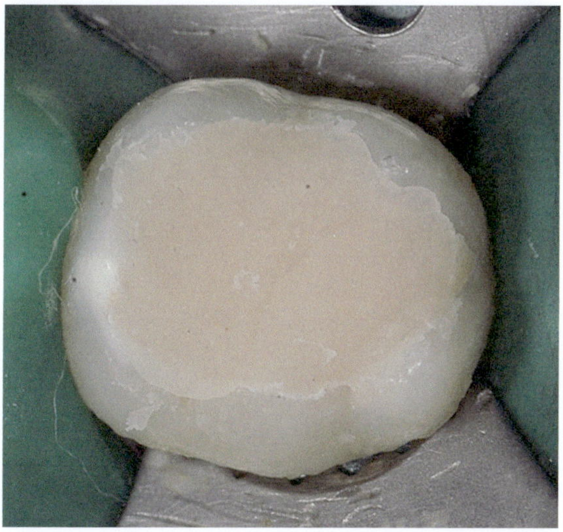

Resin-modified glass ionomer cement was placed over the MTA allowing the MTA to set underneath [14]

Clinical Notes

Since the setting time of MTA is prolonged, resin-modified glass ionomer (RMGI) restorative cement placed over the MTA protects it and does not compromise the coronal seal [14]. In the absence of RMGI, the temporary restoration placed until the MTA sets would necessitate a second appointment and risk breakdown of the coronal seal [14]. A stable restoration may be adequate if the crown structure of the tooth is intact. However, it is advisable to restore the tooth with a preformed crown for a better coronal seal especially if the tooth is expected to exfoliate after some years.

Step 9: Preformed Metal Crown

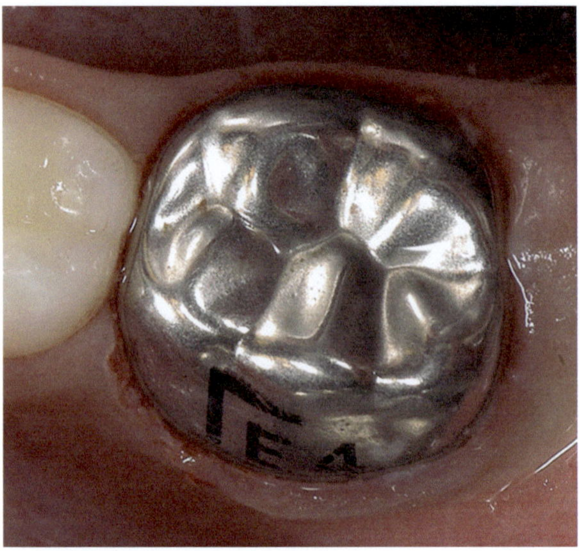

Preformed metal crown cemented for a good coronal seal

Clinical Notes

Evidence suggests a higher success rate for teeth restored with a full coronal coverage crown like a preformed metal crown [10, 15]. The crown should be placed in the same appointment or as soon as is practically possible (Chap. 4).

Step 10: Postoperative Radiograph

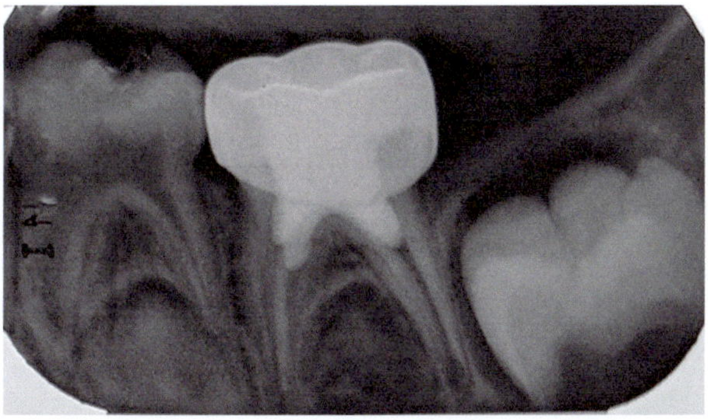

A postoperative radiograph was recorded for future reference

Step 11: One-Week Follow-Up

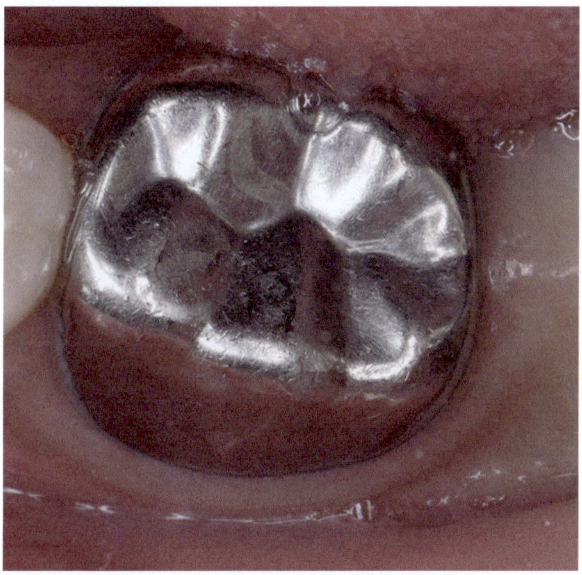

Note the excellent healing 1 week after placement of a preformed metal crown

3.2.4.3 Long-Term Follow-Up

Four-Year Follow-Up

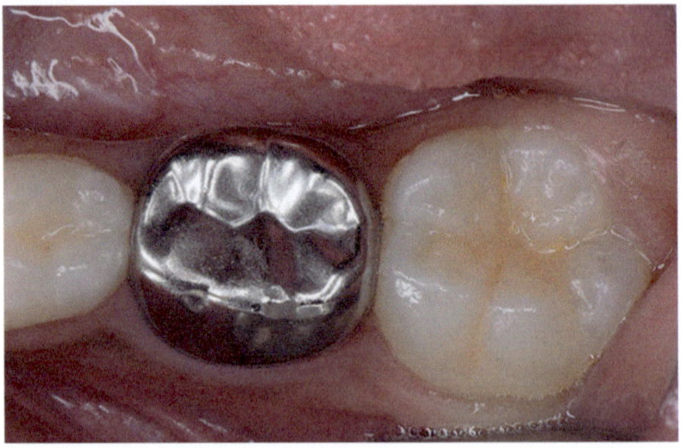

A stable crown with healthy soft tissue is seen after 4 years. Also note that the arch length is maintained with the first permanent molar, tooth 36, erupting distal to the tooth 75

Four-Year Follow-Up Radiograph

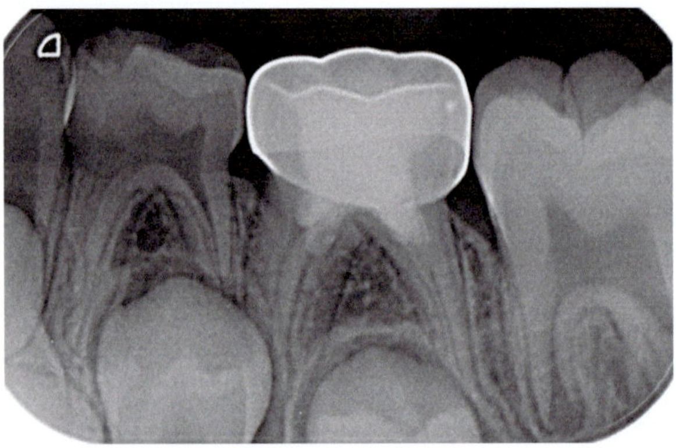

Four-year follow-up radiograph shows healthy roots, interradicular bone, and a successful outcome of the pulpotomy procedure. A coincidental finding is the further root maturation in tooth 75 as compared to the immature roots noted on the preoperative radiograph. Also note the erupting first permanent molar demonstrating how the pulpally involved tooth has acted successfully as a natural space maintainer

3.3 Single-Visit Pulpectomy

3.3.1 Introduction

Pulpectomy in primary teeth is the removal of the entire pulp tissue and the subsequent filling of the root canals with a suitable resorbable material. Pulpectomy in a primary tooth was historically considered overtreatment as compared to a traditional extraction. Torturous root canals, resorbing primary tooth roots, the effect of over obturation, potential damage to the developing succedaneous tooth [1], and behavior guidance for a young child during what was considered a lengthy and complex procedure discouraged many clinicians from attempting this useful technique. However, increasing evidence in favor of the long-term success of pulpectomies [16, 17] led to the clinical acceptance and popularity of this procedure.

3.3.2 Indications and Contraindications

Pulpectomy is indicated in a tooth [8]:

- With a diagnosis of irreversible pulpitis (criteria described in the section on pulpotomy) which is restorable with full coronal coverage post pulpectomy
- Where hemorrhage control from the root canal orifices during pulpotomy is not obtained indicative of inflamed pulp tissue in the root canals

Pulpectomy is contraindicated in children:

- With significant systemic problems like congenital heart disease, nephrotic syndrome, etc.
- Children reporting with cellulitis from the concerned tooth

Local contraindications for pulpectomy are teeth [1], which on the radiograph show:

- Advanced internal resorption
- Excessive external resorption involving more than 1/3 of the root
- Interradicular lesion involving the succedaneous tooth crypt
- Severe bone loss resulting in mobility
- Perforation in the furcation area

3.3.3 Rationale for Single-Visit Pulpectomy

Rabinowitch first published a report on endodontic procedures in primary teeth [1]. It was initially advocated as a multi-visit procedure. Pulpectomy gradually evolved into a viable single-visit procedure due to:

- Availability of long-term success data
- Development of standard anxiety management protocols like inhalation sedation

- Availability of easy-to-use obturating materials
- Clinical introduction of apex locators in primary teeth
- Rotary endodontics in primary teeth

A multiple visit pulpectomy, though not contraindicated, is best avoided. It subjects the child to multiple stress-inducing appointments leading to treatment fatigue and loss of cooperation. Extraction followed by space maintenance is a viable alternative to a multiple visit pulpectomy (Chap. 6).

3.3.4 Case Study: Single-Visit Pulpectomy in a Primary Molar

3.3.4.1 Case Selection

Why Was This Case Selected for a Single-Visit Pulpectomy?
The child reported with a deep carious lesion in tooth 85. Tooth bud of tooth 46 was visible but not yet erupted. There was no significant medical history.

- From the pain history, a diagnosis of irreversible pulpitis was made for this tooth.
- Clinically the tooth was restorable.
- There were no signs of severe mobility.
- The radiograph showed adequate root length with no signs of internal resorption or extensive furcal bone loss.

Case Selection: Preoperative Clinical View

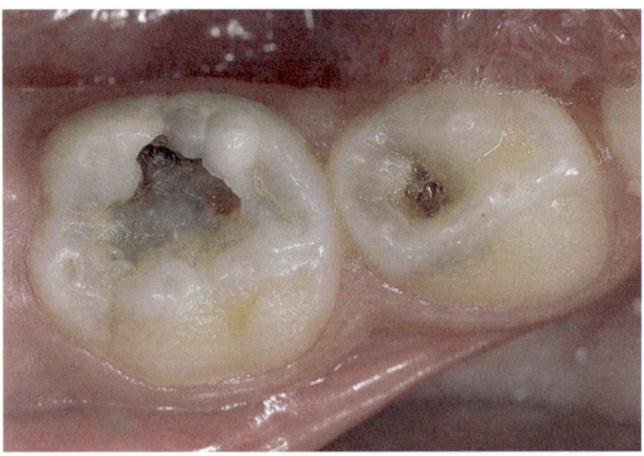

A deep carious lesion was seen in tooth 85. Tooth 84 showed an occlusal carious lesion

Case Selection: Preoperative Radiograph

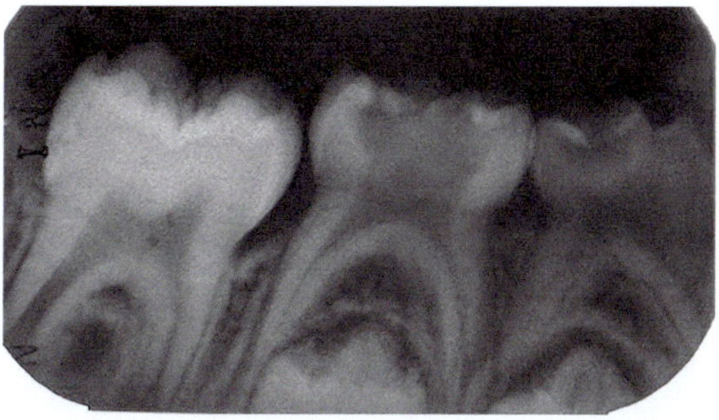

The radiograph showed a deep carious lesion in continuance with the pulp chamber. The tooth showed adequate root length with no signs of internal resorption, floor perforation, or extensive bone loss. Tooth 84 showed a moderately deep lesion, and unerupted tooth 46 was seen

3.3.4.2 Step-by-Step Guide

Step 1: Access Opening

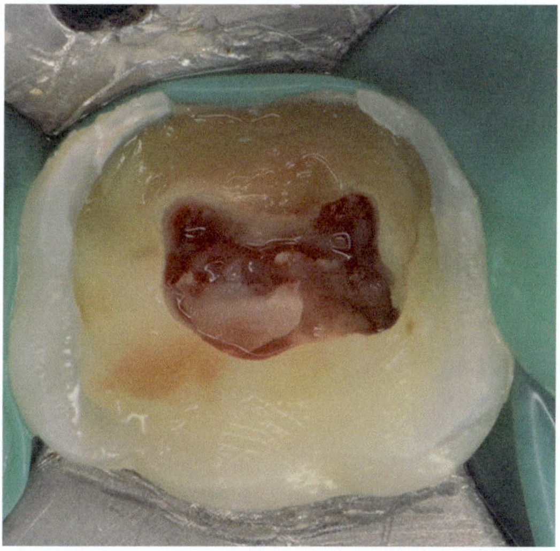

Tooth 85 was isolated with a rubber dam. Access opening was performed to expose the coronal pulp tissue in the pulp chamber

Clinical Notes

Adequate anesthesia is obtained, and carious tissue is completely removed before breaching the roof of the pulp chamber. The access cavity should not have any undercuts and should provide a straight-line access to all the canals.

Step 2: Determining the Working Length

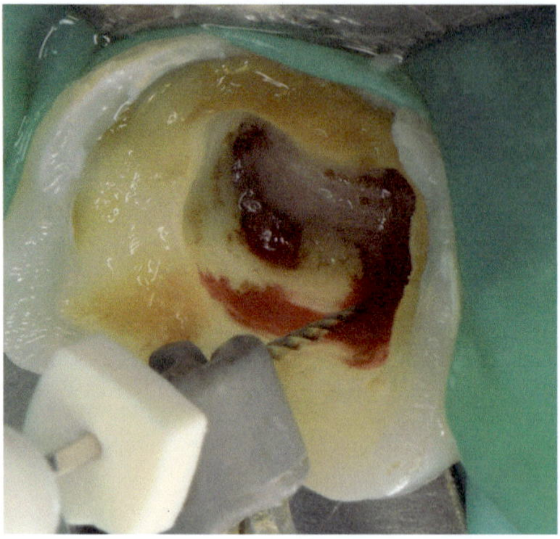

The file clip of the electronic apex locator was attached to the endodontic hand file and inserted into the canals to determine the working length

Clinical Notes

Traditionally the working length was measured from a radiograph recorded with the endodontic file in the canal. This working length was shortened 2–3 mm to prevent overextension. However, recent evidence supports the use of electronic apex locators to determine working length in primary teeth [18, 19]. Apart from accuracy the use of apex locators has the advantage of decreasing the exposure of pediatric dental patients to ionizing radiation.

Step 3: Canal Preparation

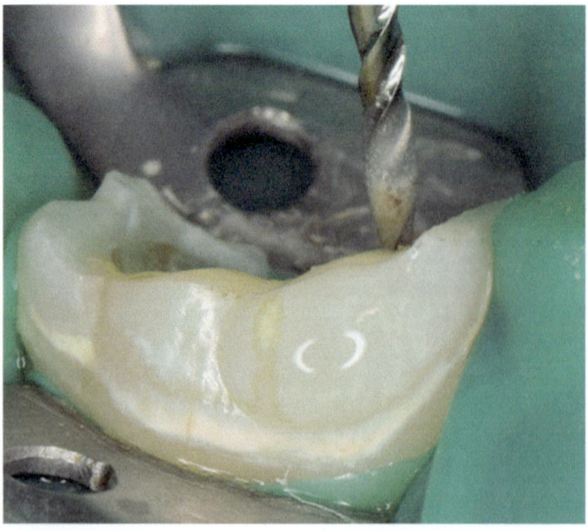

All four canals were prepared with rotary files

Clinical Notes

The thin root walls of primary teeth warrant the use of the flexible nickel titanium (NiTi) hand or rotary instruments [1], for mechanical cleansing. Though rotary instrumentation has shown a lot of promise in terms of reduced treatment time [20], there are no established protocols currently for any particular system or sequence in deciduous teeth, and the choice lies with the operator. However, for rotary instrumentation in deciduous teeth, a passive rotary system is advised.

Step 4: Irrigation

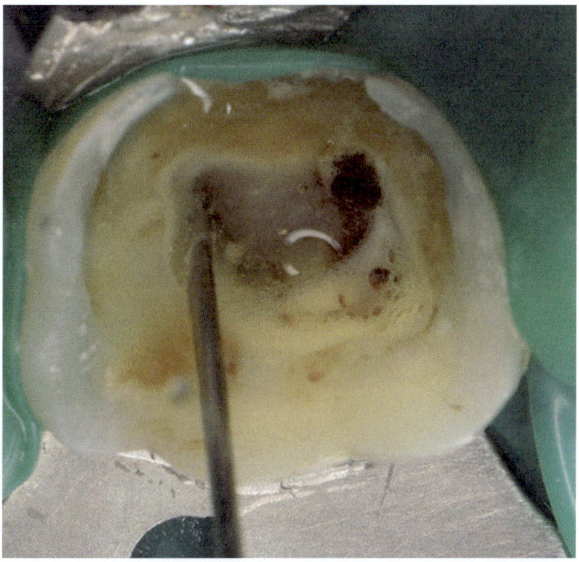

The canals were irrigated gently with 1% sodium hypochlorite

Clinical Notes

Numerous microscopic accessory canals run from the floor of the pulp chamber into the furcation area in a primary tooth. In addition due to the numerous pulpal ramifications in primary root canals, debridement is best accomplished by both mechanical and chemical means. Gentle intermediate irrigation with 1% sodium hypochlorite [8] and saline is used for chemical debridement.

Step 5: Biomechanical Preparation Complete

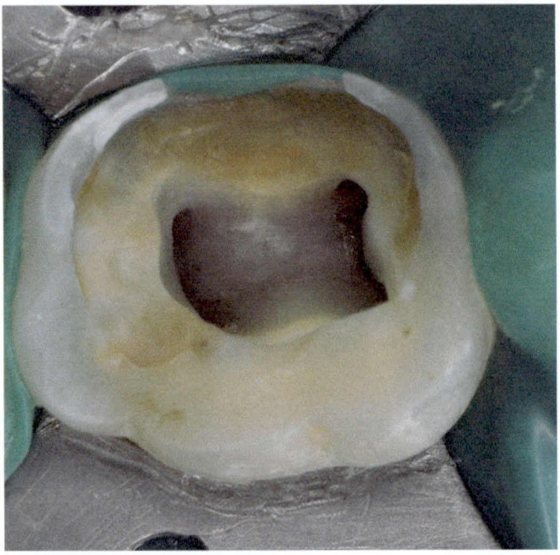

Note the enlarged and clean root canal orifices along with the convexity of the pulp chamber floor

Clinical Notes

Appropriate enlargement of the canal orifices ensures that the apical third of the root canal can be accessed for adequate cleaning and shaping. Each rotary system has dedicated files to manage the coronal third of the root canal.

Step 6: Drying the Canals

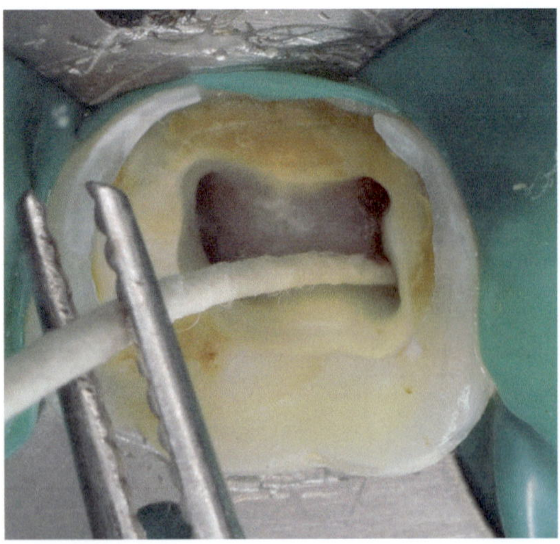

The canals were dried with paper points

Clinical Notes

Leaving the paper point in each canal for a few seconds before withdrawing it helps absorb moisture better. Obturation is carried out once dry canals, free of any exudate, are obtained.

Step 7: Obturation

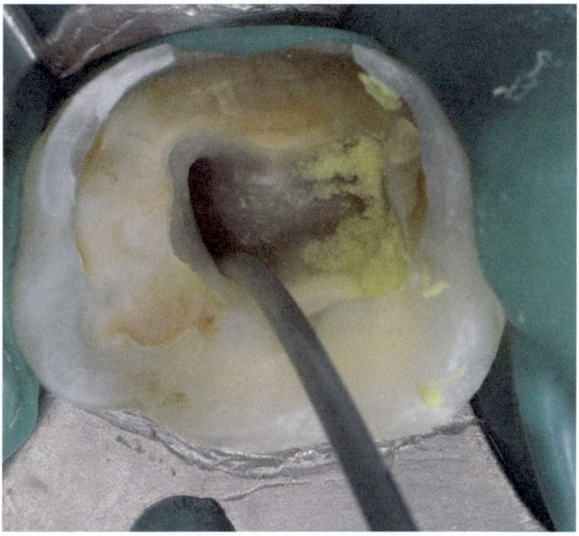

Syringe tip containing calcium hydroxide—iodoform paste inserted into the distobuccal canal. Note the mesial canals obturated

Clinical Notes

The syringe of calcium hydroxide—iodoform paste, Vitapex (J Morita Corporation, Japan) is inserted [10] into the dry canal short of working length. The syringe is withdrawn as the material is injected, leaving the material behind. A moist cotton pellet is used to compress the paste in the orifice after each canal is obturated.

Step 8: All Canals Obturated

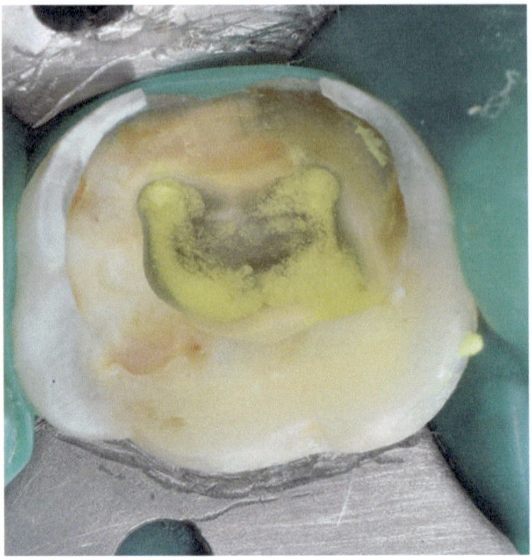

Note all four canals obturated

Clinical Notes

Though no obturation material for primary teeth has been shown superior to the other [21], the calcium hydroxide—iodoform mixture packed in a syringe—fulfils almost all the criteria of an ideal primary tooth root canal obturating material. The material has shown to have high clinical and radiographic success [22]. However the rate of resorption of the material is faster compared to the tooth root.

Step 9: Core Buildup

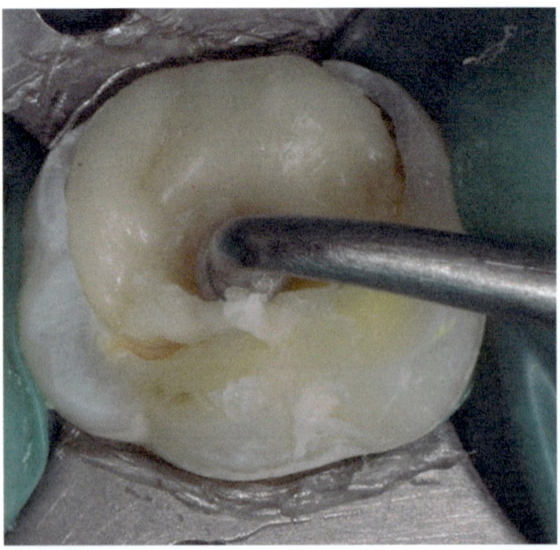

Core buildup with resin-modified glass ionomer cement

Clinical Notes

Glass ionomer cement is directly placed on the floor of the pulp chamber, which contributes to a good coronal seal. This is critical to the long-term success of the pulpectomy procedure.

Step 10: Preformed Metal Crown Cemented

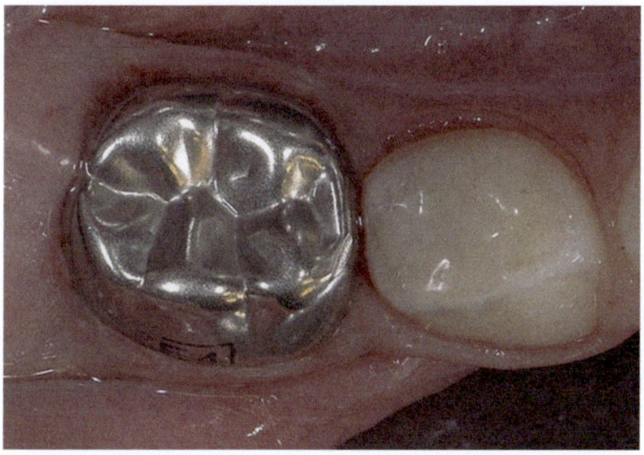

Following removal of the rubber dam clamp, a preformed metal crown was cemented

Clinical Notes

The carious lesion being extensive and multisurface, full coronal coverage reinforces the coronal seal. Hence, in addition to the glass ionomer cement core, a crown is recommended in all endodontically treated primary teeth that require to be retained in the mouth in the long term.

Step 11: Postoperative Radiograph

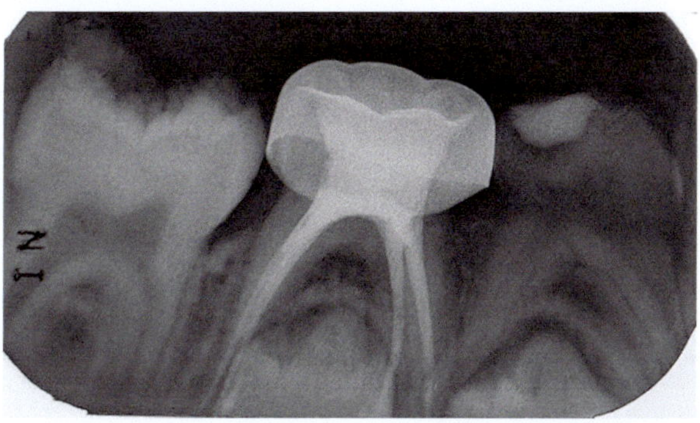

Note the four canals obturated and the well-fitting crown. Tooth 84 received a resin-modified glass ionomer restoration after selective removal of carious tissue to firm dentine (Chap. 2)

Clinical Notes
A postoperative radiograph is recorded for future reference.

3.3.4.3 Long-Term Follow-Up

Three-Year Follow-Up Radiograph

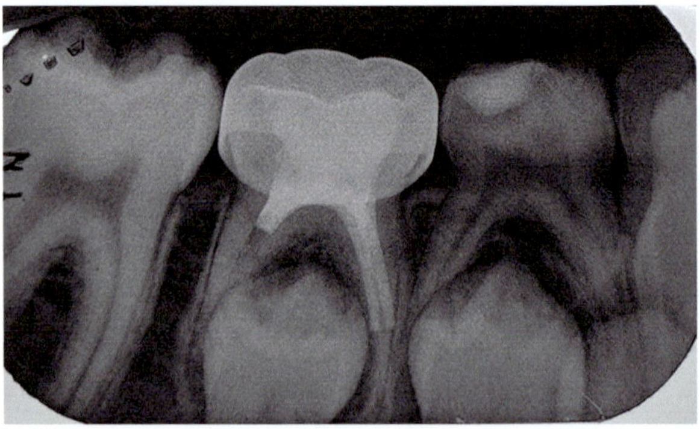

Teeth 84 and 85 show stable intracoronal and full coronal restorations, respectively. Note the healthy interradicular tissue. Note that the calcium hydroxide—iodoform paste used for obturation—is resorbing faster than the root. This is a known phenomenon and of no clinical consequence when the coronal seal is intact [23]. Tooth 46 is seen fully erupted

Five-Year Follow-Up Clinical View

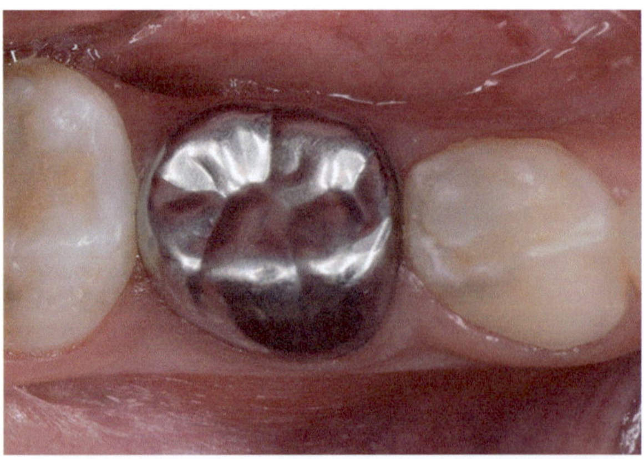

Stable restorations in teeth 84 and 85 with healthy soft tissue. The pulpectomy procedure in tooth 85 has maintained arch length and integrity by maintaining the tooth in the arch as a natural space maintainer and guiding tooth 46 into eruption distal to tooth 85

Five-Year Follow-Up Radiograph

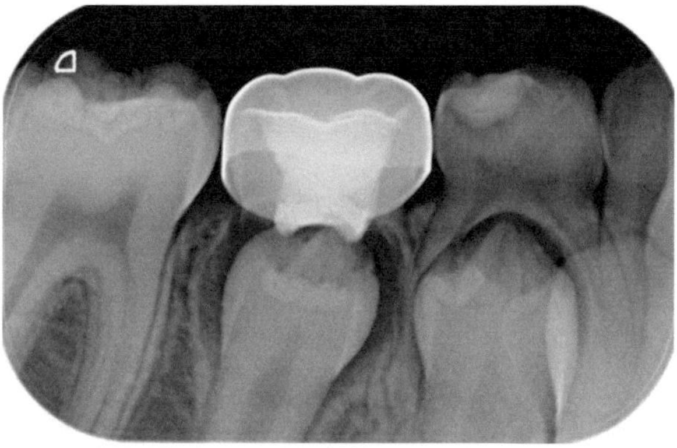

Five-year follow-up radiograph shows the roots of tooth 85 have resorbed almost completely. Tooth 45 is near eruption and at the same eruptive height as tooth 44. In tooth 84, note an increase in the zone of mineralization between the base of the carious lesion and pulp horn when compared to the preoperative and immediate postoperative radiographs. Arch length and integrity have been maintained, and tooth 46 has erupted distal to tooth 85

3.4 Conclusion

The functional primary molar fulfils all the criteria of an ideal space maintainer. Every effort must be made to preserve the pulpally involved primary molar until its natural exfoliation. Good case selection should aim at ensuring that the health and future eruption of the succedaneous tooth are not compromised. Meticulous execution of the steps discussed here will help the clinician fulfil the ultimate objective of the pulpotomy and pulpectomy procedures which is to preserve the primary tooth to natural exfoliation, thereby allowing a healthy permanent successor to take its place.

References

1. Waterhouse PJ, Whitworth JM, Camp JH, Fuks AB. Pediatric endodontics. In: Hargreaves KM, Cohen S, editors. Cohen's pathways of the pulp. St. Louis, MO: Elsevier; 2011. p. 808–56.
2. Coll JA. Indirect pulp capping and primary teeth: is the primary tooth pulpotomy out of date? Pediatr Dent. 2008;30(3):230–6.
3. BaniHani A, Toumba K, Duggal M, Deery CH. Outcomes of the conventional and biological treatment approaches for the management of caries in the primary dentition. Int J Paediatr Dent. 2018;28:12. https://doi.org/10.1111/ipd.12314.
4. Fuks AB, Kupietzki A, Guelmann M. Pulp therapy for the primary dentition. In: Casamassimo P, Fields H, Mctigue D, Nowak A, editors. Pediatric dentistry: infancy through adolescence. St. Louis, MO: Elsevier; 2013. p. 340–4.
5. Myers DR, Pashley DH, Whitford GM, McKinney RV. Tissue changes induced by the absorption of formocresol from pulpotomy sites in dogs. Pediatr Dent. 1983;5(1):6–8.

6. Çelik BN, Mutluay MS, Arıkan V, Sarı Ş. The evaluation of MTA and Biodentine as a pulpotomy materials for carious exposures in primary teeth. Clin Oral Investig. 2018; https://doi.org/10.1007/s00784-018-2472-4.
7. Steffen R, Alhamoui FA, Waes HV. Pulpotomy: is MTA/Portland cement the future? In: Splieth CH, editor. Revolutions in pediatric dentistry. Berlin: Quintessence; 2011. p. 173–83.
8. American Academy of Pediatric Dentistry. Guideline on pulp therapy for primary and young permanent teeth. Pediatr Dent. 2016;38(6):280–8.
9. Stringhini Junior E, Vitcel ME, Oliveira LB. Evidence of pulpotomy in primary teeth comparing MTA, calcium hydroxide, ferric sulphate, and electrosurgery with formocresol. Eur Arch Paediatr Dent. 2015;16(4):303–12. https://doi.org/10.1007/s40368-015-0174-z.
10. Dhar V, Marghalani AA, Crystal YO, et al. Use of vital pulp therapies in primary teeth with deep caries lesions. Pediatr Dent 2017;39(5):E146–E159.
11. Stringhini Junior E, dos Santos MGC, Oliveira LB, Mercadé M. MTA and biodentine for primary teeth pulpotomy: a systematic review and meta-analysis of clinical trials. Clin Oral Investig. 2018; https://doi.org/10.1007/s00784-018-2616-6.
12. Vargas KG, Fuks AB, Peretz B. Pulpotomy techniques: cervical (traditional) and partial. In: Fuks AB, Peretz B, editors. Pediatric endodontics: current concepts in pulp therapy for primary and young permanent teeth. New York, NY: Springer; 2016. p. 52–70.
13. Mutluay M, Arikan V, Sari S, Kisa U. Does Achievement of Hemostasis After Pulp Exposure Provide an Accurate Assessment of Pulp Inflammation? Pediatr Dent. 2018;40(1):37–42.
14. Hilton TJ. Keys to clinical success with pulp capping: a review of the literature. Oper Dent. 2009;34(5):615–25.
15. Hutcheson C, Seale NS, McWhorter A, Kerins C, Wright J. Multi-surface composite vs stainless steel crown restorations after mineral trioxide aggregate pulpotomy: a randomized controlled trial. Pediatr Dent. 2012;34(7):460–7.
16. Flaitz CM, Barr ES, Hicks MJ. Radiographic evaluation of pulpal therapy for primary anterior teeth. ASDC J Dent Child. 1989;56(3):182–5.
17. Yacobi R, Kenny DJ, Judd PL, Johnston DH. Evolving primary pulp therapy techniques. J Am Dent Assoc. 1991;122(2):83.
18. Beltrame AP, Triches TC, Sartori N, Bolan M. Electronic determination of root canal working length in primary molar teeth: an in vivo and ex vivo study. Int Endod J. 2011;44(5):402–6.
19. Odabaş ME, Bodur H, Tulunoğlu O, Alaçam A. Accuracy of an electronic apex locator: a clinical evaluation in primary molars with and without resorption. J Clin Pediatr Dent. 2011;35(3):255–8.
20. Ochoa-Romero T, Mendez-Gonzalez V, Flores-Reyes H, Pozos-Guillen AJ. Comparison between rotary and manual techniques on duration of instrumentation and obturation times in primary teeth. J Clin Pediatr Dent. 2011;35(4):359–63.
21. Smaïl-Faugeron V, Glenny AM, Courson F, Durieux P, Muller-Bolla M, Fron Chabouis H. Pulp treatment for extensive decay in primary teeth. Cochrane Database Syst Rev. 2018;5:CD003220. https://doi.org/10.1002/14651858.CD003220.
22. Nurko C, Ranly DM, García-Godoy F, Lakshmyya KN. Resorption of a calcium hydroxide/iodoform paste (Vitapex) in root canal therapy for primary teeth: a case report. Pediatr Dent. 2000;22(6):517–20.
23. Ozalp N, Saroğlu I, Sönmez H. Evaluation of various root canal filling materials in primary molar pulpectomies: an in vivo study. Am J Dent. 2005;18(6):347–50.

The Posterior Preformed Metal Crown (Stainless Steel Crown)

4

4.1 Overview

Primary molars are challenging to restore when carious lesions involve multiple surfaces. The anatomy of these teeth further reduces the retention rates of intracoronal restorations. Furthermore in vital primary teeth, large pulp spaces increase the likelihood of iatrogenic pulp exposures, when an attempt is made to increase the retention of intracoronal restorations. Consequently the most stable and durable restoration in these teeth is a full coronal coverage restoration using the stainless steel crown. This is also a gold standard for restoring immature permanent teeth with extensive carious destruction, post-endodontic restorations, and extensive developmental malformations like molar incisor hypomineralization (MIH), amelogenesis imperfecta, and dentinogenesis imperfecta.

4.2 Posterior Preformed Metal Crowns in Primary Molars

4.2.1 Introduction

Preformed metal crowns (PMC) (popularly called stainless steel crowns (SSC)) are prefabricated metal crown forms. They are selected from an assortment of sizes, adapted to individual teeth, and cemented with a biocompatible luting agent [1]. Stainless steel crowns are invaluable restorations in pediatric dentistry in terms of durability, clinical life span, and ease of use. Humphrey introduced them to the profession in 1950 [2], but they are still an essential part of a clinician's armamentarium nearly seven decades later! Contemporary steel crowns are pre-contoured, pre-crimped, and pre-festooned. They require minimal or no trimming [2]. Though newer techniques of placing an SSC, like the Hall crown (Chap. 1), are now recommended, it is useful for clinicians to familiarize themselves with the traditional technique of placing an SSC. The following is a step-by-step guide to cementing a stainless steel crown in a primary posterior tooth.

M. S. Kher, A. Rao, *Contemporary Treatment Techniques in Pediatric Dentistry*,
https://doi.org/10.1007/978-3-030-11860-0_4

4.2.2 Indications and Contraindications

PMCs are indicated in primary molars in the following situations:

- Multiple surface carious lesions [2].
- Moderate to large proximal lesions especially in first primary molars.
- Restoration of hypomineralized teeth [2].
- Restoration of teeth following pulp therapy. The outcomes for primary teeth post-pulp therapy are best when the final restoration is a PMC (Chap. 3) [3].
- As abutments for space maintainers as in a reverse crown and loop space maintainer or a distal shoe space maintainer [2] (Chap. 6).
- When placing a conventional restoration is difficult in a child due to lack of cooperation or difficulty in maintaining an isolated field.
- If a child is undergoing dental treatment under general anesthesia, then strong consideration should be given to the placement of PMCs [3].

4.2.3 Rationale

- Preformed metal crowns are invaluable restorations in pediatric dentistry in terms of their durability and clinical life span. They are also inexpensive and easy to place [2].
- Primary molars are small with thin layers of enamel and dentin. The pulp chambers are large with high pulp horns. Removal of even small amounts of tooth structure often compromises the structural and pulpal integrity of the tooth. This is even more so in interproximal carious lesions in first primary molars. The minimal tooth reduction involved in the placement of the PMC makes it a truly conservative restoration. The minimally invasive nature of the preparation also protects the pulp overriding the need for anxiety provoking pulp therapy in the child.
- The current philosophy of dental caries understands the role of the plaque biofilm in the initiation and progression of the carious lesion. If the biofilm is hermetically sealed under a restoration, the carious process gets arrested. The PMC is an invaluable tool in this approach. Examples are the Hall crown (Chap. 1), as a restoration after selective removal of carious tissue (Chap. 2) or when placing the crown after tooth preparation, as in the current section. The buccal cervical bulge of the primary molar, the flexibility of the stainless steel, and the cervical crimp contribute to a "snap fit" over the tooth. The snap fit along with a luting cement like glass ionomer cement prevents any microleakage, thereby hermetically sealing and arresting the carious lesion [4].
- In a carious molar with a large proximal lesion, the broad contact areas result in thin buccal and lingual walls lacking dentinal support. The sharp cervical constriction of primary teeth also results in minimal and sometimes no cervical

tooth structure (gingival seat) in the proximal area. This anatomy compromises the longevity of an interproximal restoration, and failures are common. Breakdown of a proximal restoration can go unnoticed leading to a compromise in the pulpal health of the tooth. This will also lead to loss of arch length. The durable PMC comprehensively covers the tooth, is stable, and restores contact, thus enabling the primary tooth to fulfill its role as a natural space maintainer.
- In a child who is at high risk, the PMC also serves to prevent new carious lesions by providing permanent full coronal coverage and not allowing access to the plaque biofilm or to fermentable carbohydrates

4.2.4 Case Study: Preformed Metal Crown for a Primary Molar

4.2.4.1 Case Selection

Why Was This Case Selected for a Posterior Preformed Metal Crown?
- A 5-year-old child presented with multisurface carious lesions in tooth 85.
- Child was judged to be at "high risk" to dental caries, and full coronal coverage was considered an ideal restoration.
- Since tooth 46 was as yet unerupted and tooth 85 was the posterior most tooth in the arch, we preferred preparing the tooth to receive a stainless steel crown to a Hall Crown (Chap. 1).

Case Selection: Preoperative Occlusal View

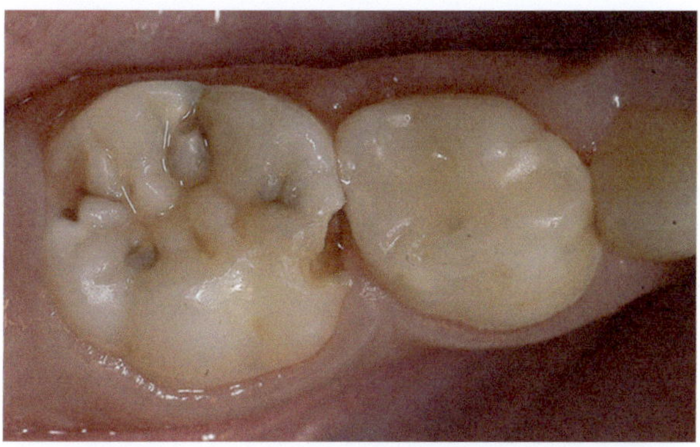

Note the multisurface carious lesions on the occlusal, lingual, mesial, and distal surfaces on tooth 85

4.2.4.2 Step-by-Step Guide

Step 1: Carious Tissue Removed

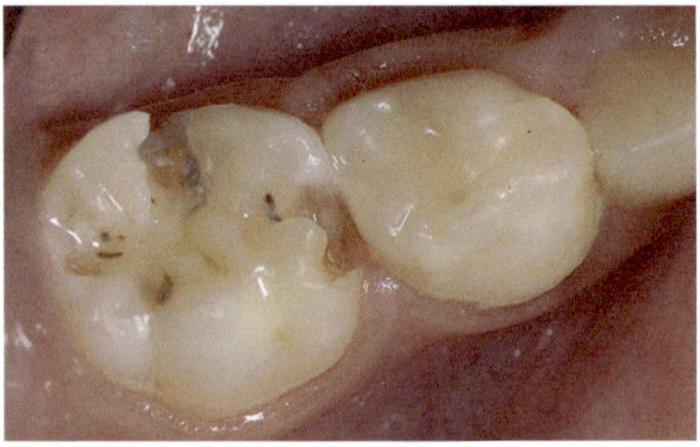

Soft carious tissue was removed before crown preparation. Alternatively, carious tissue may be sealed in under the cemented crown (Chap. 1)

Step 2: Occlusal Reduction

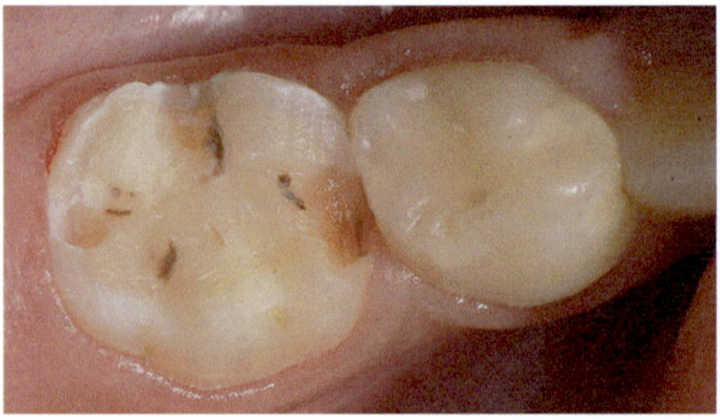

The occlusal surface was uniformly reduced by 1.5–2 mm while maintaining the cuspal inclines [2]

Step 3: Proximal Reduction

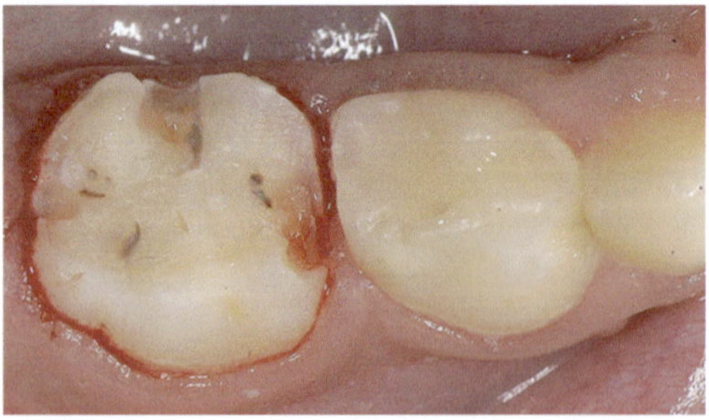

A thin tapered diamond was used to break the contacts with the adjacent tooth ending in a feather-edge gingival margin. An occlusal taper was avoided, and the proximal walls were kept as vertical as possible [2]

Step 4: Buccolingual Reduction

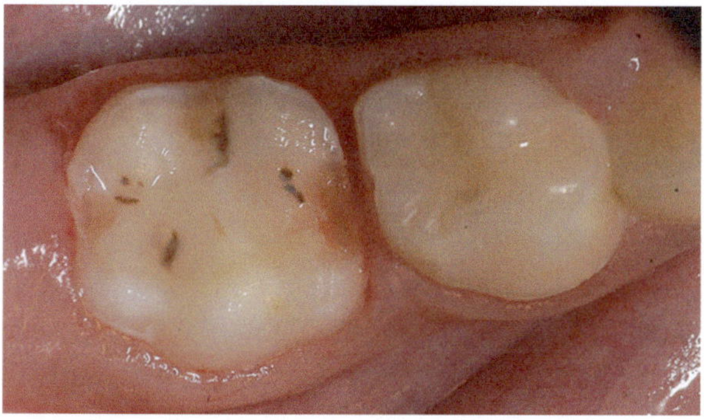

The reduction of the buccal and lingual walls was limited to beveling the occlusobuccal and occlusolingual line angles by holding the short thin diamond at a 45° angle to the occlusal surface and sweeping mesiodistally [2]

Clinical Notes

Buccal and lingual surfaces can be selectively prepared in some cases to aid crown placement.

Step 5: Rounding Line Angles

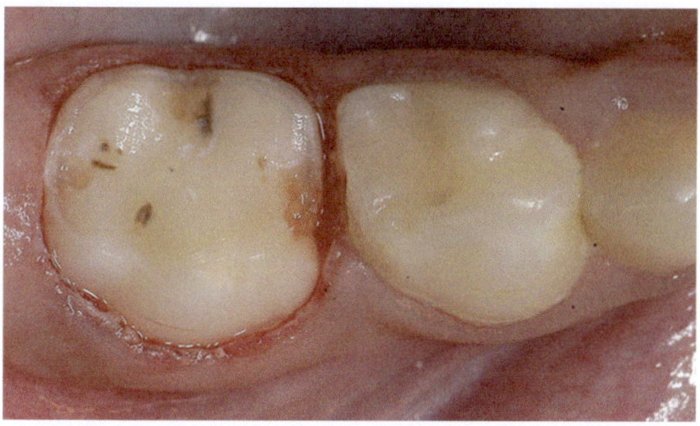

The buccal and lingual proximal line angles were rounded

Step 6: Crown Size Selection by Trial and Error—1

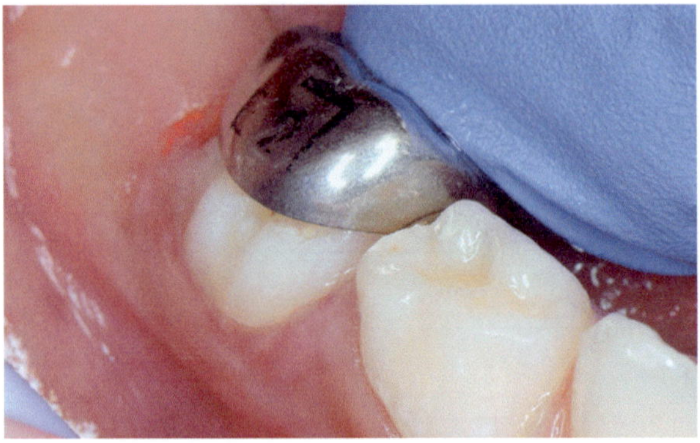

Crown size 2 (ELR 2) was tried on the prepared tooth (3M ESPE, St. Paul, MN, USA). The crown was locked on the lingual surface and rolled over the occlusal surface of the prepared tooth. Note that size 2 was too small and did not go past the upper third of the buccal surface

Clinical Notes

The correct crown size is selected by trial and error. The crown is secured with medical grade tape to prevent the crown slipping [5] (see Chap. 1, Sect. 1.6.4.2). The smallest crown that can be seated on the prepared tooth is selected from the assortment of six sizes in the kit.

Step 7: Crown Size Selection by Trial and Error—2

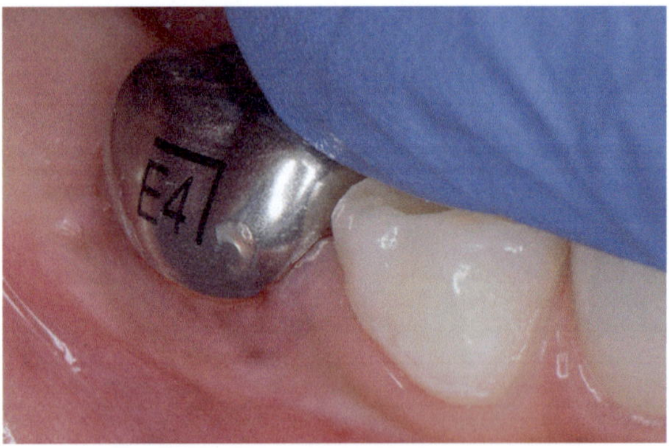

Note that crown size 4 was too large as it slid down easily on the tooth when rolled over

Clinical Notes

When size 2 is too small and size 4 too loose, it can be assumed that size 3 will offer the best fit. A well-fitting crown will offer resistance and seat with an audible click.

Step 8: Crown Size Selection by Trial and Error—3

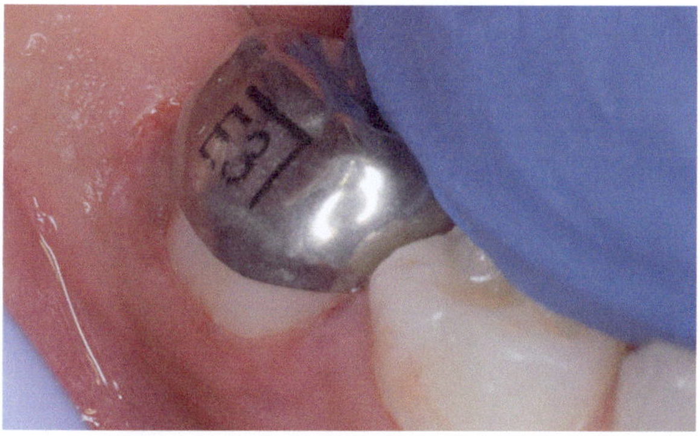

Size 3 when locked on the lingual surface and rolled over the occlusal, slid in easily up to the middle third of the buccal surface. It then offered resistance to final placement. The operator can judge at this stage that firm finger pressure will ensure that the crown seats well subgingivally

Clinical Notes

Occasionally, if selected crown size does not seat fully on the prepared tooth despite finger pressure, the tooth preparation is checked to ensure that there are no interproximal ledges and proximal contacts have been cleared completely. A slight reduction of the buccal and lingual walls may be necessary to seat the crown completely. If the crown does not seat to the same level as the adjacent tooth, further occlusal reduction may be required [2].

Step 9: Loading the Crown

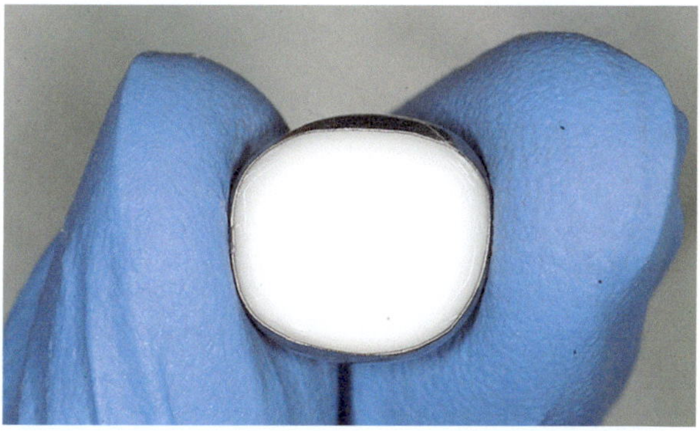

The crown form was loaded to the brim with a smooth mix of luting cement

Clinical Notes
Glass ionomer cement is the preferred luting cement. Since the steel crown is preformed and not custom made to fit the tooth, it fits tight only at the margin. Hence the crown is filled with a large volume of luting cement, and complete seating of the crown is ensured.

Step 10: Crown Seated

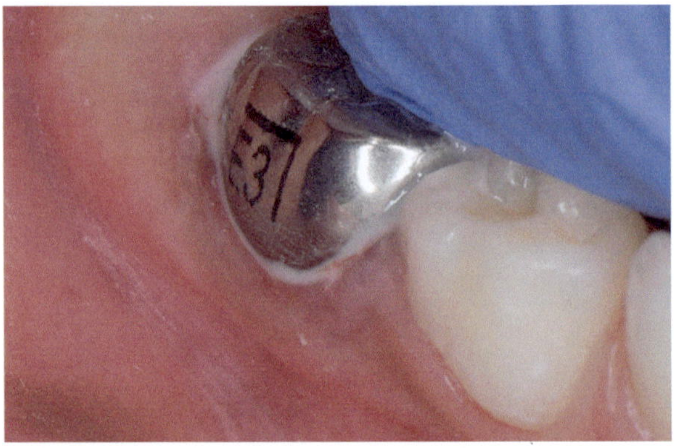

The crown loaded with luting cement was seated lingually first and then rolled over in a buccal direction using firm finger pressure. To ensure good retention and a cement seal, the crown should seat subgingivally

Clinical Notes
Excess cement in the inter proximal areas is removed with dental floss.

Crown in Occlusion

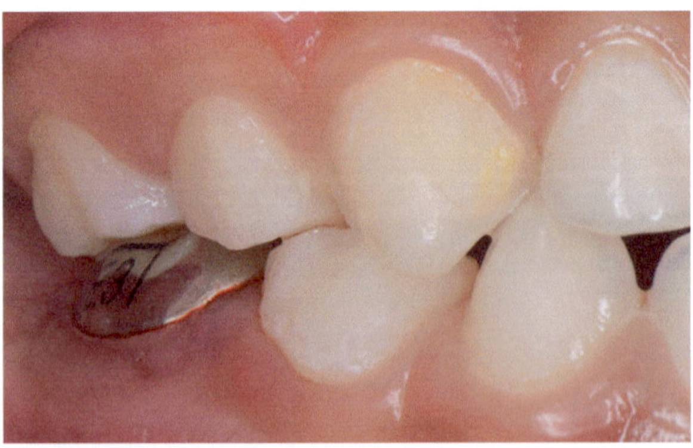

Note the occlusion in maximum intercuspation comparable with the occlusion prior to crown seating. The gingiva may blanch with a well-fitting crown as it seats

One-Week Follow-Up Occlusal View

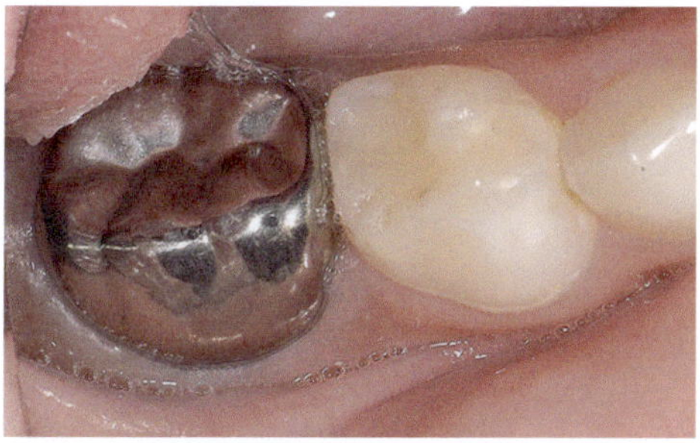

The preformed metal crown 1 week after cementation. Note the excellent tissue response and stable restoration

4.2.4.3 Long-Term Follow-Up

Four-Year Follow-Up Occlusal View

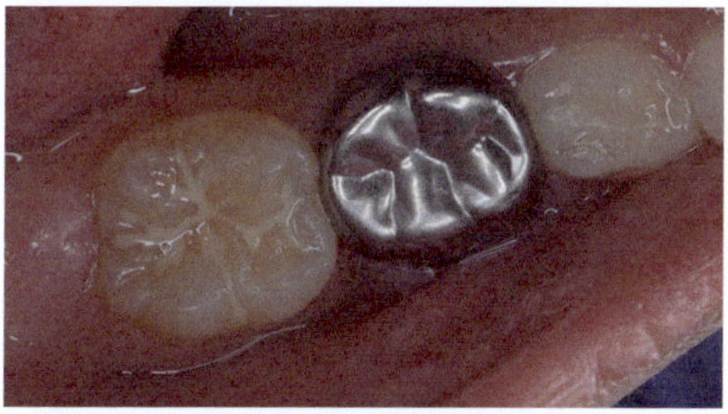

Four-year follow-up showing a stable preformed metal crown and healthy soft tissue. Note that tooth 46 has erupted distal to tooth 85

4.3 Additional Steps to Manipulate the PMC

Trimming the Crown

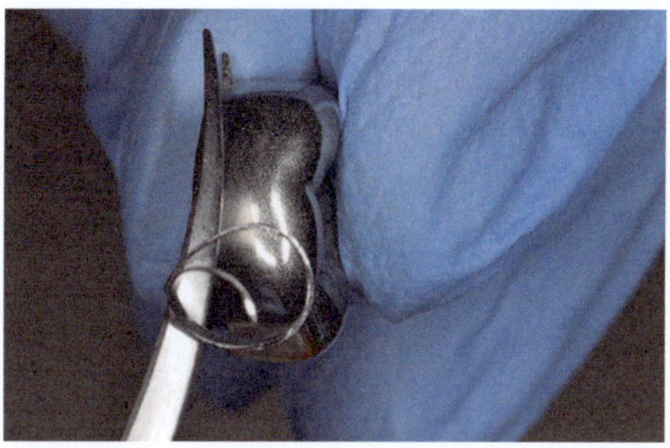

A crown-cutting scissor is used to trim the crown circumferentially following the crown margin, taking care to maintain the gingival contours of the crown

Clinical Notes

If the tooth preparation is confirmed to be adequate and the selected crown does not seat completely, it is estimated that the crown has a slightly smaller cervical diameter than required. The crown is therefore trimmed with a crown-cutting scissor or a heatless stone. Trimming the crown removes the 0.5 mm margin that is pre-crimped. There is an increase in the circumference at the crown margin thus reducing the cervical constriction of the crown. This aids in complete seating of the crown. Post seating, the occlusion should simulate the preoperative occlusion in maximum intercuspation. Trimming is generally required in teeth where there is poor remaining crown structure especially in the upper first primary molars.

Crown Crimping

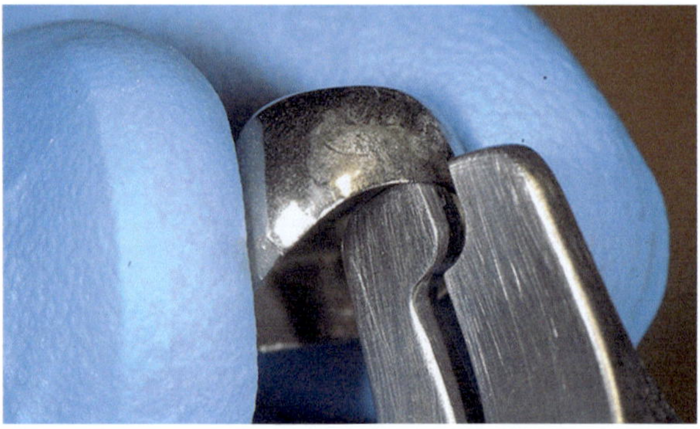

If the trimmed crown is loose, the crown is crimped with a crown-crimping plier to ensure a tight marginal fit. The convex beak of the crimping plier is placed within 0.5 mm of the margin of the crown and squeezed. The crown border gets a 0.5 mm inward bend. The crimping plier is moved circumferentially and smoothly along the cervical margin to give it an inward incline along the entire cervical margin of the crown

Clinical Notes

Following crimping, the crown will show resistance to seating. Once seated, a crimped crown has to be carefully removed by placing a finger over the crown and engaging the crown margins with a curved instrument to prevent the crown from dislodging suddenly and slipping into the oropharynx. Rarely crimping may be required in an untrimmed crown to tighten the fit.

Crown Contouring

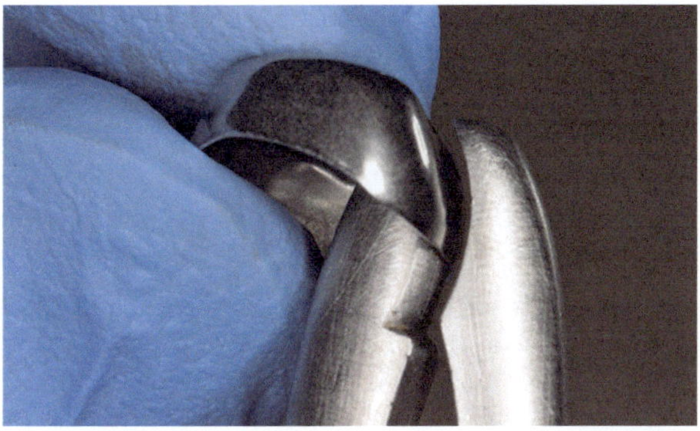

The crown is contoured with a crown contouring plier. The convex beak of the contouring plier is placed on the inner surface of the crown along its whole length, and the plier is squeezed. This action is carried out circumferentially and smoothly thus removing unwanted inward bends along the crown margin caused as a result of overzealous crimping

Clinical Notes
Since all contemporary crowns are pre-contoured, contouring is required in select cases only. It is recommended when the crown has been crimped too much and is too tight to seat. Contouring the crown involves reshaping the entire crown contour circumferentially thus reducing the degree of crimping in an over-crimped crown and allowing the tight crown to seat. It is also useful when the crown contour is distorted during manipulation.

Reducing Space Loss

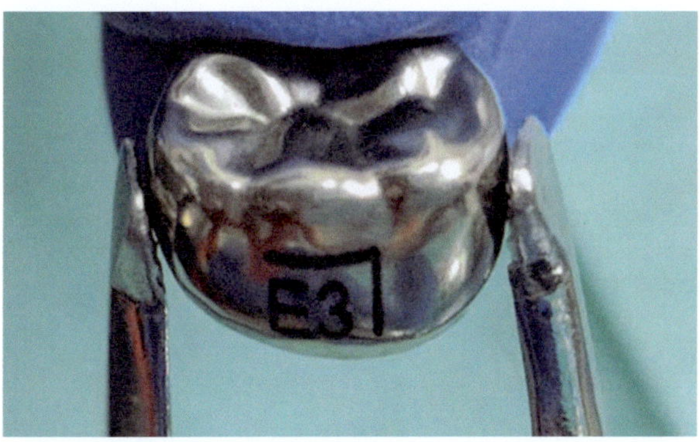

Crown flattened to reduce mesiodistal width to aid in seating

Clinical Notes
Space loss due to proximal caries makes seating of adjacent stainless steel crowns very difficult. While each crown seats when placed as a solitary crown, both crowns do not seat simultaneously. Flattening the crown with pliers reduces the mesiodistal dimension of each crown and allows adjacent crowns to seat easily [6]. This is also a helpful technique while placing a Hall Crown (Chap. 1).

4.4 A Useful Tip

4.4.1 Using a Maxillary Crown Form for a Mandibular First Primary Molar

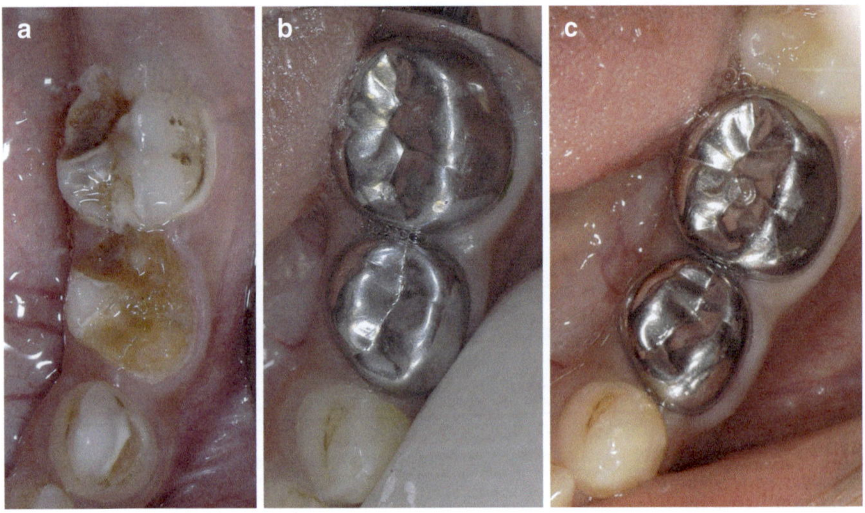

Though mandibular first molars are usually ovoid in shape, the anatomy of the carious tooth and/or the prepared tooth in many mandibular first molars may be more round than ovoid. In these situations the contralateral maxillary crown form seats best. (**a**) Tooth 74 showed extensive multisurface carious lesions and a round rather than ovoid crown anatomy. (**b**) Preformed metal crown of the contralateral maxillary arch, crown form of tooth 54, was cemented on tooth 74. (**c**) Three-year follow-up showing stable crowns on teeth 74 and 75 and erupting tooth 36

Clinical Notes
Since the maxillary crown form is narrower, this modification is also useful in cases of space loss in the lower arch due to mesial drift caused by proximal carious lesions [6].

4.5 Posterior Preformed Metal Crowns in Immature Permanent Molars

4.5.1 Introduction

The most conservative full coronal coverage restoration in an immature permanent molar is a preformed metal crown (stainless steel crown). Since young permanent molars are incompletely erupted with large pulp spaces, the conservative tooth preparation required to seat the crown is invaluable. The tooth preparation and crown adaptation are similar to placing stainless steel crowns in primary molars.

4.5.2 Indications and Contraindications

PMCs are indicated in immature permanent molars in the following situations:

- Teeth with extensive carious destruction for a stable restorative outcome
- Following pulp therapy
- Developmental malformations such as amelogenesis imperfecta and dentinogenesis imperfecta [7]
- Teeth with molar incisor hypomineralization (MIH) [8]

4.5.3 Rationale

- Since immature permanent molars have not gained complete eruptive height, they have short clinical crowns making intracoronal restorations very unstable in these teeth. Preformed metal crowns because of their ability to be cut and crimped can be placed subgingivally in these teeth with excellent retentive outcomes.
- Immature permanent teeth have large pulp spaces that increase sensitivity and the chances of iatrogenic pulp exposures when intracoronal restorations are placed in these teeth.
- The conservative tooth preparation unique to the preformed metal crown allows further tooth eruption and permits a laboratory-fabricated full coronal restoration to be placed when required in the future.
- In teeth with extensive coronal tooth destruction such as in molar incisor hypomineralization, amelogenesis imperfecta, and dentinogenesis imperfecta, a preformed metal crown protects the tooth from further wear and preserves tooth structure for a definitive full coronal coverage crown in the future.

4.5.4 Case Study 1: Preformed Metal Crown in an Immature Permanent Molar with MIH

4.5.4.1 Case Selection

Why Was This Case Selected for a Preformed Metal Crown?

- Tooth 46 displayed MIH involving all tooth surfaces.
- The tooth was at high risk to dental caries.
- Tooth 46 was partially erupted.

Case Selection: Preoperative Occlusal View

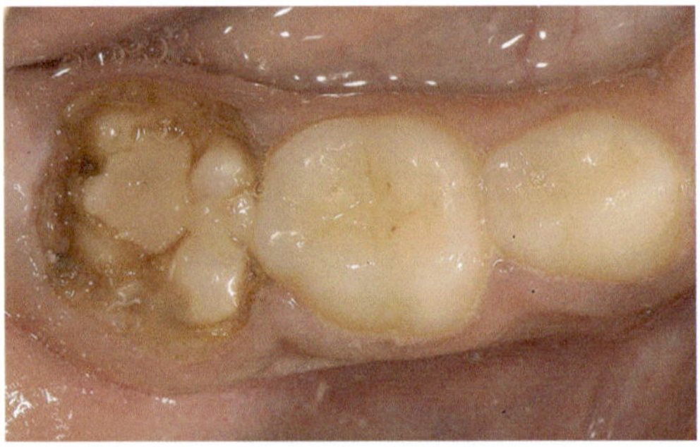

Tooth 46 displayed molar incisor hypomineralization (MIH) and had not achieved complete post-eruptive height. The hypomineralized areas involved all surfaces of the tooth. The distal wall showed extensive carious destruction, and the remaining tooth structure was below the retromolar pad. Previous attempts at restoring the tooth had resulted in failure as evident from fractured remnants of past restorations

4.5.4.2 Step-by-Step Guide

Step 1: Tooth Preparation

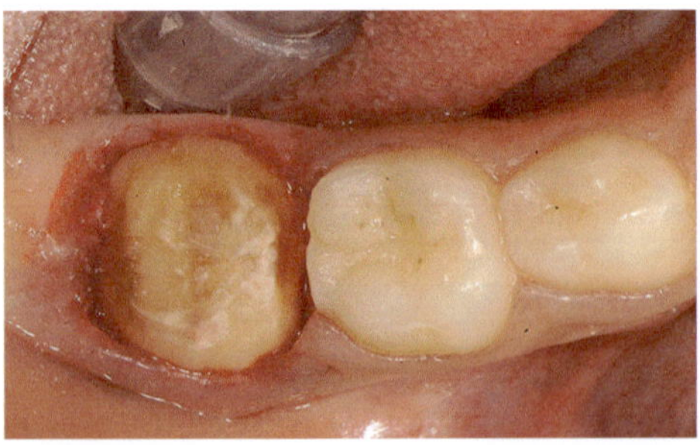

The occlusal and proximal tooth preparation in a permanent molar is similar to the tooth preparation in primary teeth. The buccal and lingual surfaces require greater reduction in permanent molars so as to allow the smallest crown to seat

Clinical Notes

Preparation needs of the future restoration should be borne in mind during tooth preparation of a PMC in a young permanent molar [9]. Since the immature permanent tooth does not have an anatomy that is especially amenable to placing stainless steel crowns (buccal bulge and sharp cervical constriction), all retention is achieved by crimping the crown.

Step 2: Stainless Steel Crown Cemented

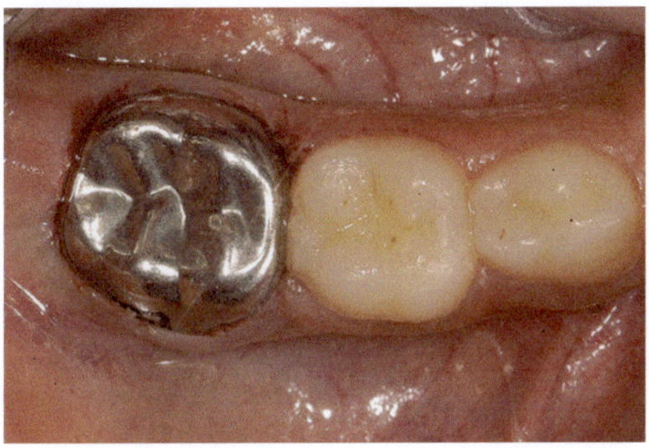

Note the crown (3M ESPE, St. Paul, MN, USA) seated well subgingivally and the excellent contact with tooth 85

Clinical Notes

The permanent stainless steel crown form is much longer in height than the tooth and requires to be trimmed to height and crimped for every case. Accurate circumferential crimping makes the crown extremely retentive and allows the crown to seat with a snap fit.

Crown in Occlusion

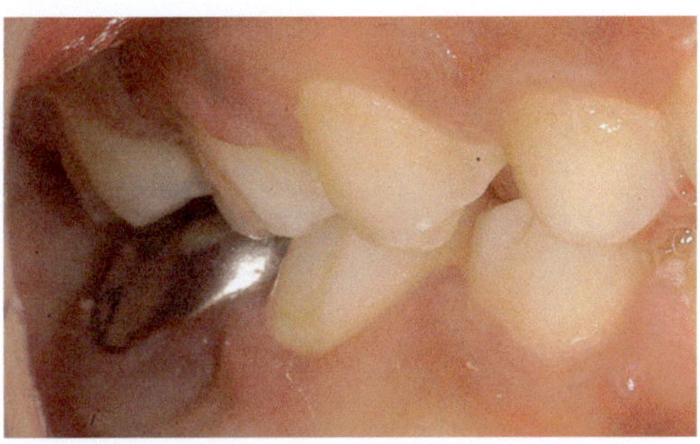

Occlusion in maximum intercuspal position should match the pretreatment occlusion

Clinical Notes

Unlike primary molar crowns where an occlusal discrepancy of 1–1.5 mm settles in a few weeks [6], permanent molar crowns cannot be left in hyper occlusion [7]. The occlusion has to be adjusted to pretreatment occlusion.

4.5.4.3 Long-Term Follow-Up

Three-Year Follow-Up

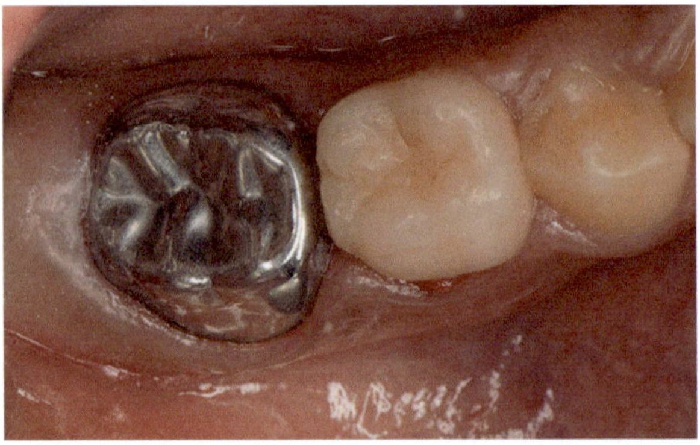

Three-year follow-up shows excellent soft tissue and a stable restoration. Note the exfoliation of tooth 84 and eruption of tooth 44. Also tooth 85 is mobile and ready to exfoliate

4.5.5 Case Study 2: Immature Permanent Molars with Amelogenesis Imperfecta

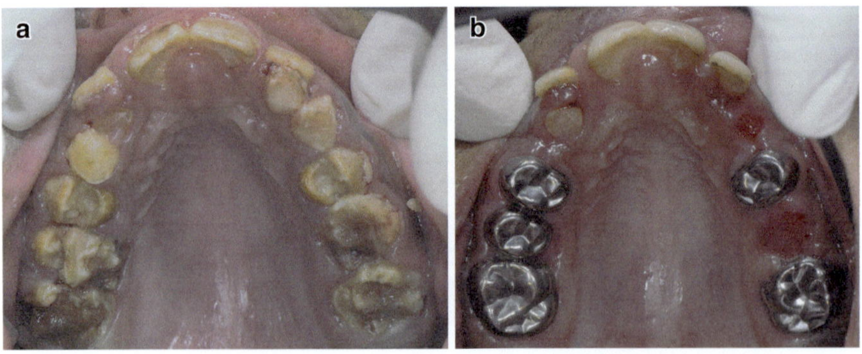

A 10-year-old girl with amelogenesis imperfecta received restorations using preformed metal crowns. (**a**) Preoperative occlusal view of maxillary arch showed extensive destruction of crown structure in the newly erupted permanent posterior teeth. (**b**) Preformed metal crowns are cemented on teeth 14, 15, 16, 24, and 26. Note that in teeth 14, 15, and 24, due to nonavailability of premolar crowns, lower first primary molar crowns were trimmed, recontoured, crimped, and rotated so that the buccal and lingual crown surfaces were placed mesially and distally on the premolar teeth

4.5.6 Case Study 3: Fifteen-Year Follow-Up of a Stainless Steel Crown Placed on an Endodontically Treated Young Permanent Molar

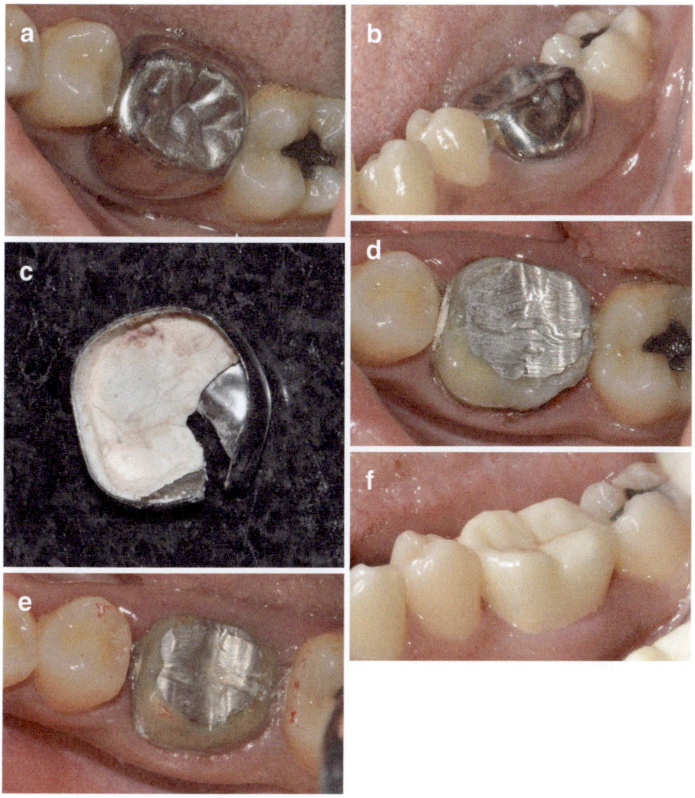

This young adult requested an aesthetic replacement to a stainless steel crown (3M ESPE, St. Paul, MN, USA) that the author placed 15 years ago following endodontic treatment on tooth 36 when the child was 9 years of age. (**a**) Fifteen-year follow-up occlusal view of tooth 36 shows a stable full coronal restoration, excellent retention, and good proximal contacts. (**b**) Note the buccal view at 15-year follow-up of tooth 36 and the excellent soft tissue response. (**c**) The crown is cut to remove it. Note the intact zinc phosphate luting cement in the crown cemented 15 years earlier, indicative of excellent marginal seal and no leakage. (**d**) On removal of the crown, note the bare minimal conservative tooth preparation. No underlying caries was seen indicative of impeccable marginal integrity and retention. (**e**) Tooth is prepared by the restorative dentist to receive a laboratory-fabricated monolithic zirconia crown. (**f**) Zirconia crown is cemented

Clinical Notes

Full coronal coverage restorations using preformed metal crowns can significantly improve the life span of an immature permanent tooth and provide a reliable and durable long-term restoration.

4.6 Conclusion

Preformed metal crowns continue to remain an indispensible and valuable part of the armamentarium of a clinician treating children. While they have been in routine use in primary teeth, a clear understanding of the manipulation of these amenable restorations guarantees long-term restorative success. Their value as full coronal restorations in the immature permanent tooth has largely been overlooked. This underutilization stems from the lack of understanding of their advantages as compared to laboratory-fabricated custom-made crowns. A clear understanding of the principles, the numerous clinical indications, and clinical manipulation of stainless steel crowns will increase the clinician's confidence and utilization of this beneficial, convenient, durable, and predictable mode of treatment in pediatric practice.

References

1. American Academy of Pediatric Dentistry. Pediatric restorative dentistry. Pediatr Dent. 2017;39(6):312–24.
2. Waggoner WF. Restorative dentistry for the primary dentition. In: Casamassimo P, Fields H, Mctigue D, Nowak A, editors. Pediatric dentistry: infancy through adolescence. St. Louis, MO: Elsevier; 2013. p. 304–32.
3. Seale NS, Randall R. The use of stainless steel crowns: a systematic literature review. Pediatr Dent. 2015;37(2):145–60.
4. Ricketts DNJ, Innes NPT. To drill or not to drill? How much caries removal do we need? In: Splieth CH, editor. Revolutions in pediatric dentistry. Berlin: Quintessence; 2011. p. 119–34.
5. Evans D, Innes N. The Hall Technique a minimal intervention, child centred approach to managing the carious primary molar: a users manual. November 11, 2010. 3rd ed. Dundee: University of Dundee; 2010. https://dentistry.dundee.ac.uk/files/3M_93C%20HallTechGuide2191110.pdf Accessed 15 Sep 2018.
6. Kindelan SA, Day P, Nichol R, Willmott N, Fayle SA, British Society of Paediatric Dentistry. UK National Clinical Guidelines in paediatric dentistry: stainless steel preformed crowns for primary molars. Int J Paediatr Dent. 2008;18(Suppl 1):20–8. https://doi.org/10.1111/j.1365-263X.2008.00935.x.
7. Randall RC. Preformed metal crowns for primary and permanent molar teeth: review of the literature. Pediatr Dent. 2002;24(5):489–500.
8. Koleventi A, Sakellari D, Arapostathis KN, Kotsanos N. Periodontal impact of preformed metal crowns on permanent molars of children and adolescents: a pilot study. Pediatr Dent. 2018;40(2):117–21.
9. Radcliffe RM, Cullen CL. Preservation of future options: restorative procedures on first permanent molars in children. ASDC J Dent Child. 1991;58(2):104–8.

Aesthetic Full Coronal Coverage Restorations

5

5.1 Overview

Where aesthetics is the prerequisite, full coronal coverage restorations have increased stability and durability in primary teeth. Extensive loss of tooth structure due to trauma or dental caries challenges intracoronal restorative outcomes in these teeth. In primary incisors, resin-based strip crowns fulfil the requirements of a good full coronal coverage aesthetic restoration. Its advantages include ease of use, cost-effectiveness, and excellent visual outcomes. However being resin based, the long-term stability of the strip crown in terms of aesthetics and retention continues to pose a challenge. The advent of preformed zirconia crowns offers an exciting alternative for full coronal coverage in both anterior and posterior primary teeth because of their aesthetics, biocompatibility, stability, and durability.

This chapter elucidates, with the help of clinical tips, high-resolution clinical pictures, and long-term follow-ups, the step-by-step use of "strip crowns" and "anterior and posterior prefabricated zirconia crowns."

5.2 Composite Strip Crowns

5.2.1 Introduction

Direct composite restorations in maxillary primary incisors using prefabricated plastic crown forms are popularly called strip crowns. The name "strip crown" originates from the clinical manipulation of these crown forms. The crown form is filled with composite resin, positioned accurately on the prepared tooth surface and light cured. This is followed by peeling or stripping of the crown form from the tooth surface leaving behind the composite resin restoration to provide full coronal coverage. Strip crown forms allow for an automatic, aesthetic, and life-like contouring of the anterior buildup which would otherwise be a tedious and time-consuming

M. S. Kher, A. Rao, *Contemporary Treatment Techniques in Pediatric Dentistry*,
https://doi.org/10.1007/978-3-030-11860-0_5

procedure in a child. The crown forms are available in an assortment of sizes for the maxillary central and lateral incisors. The following is a step-by-step guide to restoring a primary anterior tooth with a strip crown form.

5.2.2 Indications and Contraindications

Strip crowns are aesthetic full coronal coverage restorations for primary maxillary incisors. They are indicated in [1]:

- Teeth with multisurface carious lesions with or without pulp therapy
- Teeth with loss of tooth structure due to developmental defects or trauma

Since they are direct composite restorations, strip crowns are technique sensitive to place [6].

- They are contraindicated in situations where isolation is a challenge due to age, behavior, or gingival hemorrhage [2].
- They are contraindicated in teeth where inadequate tooth structure remains for retention from acid etching and bonding [2].

5.2.3 Rationale

Anterior restorations in primary teeth should be durable and esthetic. These ideals are challenging to meet due to the small size of primary teeth and the multisurface nature of carious lesions in primary incisors.

The superior aesthetic properties of composite resins make them an ideal choice of material to restore primary incisors. In addition, composite resins have adequate strength and good wear resistance in anterior teeth restorations [3]. A freehand buildup in direct composite resin is a technique-sensitive procedure and time-consuming and requires exceptional cooperation from the patient. These requirements are challenging to meet in children.

Strip crowns facilitate quick placement of a direct composite resin restoration utilizing the entire coronal tooth surface for bonding thereby improving the retention and stability of the restoration. The preformed strip crown form enables a superior aesthetic outcome by providing an automatic contour and finish to the restoration. Strip crowns have shown approximately 80% retention rates over 24–36 months [4].

They are cost-effective and easy of repair, can be placed in crowded dentitions, and are an excellent choice as a full coronal coverage restoration for primary maxillary incisors.

5.2.4 Case Study: Composite Strip Crowns for Anterior Full Coronal Coverage

5.2.4.1 Case Selection

Why Was This Case Selected for Anterior Restorations Using Strip Crowns?

- Child was 5.5 years old and presented with multisurface lesions in the upper incisor teeth.
- There was adequate tooth structure for bonding and retaining composite strip crowns.
- There were no signs or symptoms of pulp pathology.
- Parents wanted improved aesthetics, and child cooperation allowed the use of this technique-sensitive procedure.

Case Selection: Preoperative View

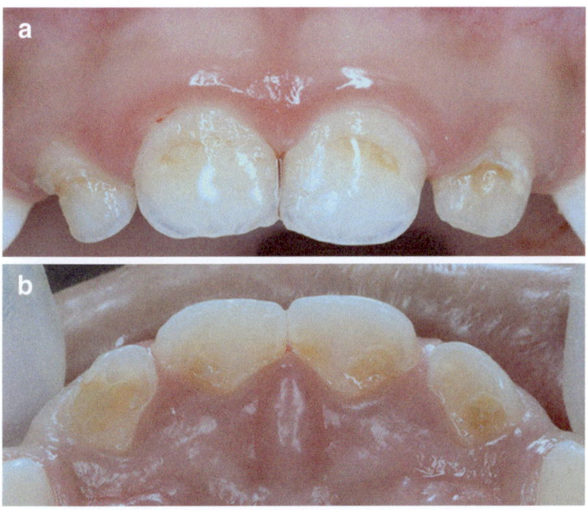

(**a**) Upper incisors showed labial carious lesions and large areas of demineralization. (**b**) Palatal surfaces of incisors showed large carious lesions and breakdown of tooth structure

5.2.4.2 Step-by-Step Guide

Step 1: Isolation

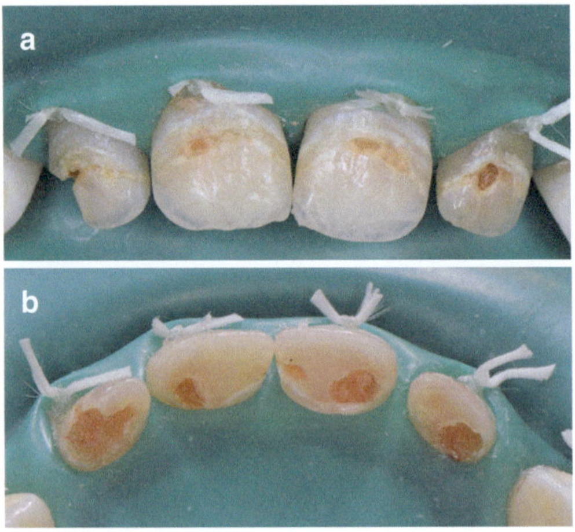

(**a**) Labial view of teeth 51, 52, 61, and 62 after placement of dental dam. (**b**) The widespread palatal lesions clearly visualized following placement of the dental dam

> **Clinical Notes**
> The slit-dam method could also be used for rubber dam isolation as ligature ties can induce gingival bleeding if not placed with care [5].

Step 2: Crown Form Selection

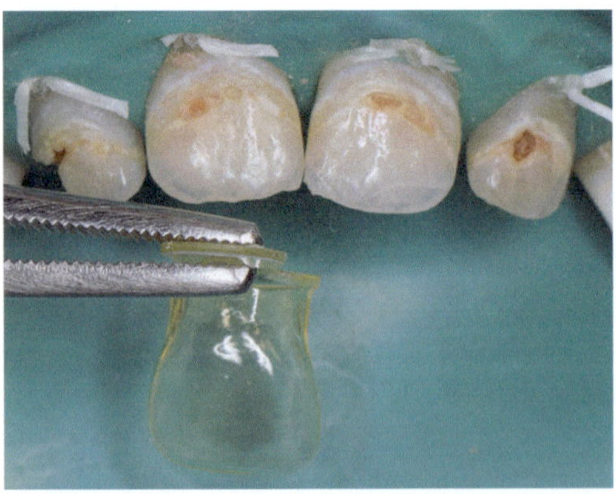

The crown form (3M ESPE, St. Paul, MN, USA) was selected by comparing the mesiodistal width of the incisal edge of the tooth to be restored with that of the crown form

Step 3: Preparation of Tooth

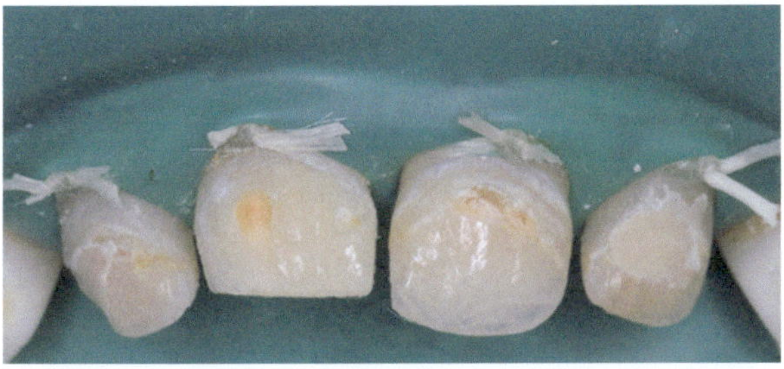

Tooth 51 was prepared to receive a strip crown. Interproximal disking with a fine tapered bur was followed by incisal reduction of approximately by 1–2 mm. The labial and lingual surfaces were prepared minimally to roughen the enamel surface

Clinical Notes

Care must be taken to preserve as much tooth structure as possible to increase efficiency of acid etching. Note the soft carious tissue removed from tooth 51, 52, 61, and 62. The distal surface of tooth 52 and the labial surface of tooth 62 with deep carious lesions are lined with resin-modified glass ionomer cement restoration.

Step 4: Trimming the Crown Form

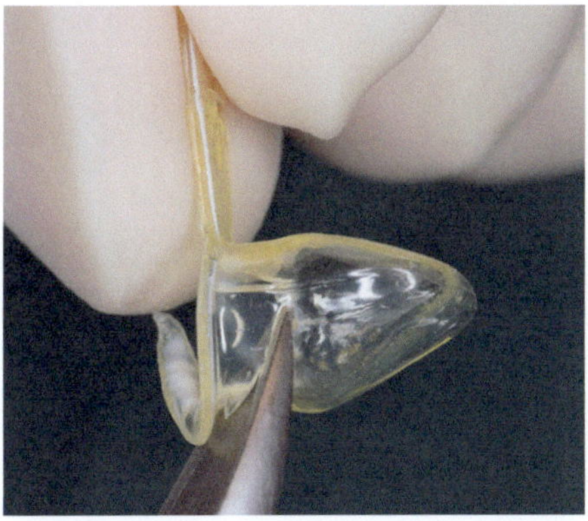

The crown forms have a narrow/constricted cervical collar. The cervical collar and tab of the selected crown form were trimmed with fine curved scissors

Step 5: Contouring the Cervical Margin

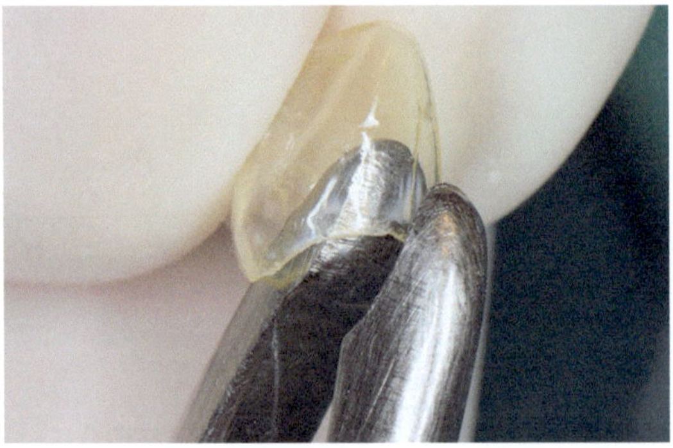

After trimming the crown form, the rough cervical margin was smoothened with a contouring plier (Chap. 4). This removed any ragged margins caused during trimming

Step 6: Trimmed Strip Crown Form

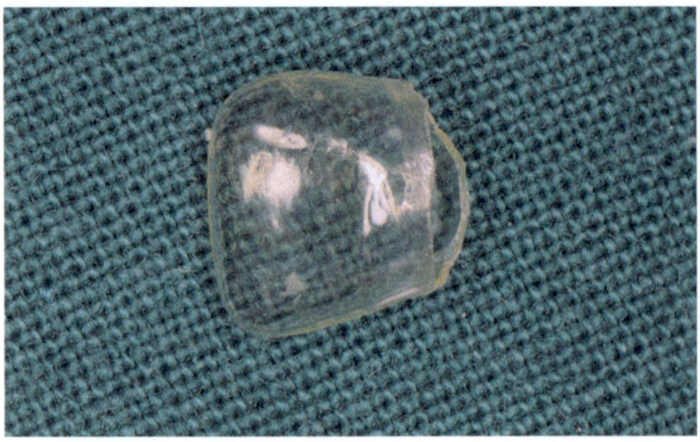

The trimmed crown form ready to be tried on the tooth

Step 7: Slitting the Crown Form: A Novel Modification

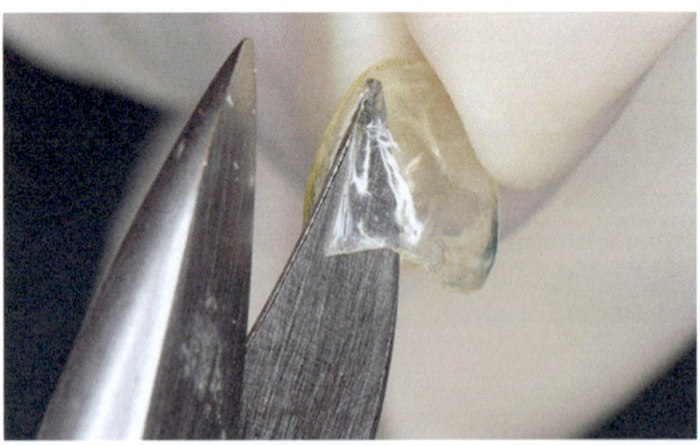

A slit was placed on the distal surface of the crown form instead of the traditional vent hole

Clinical Notes
The slit in addition to preventing air entrapment and allowing flow of excess composite opens up the crown form and aids in moving it subgingivally. This gives the completed restoration a neat emergence profile. The slit also helps to peal the crown form off easily at the end of the procedure.

Step 8: Trial Fitting the Crown Form

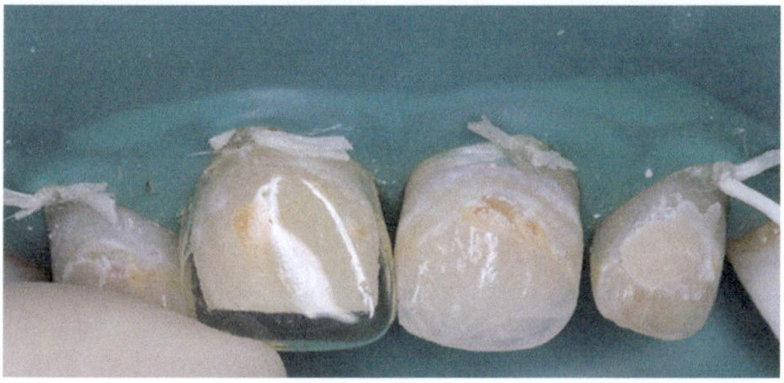

The prepared strip crown form was tried on the tooth to ensure adequate seating

Clinical Notes
The gingival margin of the crown form should extend about 0.5 mm subgingivally. Its height should also match the adjacent tooth.

Step 9: Tooth Surface Prepared for Bonding

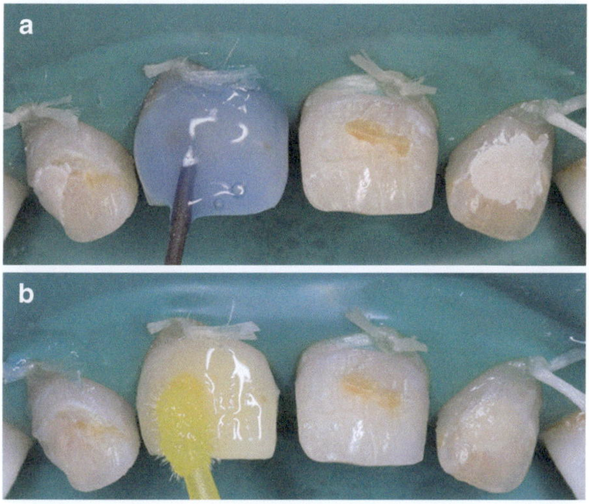

The tooth surface was prepared to receive the composite strip crown. (**a**) The tooth surface was acid etched circumferentially. (**b**) Bonding agent was applied and light cured after washing and gentle air drying

Step 10: Loading the Crown Form

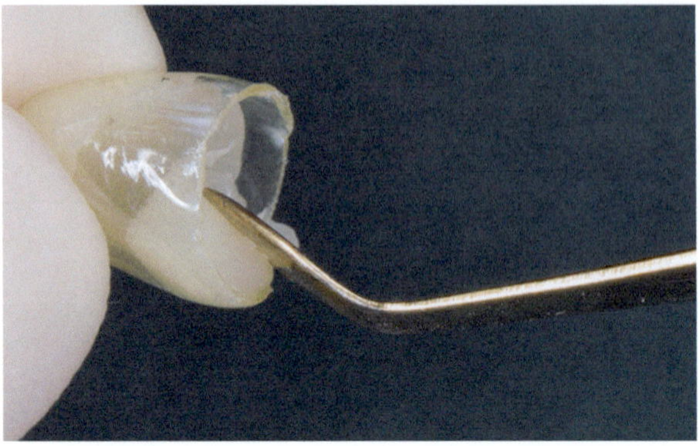

Composite resin was loaded into the crown form

Clinical Notes
Composite resin is loaded taking care to avoid air bubbles. The resin is hollowed out in the center to avoid excess and allow ease of insertion.

Step 11: Seating the Crown Form

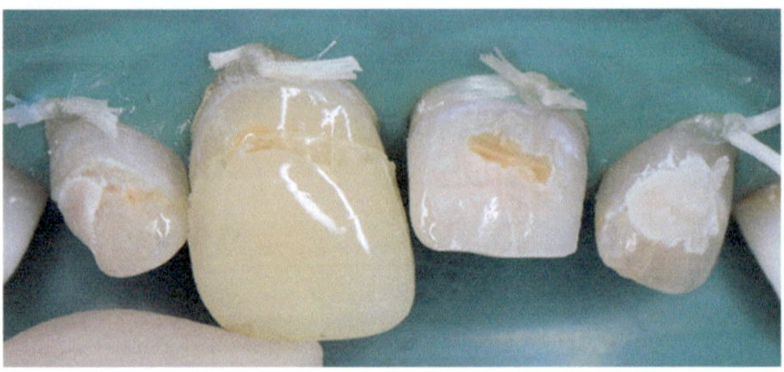

The crown form packed with composite resin was firmly seated over the prepared tooth

Clinical Notes
The excess composite resin escaping from the distal slit is removed before curing. The gingival margin is also cleared of any excess.

Step 12: Light Curing the Resin

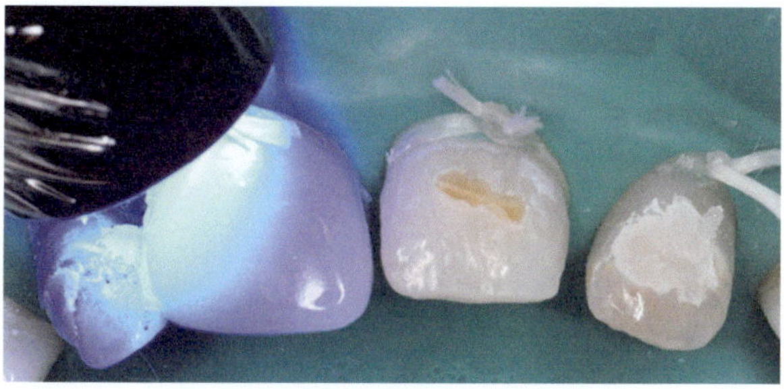

The strip crown form was cured labially, incisally, and palatally

Clinical Notes
Since the resin material is bulk packed into the crown form, bulk-fill composite resin materials are preferred.

Step 13: Stripping the Crown Form

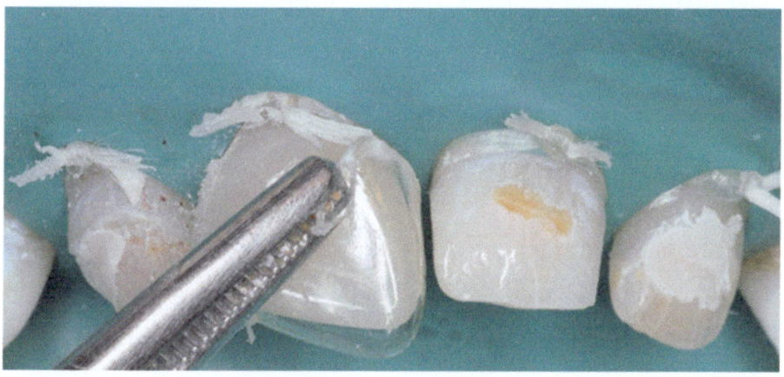

The cut distal edge of the crown form was located with a fine probe, and the crown form was stripped or peeled out—hence the name "strip crown"

Clinical Notes
The crown form strips off easily leaving behind a smooth resin surface.

Immediate Postoperative View

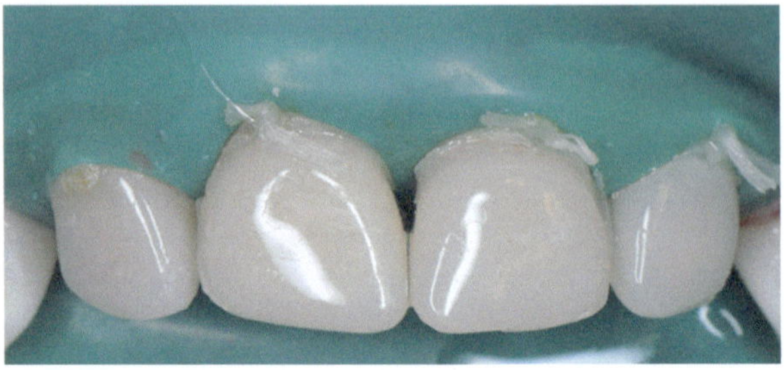

Postoperative view of composite strip crowns in teeth 51, 52, 61, and 62

Clinical Notes
Following peeling of the strip crown forms, the occlusion is checked, and the restorations are finished and polished to remove any subgingival flash.

5.2.4.3 Long-Term Follow-Up

Eighteen-Month Follow-Up: Labial View

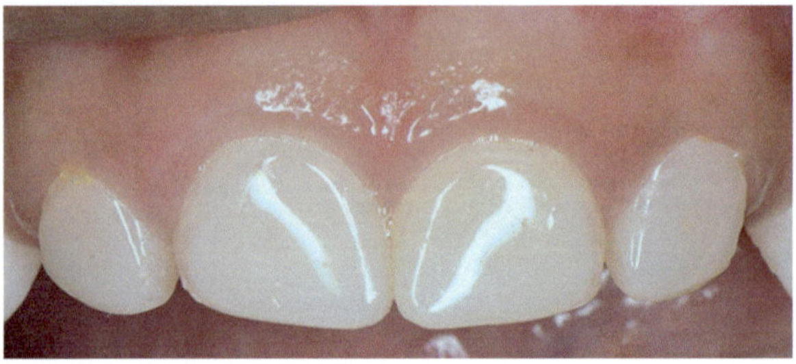

Follow-up labial view at 18 months shows aesthetically pleasing and stable composite strip crowns in teeth 51, 52, 61, and 62. Note the healthy soft tissue response to the well-finished restorations

Eighteen-Month Follow-Up: Palatal View

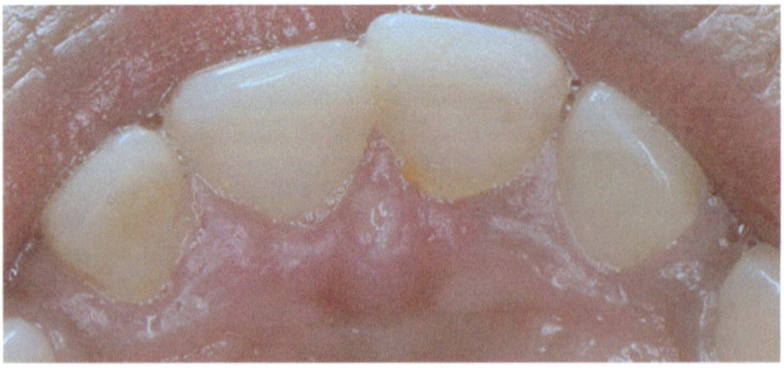

Palatal view at 18-month follow-up shows stable composite strip crowns in teeth 51, 52, 61, and 62. Note the healthy soft tissue response

5.3 Preformed Zirconia Crowns

5.3.1 Introduction

Zirconia has found numerous applications in general dentistry in the last 15 years from its use in prosthetic crowns and bridges and endodontic posts to implant abutments [6]. Zirconia crowns are the most contemporary addition to the restorative armamentarium in pediatric dentistry. Introduced in 2010, monolithic preformed zirconia primary crowns are full-coverage restorations that offer life-like aesthetics combined with high color stability, biocompatibility, strength, and durability [4]. The following is a step-by-step guide to placing zirconia primary anterior and posterior crowns.

5.3.2 Indications and Contraindications

Preformed zirconia crowns are available for both anterior and posterior primary teeth. They are indicated in:

- Teeth with multisurface carious lesions with or without pulp therapy
- Teeth with developmental defects
- Crown discolored or fractured due to traumatic injury
- Lower mandibular primary incisors that require full coronal coverage [4]
- Children allergic to nickel and hence contraindicated for preformed metal crowns

They are contraindicated:

- In a crowded arch [6].
- Placing a zirconia crown requires adequate patient cooperation and is not indicated in children where cooperation is compromised by age, behavior, or disabilities.
- Zirconia crowns are expensive [4] making them unaffordable for many families.
- In grossly decayed teeth where there is less than 2 mm of healthy supragingival tooth structure,
- If the tooth requiring full coronal coverage is planned as an abutment for a space maintainer.

5.3.3 Rationale

Restorations using composite resin in primary anterior teeth are challenged by the lack of color stability and retention. In posterior teeth, though preformed metal crowns fulfil most of the prerequisites of an ideal full coronal restoration, the lack of aesthetics is a major deterrent for some parents. Anterior and posterior zirconia crowns exhibit natural aesthetics, tissue compatibility, durability, color stability, and lack of wear on opposing teeth, making them a very useful addition to the repertoire of full coronal coverage restorations for primary teeth [7].

5.3.4 Case Study 1: Preformed Zirconia Crowns for Anterior Full Coronal Coverage

5.3.4.1 Case Selection

Why Was This Case Selected for Restoration with Preformed Zirconia Crowns?

- Parents of a 5-year-old child presented with a chief complaint of unaesthetic anterior incisors.
- Aesthetic expectations of the parents were very high.
- There were no signs or symptoms of pulp pathology.

Case Selection: Preoperative View

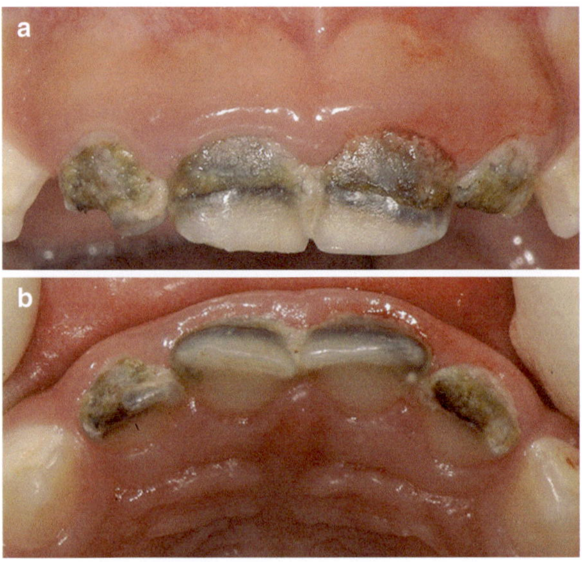

(**a**) Preoperative labial view of upper incisors showed extensive carious destruction of the labial surfaces of teeth 51, 52, 61, and 62. Incisal edges of teeth 52 and 62 were also completely destroyed. There were no clinical signs of pulp pathology, and the soft tissue appeared healthy. Marginal gingivitis was seen in response to the plaque stagnation areas on all four incisors. (**b**) Palatal view of upper incisors showed that palatal surfaces were intact and free of carious lesions

Clinical Notes

The best aesthetic result is achieved when crowns are placed on all incisors or all six anterior teeth.

Case Selection: Preoperative Radiograph

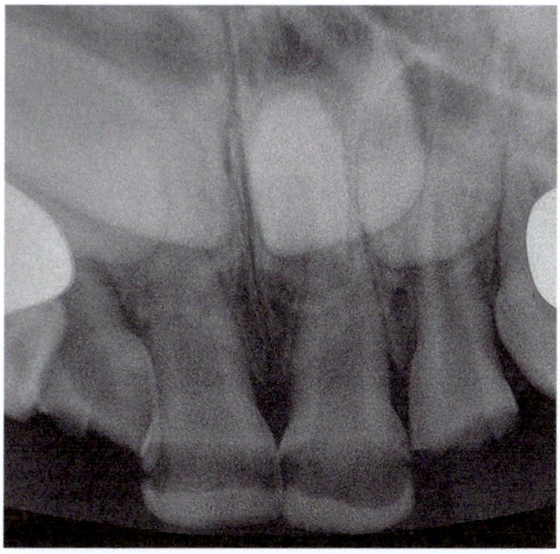

Periapical radiograph of teeth 51, 52, 61, and 62 showed carious lesions in all four teeth. The labial lesions in teeth 51 and 61 superimposed on the pulp chamber of those teeth; however the radicular bone and roots appeared healthy. In teeth 52 and 62, the carious lesions were in close proximity to the pulp, but a clear layer of dentinal tissue separated the pulp tissue from the carious lesions. The radicular tissue and roots appeared healthy. A coincidental finding was the presence of a developing mesiodens near the apical third of tooth 61

5.3.4.2 Step-by-Step Guide

Step 1: Incisal Depth Grooves

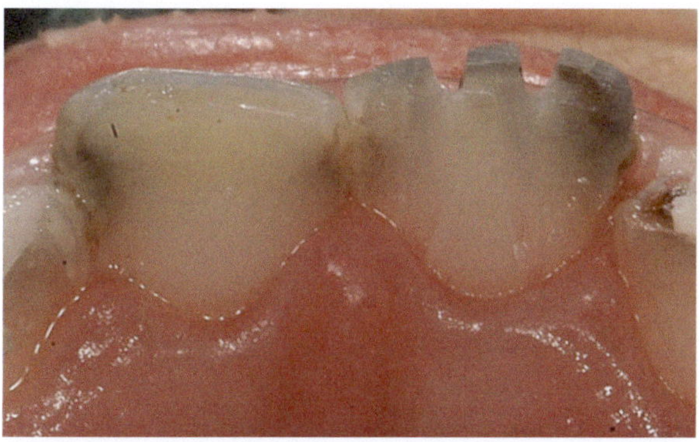

Incisal depth groves or notches to the depth of 2 mm were made in tooth 61. These aided as a guide for incisal reduction

Clinical Notes

Depending on the merits of the tooth receiving the crown, carious tissue is removed, and a restoration is placed, or pulp therapy is performed prior to tooth preparation.

Step 2: Incisal Reduction and Labial Grooves

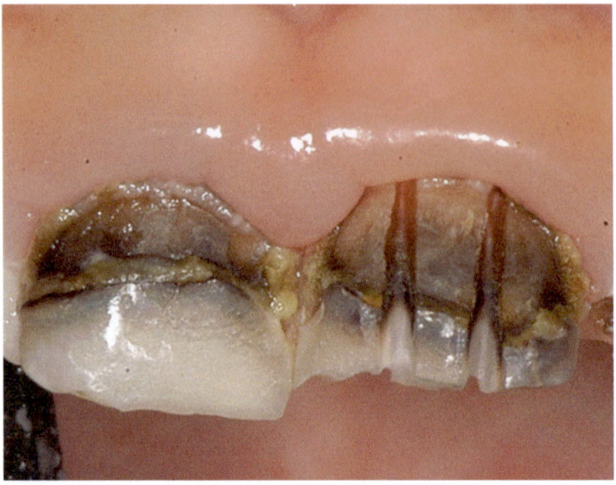

Incisal edge of tooth 61 was reduced by 2 mm guided by the notches. Labial depth groves were made to a depth of 2 mm to aid in labial reduction

Clinical Notes

Carious tissue in the lesions in teeth 51, 52, and 61 was firm to tactile pressure with a hand instrument. Hence no carious tissue was intentionally removed other than which was removed with the crown preparation. The cemented crowns would provide an excellent coronal seal, remineralize carious tissue, and maintain health of the tooth pulp thus preserving tooth structure.

Step 3: Proximal Reduction

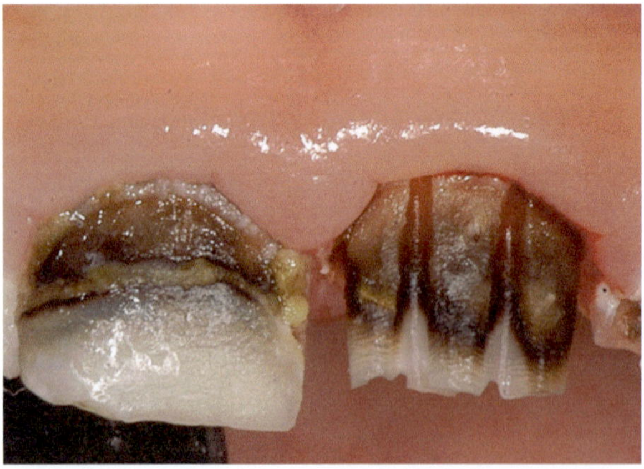

Interproximal reduction was carried out ensuring that the line angles were kept as parallel as possible to the long axis of the tooth. Proximal reduction should be up to 2 mm

Step 4: Labial and Palatal Reduction

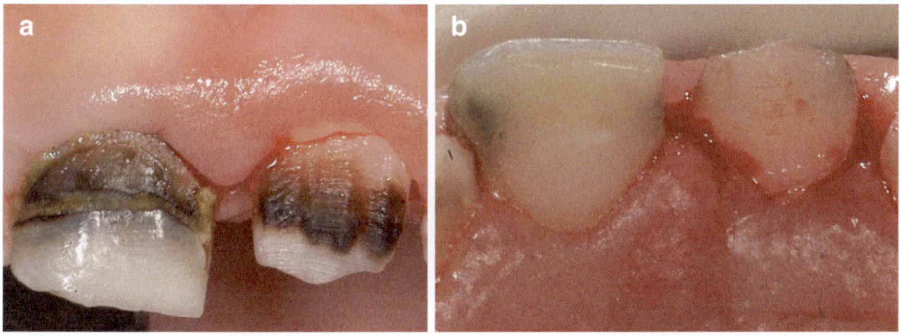

The depth grooves were leveled facially. The palatal surface was prepared to create a knife-edge incisally. The preparation was extended subgingivally to create a featheredge margin 1–2 mm subgingivally ensuring that all subgingival ledges were removed. The line and point angles were rounded leaving no undercuts in the preparation

Step 5: Tooth Preparation in All Incisors

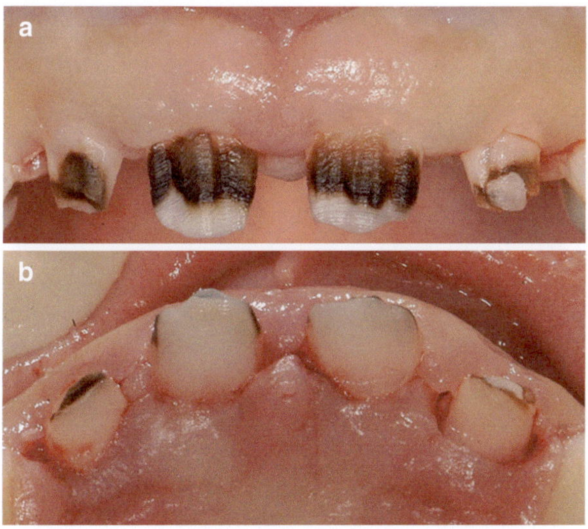

(**a**) Labial view of incisors prepared to receive preformed zirconia crowns. In tooth 62, a small labial lesion on tooth 62 was restored with resin-modified glass ionomer cement restoration after removing carious tissue selectively to firm dentine (Chap. 2). Striations left behind by the depth grooves aid in retention. (**b**) Palatal view of the tooth preparations

> **Clinical Notes**
> The featheredge margin in the tooth preparation compliments the margin prebuilt into the zirconia crown. The inability to crimp the zirconia crowns dictates that the tooth is prepared to fit the crown [4].

Step 6: Try-In Crowns Selected

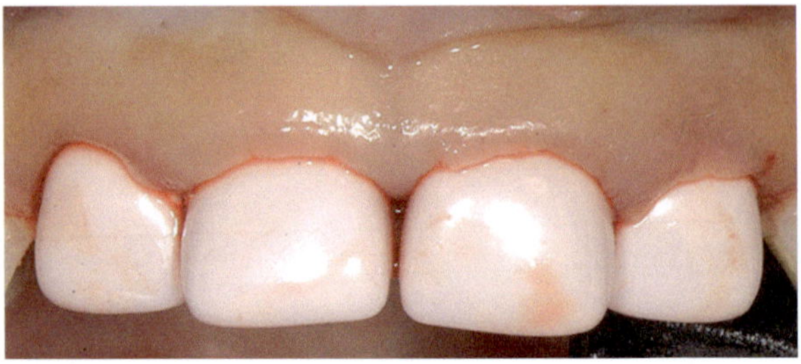

The pink autoclavable try-in crowns (NuSmile Ltd, Houston, TX, USA) were selected by trial and error to fit all four prepared teeth

Clinical Notes

The crowns should fit passively and seat subgingivally on sound tooth structure. If there is resistance to crown seating, the tooth preparation has to be refined further to fit the crown. When crowns are placed on multiple adjacent teeth, the crowns are best tried onto the preparations at the same time to ensure correct size selection and a passive fit. The try-in crowns prevent contamination of the final zirconia crowns to be cemented [8].

Step 7: Tack Cure

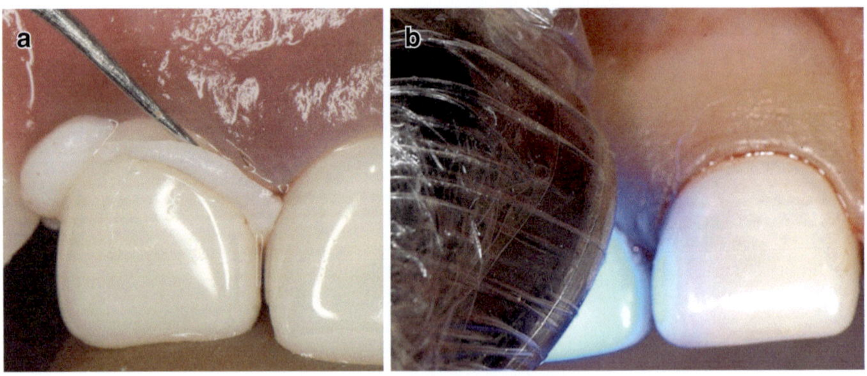

(**a**) A zirconia crown (NuSmile Ltd, Houston, TX, USA) of the same size as the selected try-in crown was loaded with resin-modified glass ionomer luting cement, positioned on the preparation, and tack cured and the excess cement cleared. (**b**) Final cure

Clinical Notes

Dual-cured resin cements and bioactive cements can also be used for luting the crown.

Step 8: Crowns Cemented

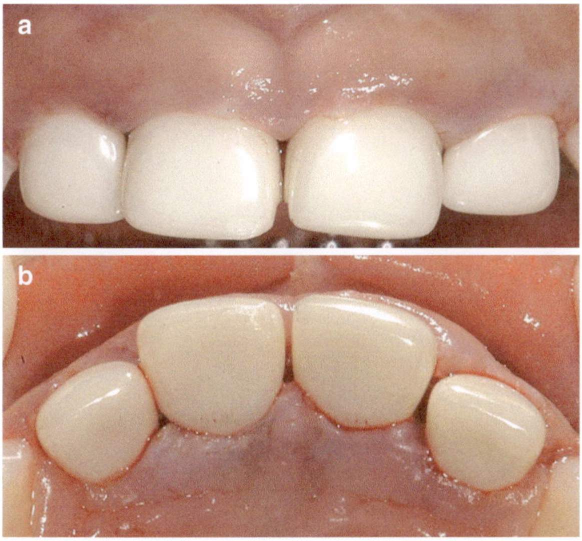

(**a**) Labial view of zirconia crowns (NuSmile Ltd, Houston, TX, USA) cemented on teeth 51, 52, 61, and 62. (**b**) Palatal view of zirconia crowns cemented on teeth 51, 52, 61, and 62

Step 9: Postoperative Radiograph

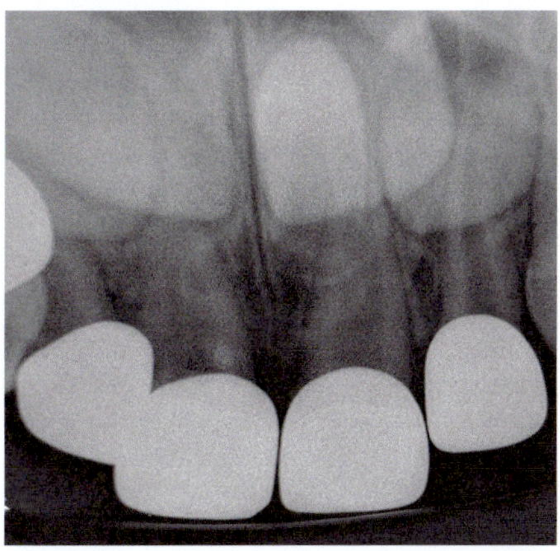

Postoperative radiograph was recorded to confirm the absence of excess subgingival luting cement

Ten-Day Follow-Up

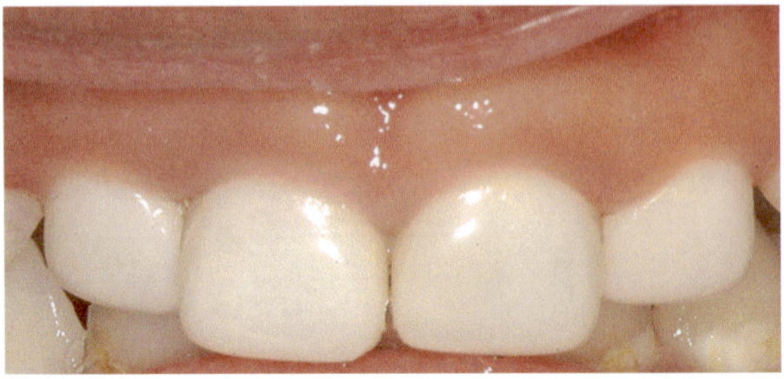

Follow-up at 10 days showed excellent soft tissue response and gingival healing. The smooth zirconia surface prevented biofilm formation, which encouraged a positive tissue response

5.3.4.3 Long-Term Follow-Up

Two-Year Follow-Up

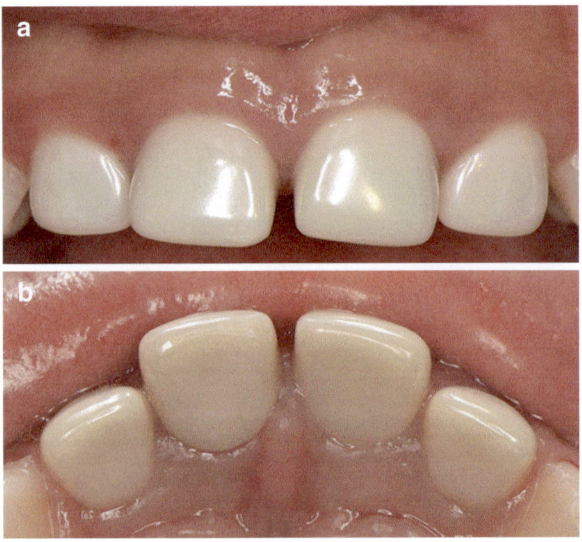

Two-year follow-up shows stable zirconia crowns in all four incisor teeth. Note the superior aesthetics and excellent soft tissue response in (**a**) labial and (**b**) palatal views in all four incisors

Two-Year Follow-Up Radiograph

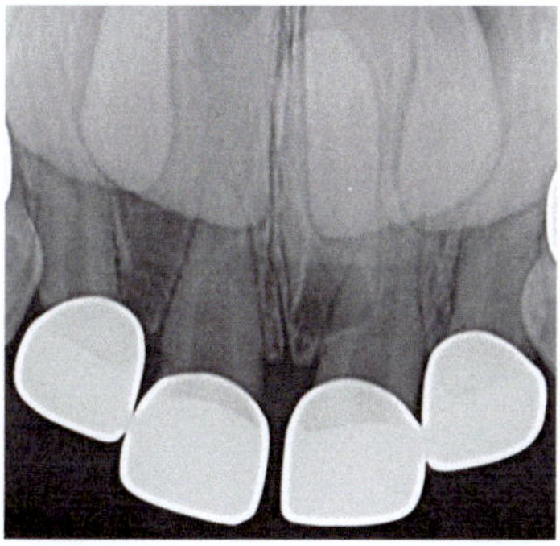

Two-year follow-up radiograph shows healthy radicular bone and stable full coronal restorations

5.3.5 Case Study 2: Preformed Zirconia Crowns for Posterior Full Coronal Coverage

The principles of tooth preparation, crown selection, and cementation for posterior primary teeth are similar to that of anterior teeth. A long-term follow-up of posterior primary teeth following pulp therapy, restored with preformed zirconia crowns, is presented.

5.3.5.1 Case Selection

Why Was This Case Selected for Restoration with Preformed Zirconia Crowns?

- Tooth 74 and 75 required full coronal coverage following pulp therapy.
- Parents had high aesthetic expectations and opted for zirconia crowns.

Preoperative View

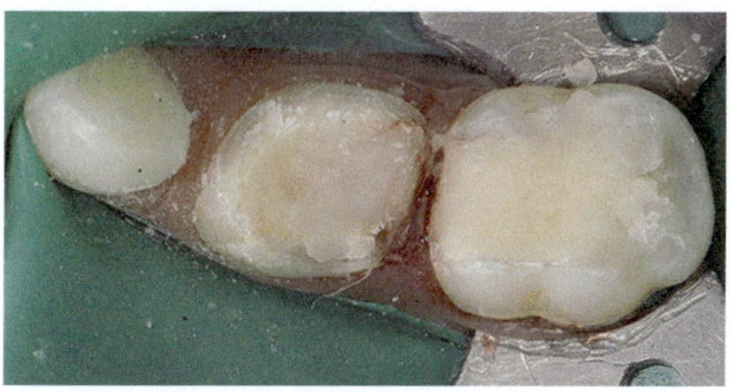

Tooth 74 and 75 underwent pulp therapy and received a core buildup with resin-modified glass ionomer restorative cement

5.3.5.2 Step-by-Step Guide

Step 1: Tooth Preparation

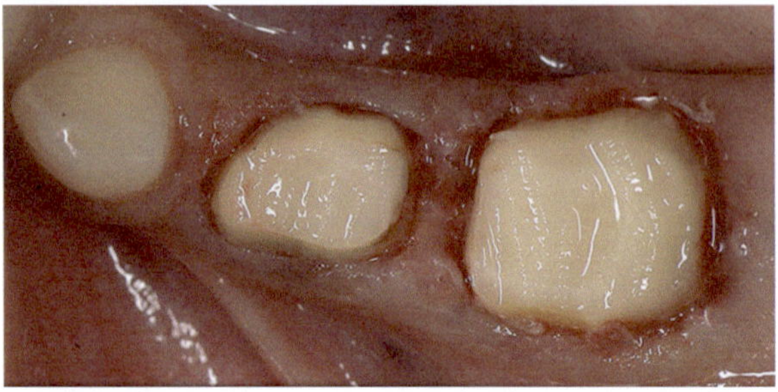

Teeth 74 and 74 were prepared to receive preformed zirconia crowns. Since zirconia crowns cannot be cut or crimped, the teeth have to be prepared to receive the crowns, making the tooth preparation more aggressive

Step 2: Try-In Crowns Selected

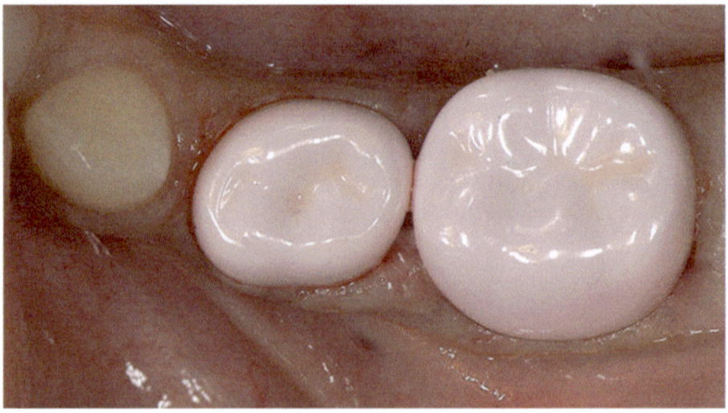

The pink try-in crowns were selected by trial and error to seat appropriately (NuSmile Ltd, Houston, TX, USA)

Step 3: Zirconia Crowns Cemented

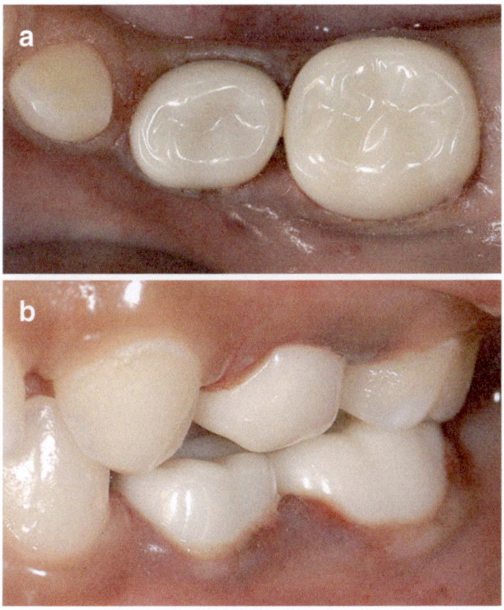

Zirconia crowns (NuSmile Ltd, Houston, TX, USA) of the same size as the selected try-in crowns cemented. (**a**) Occlusal view post cementation. (**b**) Buccal view in occlusion

Fifteen-Day Follow-Up

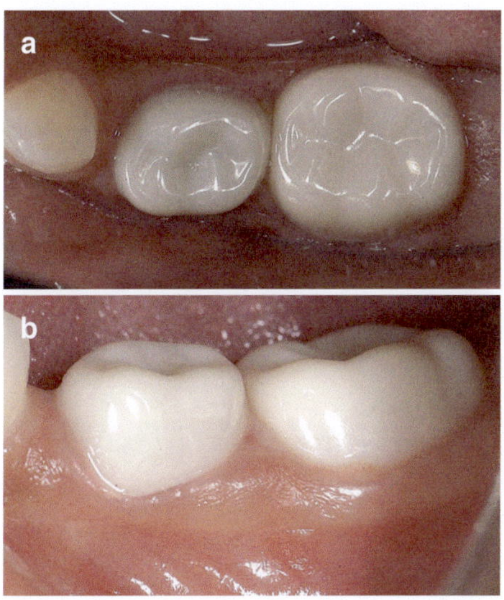

Fifteen-day follow-up of teeth 74 and 75 showed excellent soft tissue response and stippled gingiva in (**a**) occlusal and (**b**) buccal views

5.3.5.3 Long-Term Follow-Up

Two-Year Follow-Up

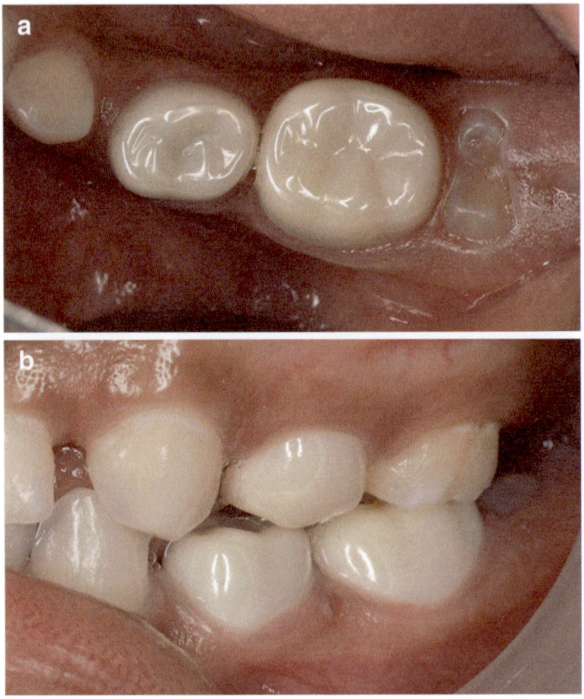

At the end of 2 years, the zirconia crowns in teeth 74 and 75 are stable, and soft tissue is healthy. Note tooth 36 erupting distal to tooth 75 in (**a**) occlusal view and (**b**) buccal view in occlusion

Four-Year Follow-Up

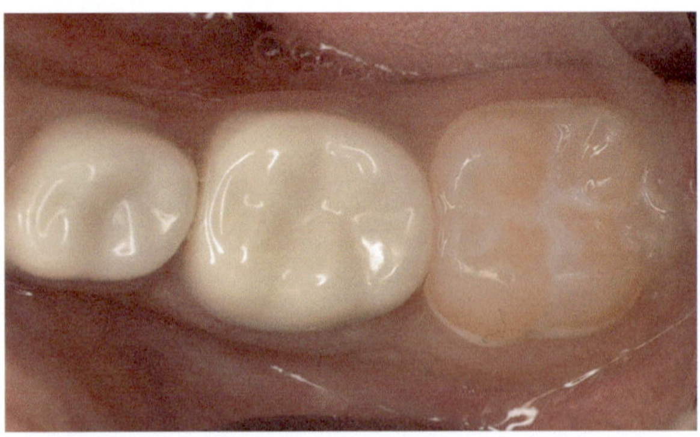

Note tooth 36 fully erupted on 4-year follow-up, stable crowns in teeth 74 and 75, and healthy gingiva

5.4 Conclusion

Multisurface carious lesions, relatively small tooth size, a large pulp chamber, and challenges related to age, behavior, and disabilities can negatively impact the longevity of intracoronal restorations in primary teeth. Though preformed metal crowns are still the gold standard in primary molars, preformed zirconia crowns offer an alternative to parents who prioritize aesthetics. In anterior restorations, the resin-based strip crowns provide optimum aesthetics. However, preformed zirconia crowns offer long-term stability and tissue compatibility. Increased costs and aggressive tooth preparation not withstanding, zirconia crowns have become the preferred choice for many parents and clinicians, as full coronal coverage restorations in children.

References

1. Waggoner WF. Restorative dentistry for the primary dentition. In: Casamassimo P, Fields H, Mctigue D, Nowak A, editors. Pediatric dentistry: infancy through adolescence. St. Louis, MO: Elsevier; 2013. p. 304–32.
2. Croll TP. Restorative dentistry for preschool children. Dent Clin N Am. 1995;39:737–70.
3. Waggoner WF. Restoring primary anterior teeth. Pediatr Dent. 2002;24(5):511–6.
4. Waggoner WF. Restoring primary anterior teeth: updated for 2014. Pediatr Dent. 2015;37(2):163–70.
5. Kupietzky A. Bonded resin composite strip crowns for primary incisors: clinical tips for a successful outcome. Pediatr Dent. 2002;24(2):145–8.
6. William F. Waggoner. Pediatric zirconia crowns: changing pediatric restorative dentistry. In: Dental economics. March 22, 2018; 2018. https://www.dentaleconomics.com/articles/print/volume-106/issue-3/science-tech/pediatric-zirconia-crowns-changing-pediatric-restorative-dentistry.html. Accessed 13 Oct 2018.
7. Lopez Cazaux S, Hyon I, Prud'homme T, Dajean Trutaud S. Twenty-nine-month follow-up of a paediatric zirconia dental crown. BMJ Case Rep. 2017;2017 https://doi.org/10.1136/bcr-2017-219891.
8. Planells del Pozo P, Fuks AB. Zirconia crowns--an esthetic and resistant restorative alternative for ECC affected primary teeth. J Clin Pediatr Dent. 2014;38(3):193–5.

Space Maintenance in the Primary Dentition: Custom Made and Prefabricated

6

6.1 Overview

One of the most important roles of primary teeth is to maintain space for the unerupted succedaneous teeth. Primary teeth are therefore considered the best space maintainers fulfilling all the prerequisites of an ideal space maintainer. The premature extraction of posterior primary teeth leads to space loss in the mixed and permanent dentitions [1]. It also compromises the subsequent eruption of the succedaneous teeth [2]. In the mixed dentition, some of the dynamics that influence treatment planning for space maintenance include the developmental stage of the underlying permanent tooth, the expected time of exfoliation of the primary tooth, and the presence of crowding among others. Unlike the mixed dentition, however, the premature loss of a posterior primary tooth in the primary dentition is a nearly immediate universal recommendation for space maintenance [3]. A space maintainer may reduce the need to extract permanent teeth during future corrective orthodontic treatment. It could also obviate the need for complex orthodontics all together [4].

The knowledge and ability to provide space maintenance increases the chances of the clinician making the right judgment call when faced with a primary molar that has poor endodontic prognosis. Endodontics in such teeth can compromise the health of the permanent tooth bud and is very demanding on both the child and the operator. Extraction followed by space maintenance not only removes the infected tooth but is also very quick, easy, and less challenging for the both the child and clinician.

The following chapter will discuss space maintainers commonly used in the primary dentition, namely, the band and loop, the reverse band/crown and loop, and the distal shoe space maintainer. All the clinical steps required to place a laboratory fabricated custom-made space maintainer and the prefabricated variation of each of these space maintainers are discussed.

M. S. Kher, A. Rao, *Contemporary Treatment Techniques in Pediatric Dentistry*,
https://doi.org/10.1007/978-3-030-11860-0_6

6.2 Band and Loop Space Maintainers

6.2.1 Introduction

The band and loop space maintainer is a unilateral, nonfunctional, passive fixed space maintainer commonly used in the primary dentition. It has a cantilever design with the band on the abutment tooth and the loop traversing the space of the prematurely lost tooth to contact the next tooth in the arch. This simple design is also versatile and can be modified according to the clinical situation as in a reverse crown and loop, which is subsequently explained.

6.2.2 Indications and Contraindications

It is indicated during the:

- Unilateral premature loss of the primary first molar prior to eruption of the first permanent molar [2]
- Unilateral premature loss of the second primary molar after the eruption of the first permanent molar
- Bilateral premature loss of lower primary first molars before the eruption of the permanent incisors and first permanent molars [2]
- Bilateral premature loss of lower primary second molars after the eruption of the permanent first molars but before the complete eruption of the permanent incisors
- In the two clinical situations of bilateral premature loss described above, a lingual arch is not indicated because it can interfere with the eruption of the permanent incisor tooth buds placed lingual to the primary incisors [2].
- Evidence in literature reports clinically insignificant space loss following the premature loss of the primary first molar after the full eruption of the permanent first molar [5]. This has been reported in both the maxillary [6] and mandibular arches [7]. However, the final decision to place a band and loop space maintainer following premature extraction of the first primary molar when the first permanent molar is fully erupted should comprehensively consider the prevailing clinical situation. The degree of clinical interdigitation, lip and incisor protrusion, and a steep curve of spee are factors which can accentuate space loss in the above clinical situation and must be taken into account [5].

6.2.3 Rationale

In the primary dentition, where indicated, the band and loop space maintainer fulfils most requisites of an ideal space maintainer:

- It predictably maintains the mesiodistal dimension of the space occupied by the prematurely lost tooth.

- It remains passive without exerting forces on the adjacent teeth and does not restrict normal growth and development.
- It has sufficient strength to withstand occlusal forces.
- It has a simple design and is easy to fabricate and maintain.
- It is durable and has fewer problems compared to other space maintainers [8].

6.2.4 Case Study 1: Custom-Made Band and Loop Space Maintainer

6.2.4.1 Case Selection

Why Was This Case Selected for a Band and Loop Space Maintainer?

- A 5-year-old child presented with a deep carious lesion in tooth 64. Parent gave a history of many episodes of spontaneous pain and two episodes of extraoral swelling in relation to tooth 64.
- The crown was non-restorable, and the opening of a chronic draining sinus tract buccally was observed.
- Radiograph showed a deep carious lesion in tooth 64 extending beyond the cementoenamel junction. There was periapical radiolucency around the palatal root and root resorption in tooth 64. Tooth 26 was yet to erupt.
- Hence placement of a band and loop space maintainer was planned since tooth 64 required to be extracted well before the eruption of tooth 26 [6].

Case Selection: Preoperative Occlusal View

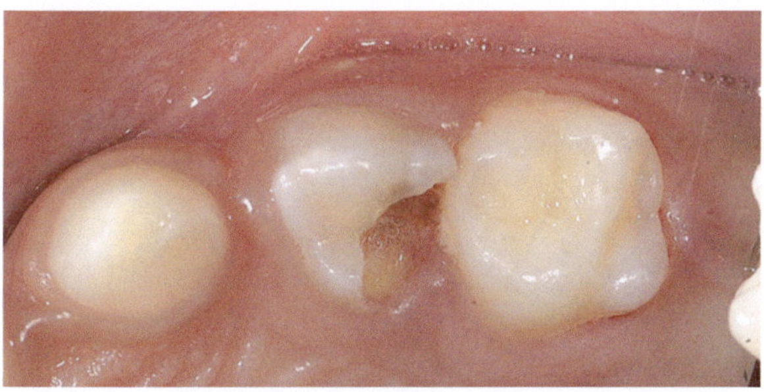

Tooth 64 showed the opening of a chronic fistulous tract buccally. The tooth had poor clinical crown structure and was non-restorable. There was no clinical evidence of the eruption of tooth 26 distal to tooth 65

Case Selection: Preoperative Radiograph

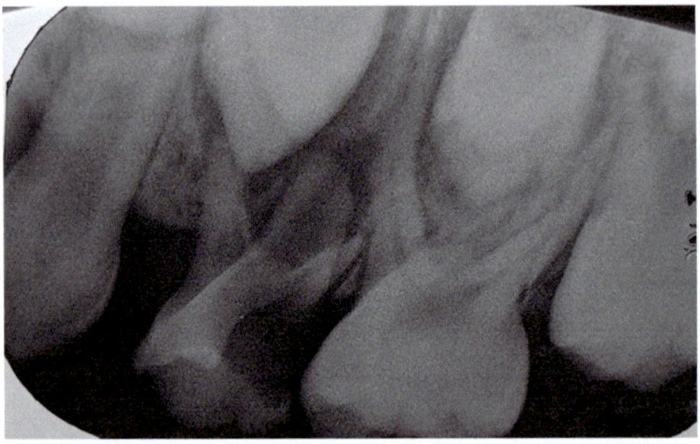

The radiograph demonstrated a deep carious lesion extending beyond the cementoenamel junction. Periapical radiolucency and root resorption were evident. Tooth 26 was seen developing and unerupted on the radiograph

Clinical Notes

In this 5-year-old child, there were no clinical or radiographic signs of the first permanent molar erupting for at least 12–24 months. In the mixed dentition, space loss following the premature loss of the mandibular first primary molar, after the first permanent molar has erupted, occurs due to a distal drift of the cuspid and does not result in loss of arch length or perimeter [5–7].

6.2.4.2 Step-by-Step Guide to Fabrication

Step 1: Molar Band Seated

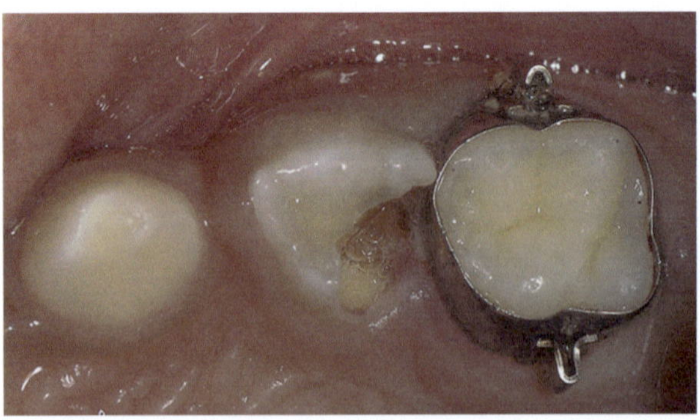

A preformed molar band was selected through trial and error and fitted onto the abutment tooth

Clinical Notes
Note that brackets have been spot welded on buccal and lingual sides of the selected preformed band. The brackets help the clinician position the band accurately in the impression and also stabilize the band during impression pouring.

Step 2: Impression Made

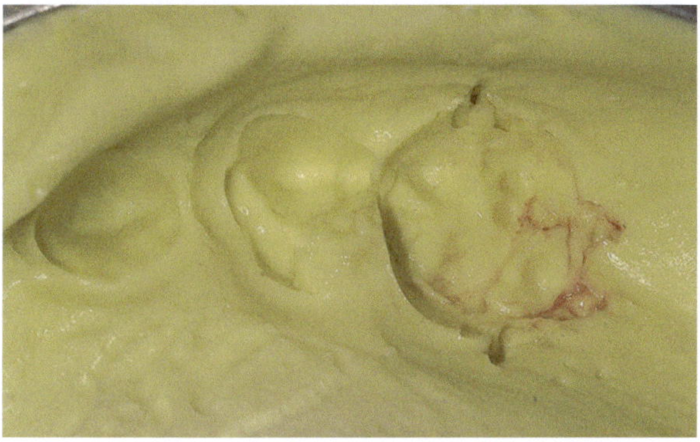

A sectional impression was recorded in alginate with the band positioned on the abutment tooth. Note the indentation made by the brackets in the center of the buccal and palatal surface of the impression

Clinical Notes
The impression should include the abutment tooth, site of extraction, and the tooth anterior to the extracted tooth.

Step 3: Band Positioned and Stabilized

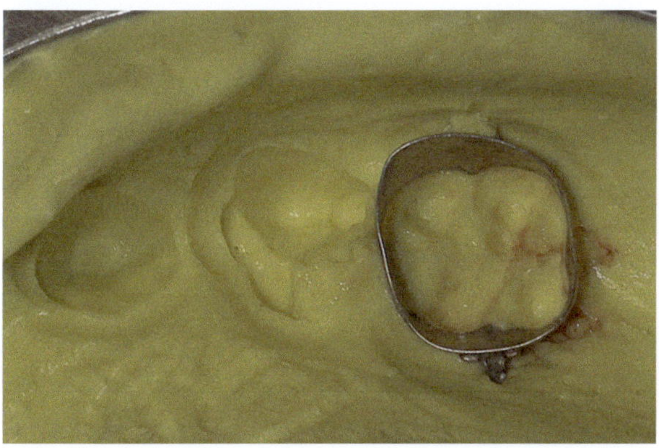

The band was removed from the abutment tooth and correctly positioned and stabilized in the impression

Clinical Notes

The markings made on the impression surface by the occlusal margin of the band and welded brackets aid in the positioning and stabilization of the band.

Step 4: Pouring the Impression in Stone

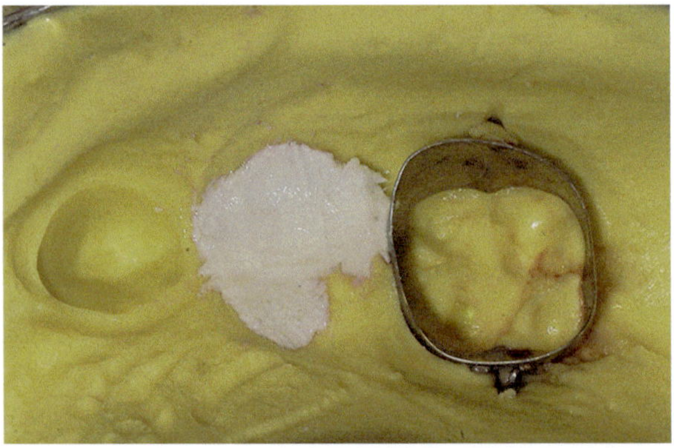

The impression space of the tooth to be extracted was blocked out with an intermediate restorative material (IRM) before the impression was poured in stone to produce the working model

Clinical Notes

Placing IRM in the impression space of the tooth to be extracted saves the time involved in subsequently scrapping the extracted tooth off the cast and also prevents damage to the cast. Alternatively, the tooth can be extracted first and the impression recorded in the same appointment.

Step 5: Working Model

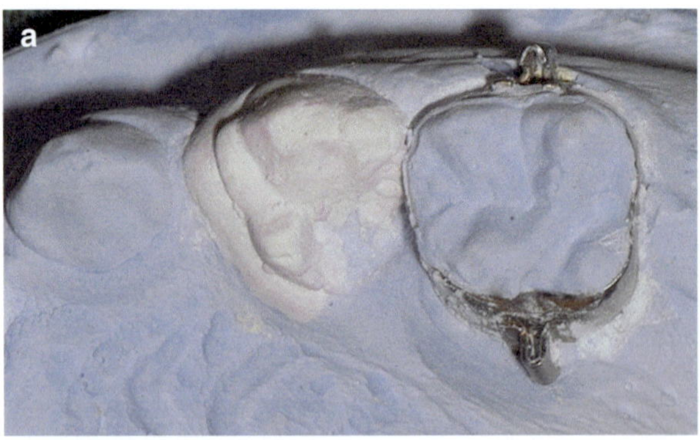

(**a**) Working model was poured in dental stone. Note the tooth to be extracted in IRM. (**b**) The IRM can be scraped off cleanly

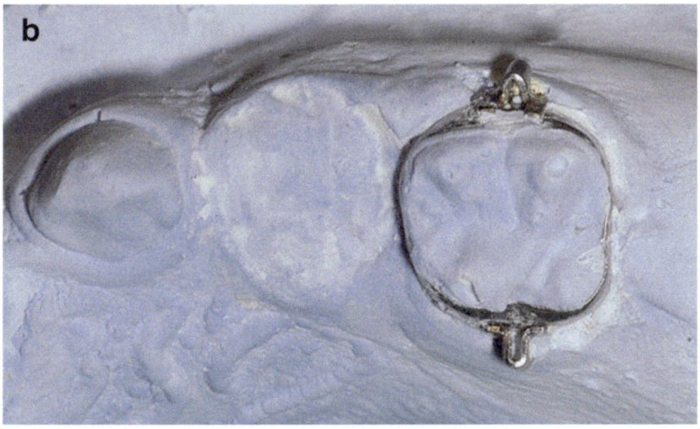

Clinical Notes
Care should be taken to see that the band does not move when the working model is made. There should be no air bubbles especially in the region where the loop will rest. The brackets can be sheared off easily from the band with a plier.

Step 6: Band and Loop Space Maintainer Fabricated

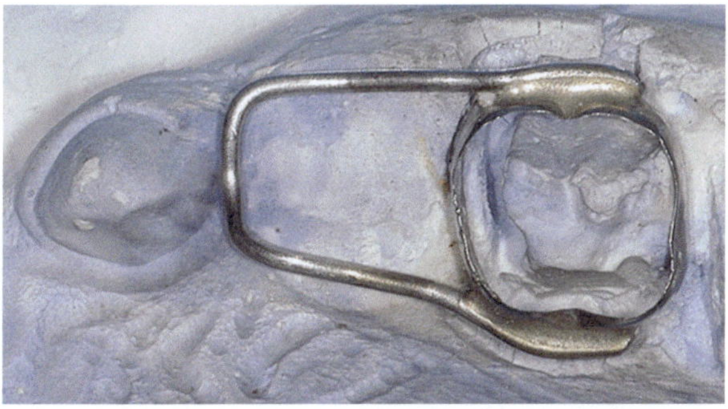

The loop was fabricated with a 0.9 mm wire and soldered to the buccal and lingual surfaces of the band. The loop should run parallel to the edentulous ridge, rest just below the contact point, and be approximately 8 mm wide so as to allow free eruption of the premolar [2]

Clinical Notes
In cases where the abutment tooth requires full coronal coverage, it is recommended that the band and loop space maintainer be cemented on the preformed metal crown rather than placing a crown and loop space maintainer [4, 9, 10]. Fractures of the solder joint are known to occur though not common. While a repair is easy when the abutment tooth has a band placed on it, repair

of a fractured crown and loop space maintainer is difficult, and hence such space maintainers are best avoided. Also, many teeth requiring full coronal coverage have received pulp therapy, and it is best to cement the preformed metal crown immediately following treatment.

Step 7: Band and Loop Space Maintainer Cemented

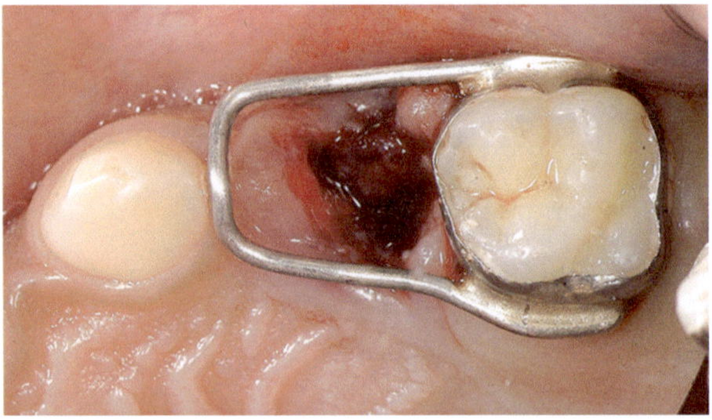

The space maintainer was cemented using glass ionomer luting cement following extraction of tooth 64

Clinical Notes
The space maintainer should rest passively without applying any active force on adjacent teeth. This design maintains critical arch length until the first permanent molar erupts distal to the abutment tooth. The child is put on a 6-month follow-up and cautioned against eating foods that are excessively tacky and sticky in consistency.

6.2.4.3 Long-Term Follow-Up

Two-Year Follow-Up

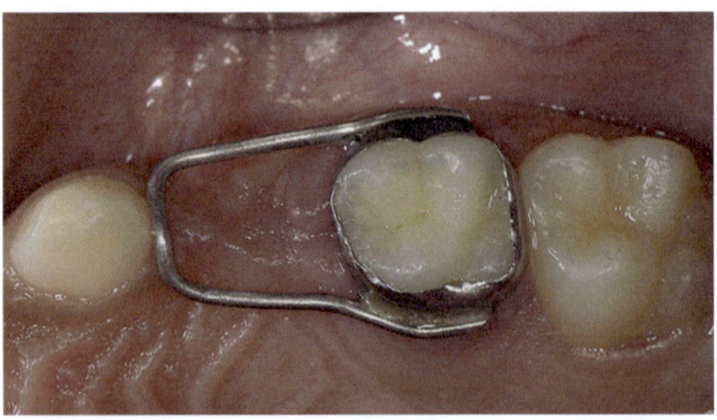

Follow-up at 2 years showed the first permanent molar guided into correct position with no loss of arch length and space maintained for the first premolar when it erupts

Three and Half-Year Follow-Up

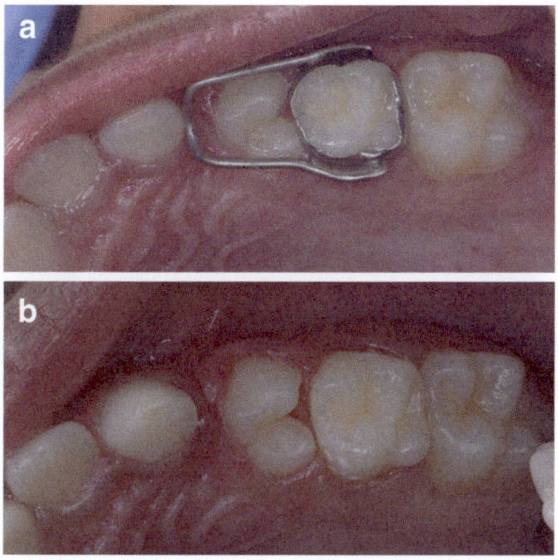

Follow-up at three and half years shows (**a**) tooth 24 erupting through the loop. (**b**) Space maintainer removed

6.2.5 Case Study 2: Prefabricated Band and Loop Space Maintainer

6.2.5.1 Case Selection

Why Was This Case Selected for a Band and Loop Space Maintainer?

- Tooth 54 showed poor prognosis clinically and radiographically and was indicated for extraction.
- Tooth 16 had not erupted.

Preoperative Occlusal Image

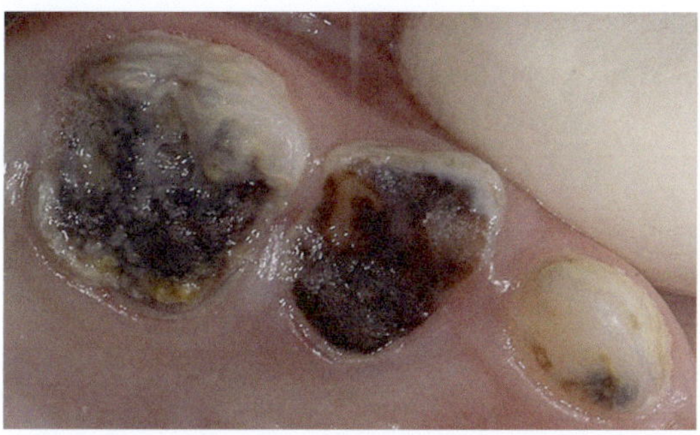

Tooth 54 indicated for extraction showed a chronic draining sinus, pathological mobility, and inadequate coronal tooth structure. Tooth 55 showed a large multisurface carious lesion. Tooth 16 had not erupted

Preoperative Radiograph

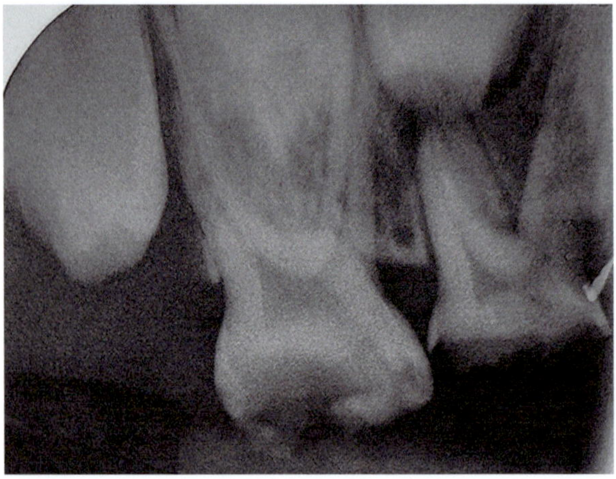

Tooth 54 showed periapical radiolucency and poor coronal tooth structure. Tooth 55 showed a deep carious lesion with adequate layer of dentine separating the lesion from the pulp. Tooth 16 was yet to erupt

6.2.5.2 Step-by-Step Guide to Placement

Step 1: Tooth Extracted

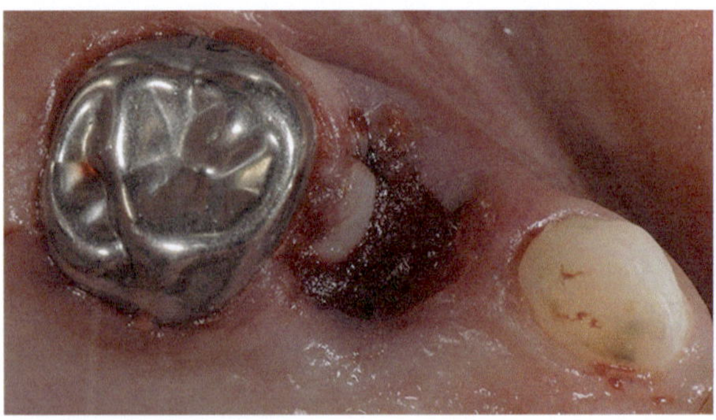

Tooth 54 was extracted, and the abutment tooth 55 was restored with a preformed metal crown (PMC) (Chap. 4)

Components of a Prefabricated Band and Loop

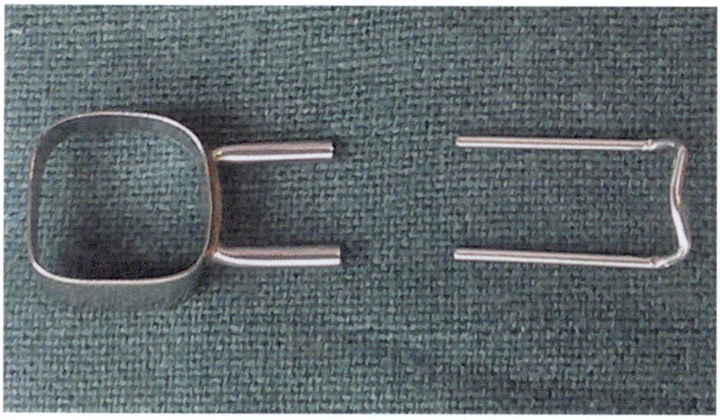

The appropriate sized band with the tubes attached was selected by trial and error from a variety of sizes (Denovo Dental, CA, USA). The loop to be inserted into the tubes was also selected from the kit

Clinical Notes

Prefabricated space maintainers have the advantage of being adjusted and cemented in a single chairside visit. They can be cemented on the day of the extraction without the need for an impression. This is especially useful in the absence of adequate laboratory support or when an additional visit for cementation of the space maintainer is not possible. It is also very useful when treating the child under general anesthesia.

Step 2: Band Placed

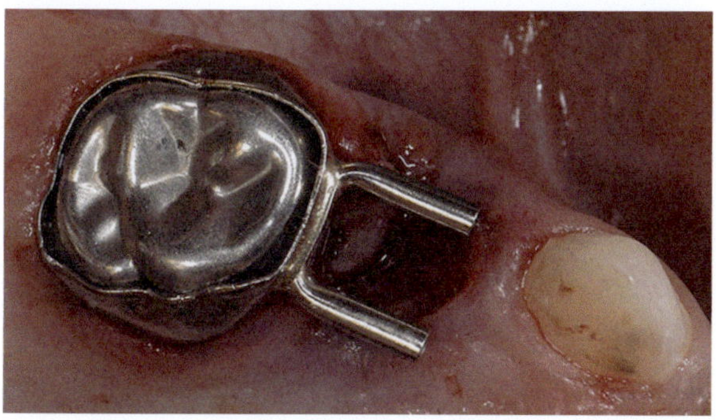

The band with the space maintainer tube attached was selected by trial and error and adapted on the abutment tooth

Clinical Notes

The loop is inserted fully into the tube and the length adjusted. It is cut to size with a wire cutter so that the contact of the loop with the tooth anterior to the extraction space is satisfactory.

Step 3: Tube with Loop Crimped

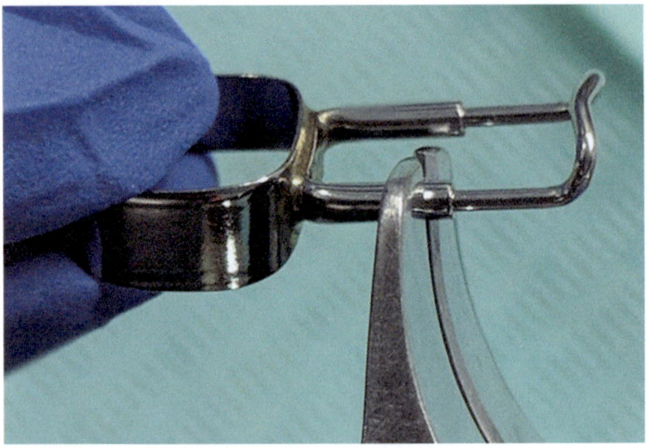

The tube with the adjusted loop inserted into it was crimped with a wire-crimping plier. This locked the loop into the tube

> **Clinical Notes**
> The tube is tugged manually to confirm that it is firmly secure inside the tube.

Step 4: Cementation

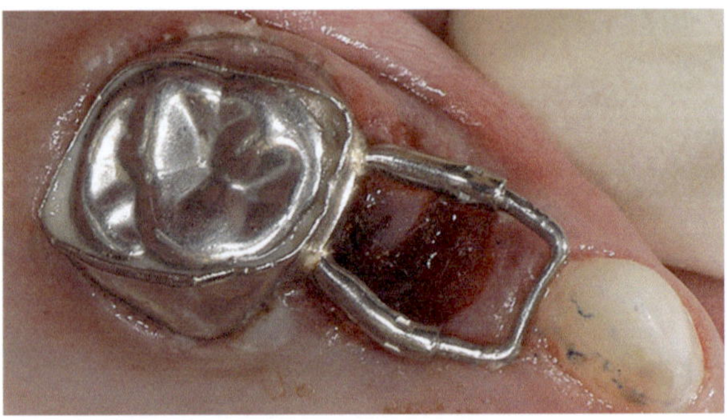

The band and loop space maintainer was cemented in place. Note that the loop has been contoured with a three-prong plier for a superior fit

6.2.5.3 Long-Term Follow-Up

Two-Year Follow-Up

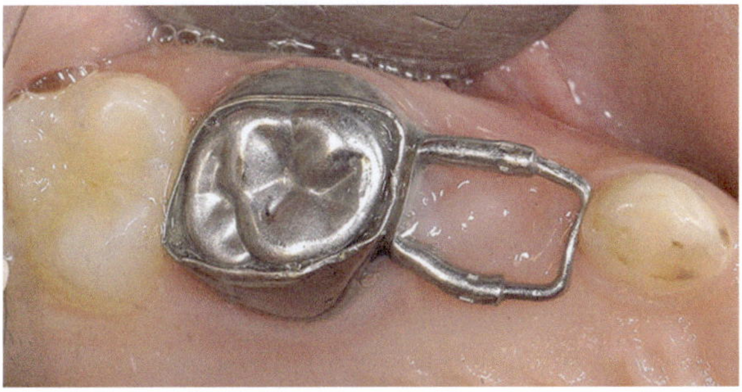

Two-year follow-up image showed the 6-year molar guided into occlusion with no space loss at the sight of extraction

Four-Year Follow-Up

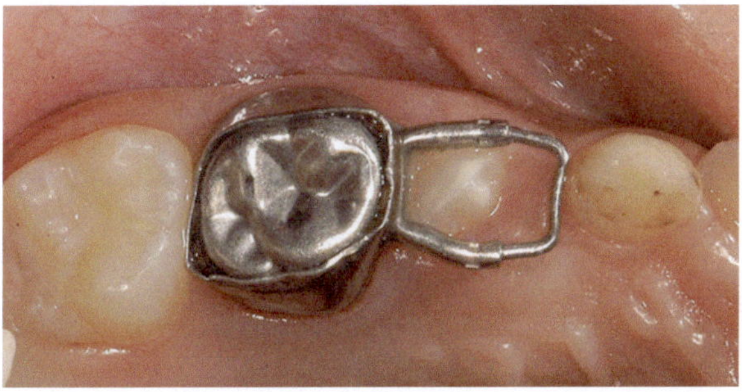

Follow-up at 4 years shows the tooth 14 erupting. The arch length has been maintained successfully

6.3 Reverse Crown and Loop Space Maintainers

6.3.1 Introduction

The reverse crown and loop space maintainer, as the name suggests, is placed when the extraction site is posterior to the abutment tooth. Since it holds space created by the premature loss of the tooth posterior to the abutment tooth, the loop travels in the reverse direction. Classically this space maintainer design is of value when the second primary molar needs to be extracted prematurely and the first permanent molar has just started to erupt and is still embedded in gingival tissue. The following is a step-by-step description of the clinical steps involved in the fabrication of both the custom-made and prefabricated reverse crown and loop space maintainer.

6.3.2 Indications and Contraindications

- The reverse band/crown and loop space maintainer is most commonly used to guide the partially erupted first permanent molar when the second primary molar requires to be extracted prematurely.

6.3.3 Rationale

The age of eruption of the first permanent molar can have variations in the population [11]. Of equal significance is the duration of eruption, which is the period from the time the first permanent molar is seen in the oral cavity, covered largely by gingival tissue, to the time the tooth reaches functional occlusion. Ekstrand KR et al. [11] showed the duration of eruption of the first permanent molar to be 5–32 months (mean 15.4 months) in girls and from 7 to 28 months (mean 15.0) in boys. Loss of the second primary molar during this stage of eruption would have significant detrimental consequences in terms of space and arch length loss. When extraction of the second primary molar during this phase of active eruption of the first permanent molar becomes unavoidable, a reverse band/crown and loop space maintainer passively holds space preventing mesial migration of the first permanent molar.

6.3.4 Case Study 1: Custom-Made Reverse Crown and Loop Space Maintainer

6.3.4.1 Case Selection

Why Was This Case Selected for a Reverse Crown and Loop Space Maintainer?

- A 6-year-old child presented with a few episodes of spontaneous pain in relation to tooth 75. There was one episode of an extraoral swelling in relation to tooth 75.
- Clinical examination revealed a deep carious lesion involving the pulp in tooth 75. The tooth was non-restorable with loss of the distal half of the clinical crown.
- The child had difficulty chewing on solid food on the left side that was also evident from the accumulation of plaque and calculus on that side.
- Tooth 74 had a large restoration on the mesial surface that appeared to have chipped and hence required full coronal coverage.
- Tooth 36 was partially erupted with the mesial marginal ridge visible.

Case Selection: Preoperative Occlusal View

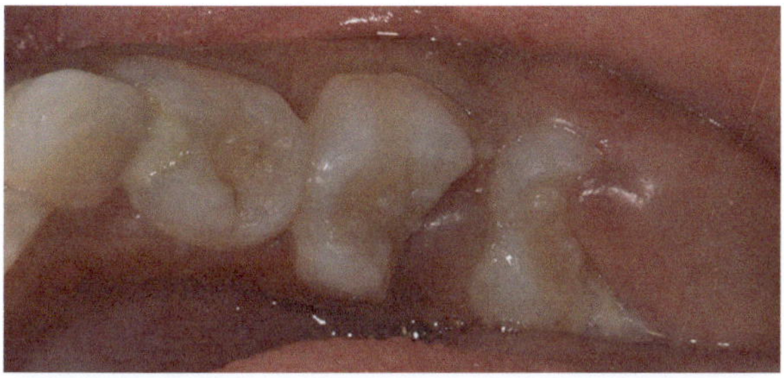

Tooth 85 had a deep carious lesion on the distal surface involving the entire distal half of the clinical crown. Note the gingival growth into the lesion. Tooth 84 had a restoration on the mesial surface with a fracture of the mesiobuccal line angle. Tooth 46 was partially erupted and had plaque and calculus accumulation on the occlusal surface

> **Clinical Notes**
> Since tooth 46 would take on an average 15 months to erupt to complete functional occlusion [11], tooth 85 could not have been retained for that length of time and would require to be extracted.

Case Selection: Preoperative Radiograph

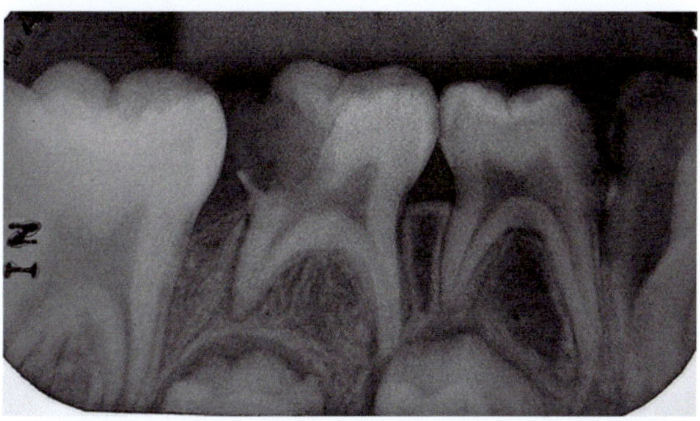

The radiograph showed a deep carious lesion involving the pulp in tooth 85. The lesion extended subgingivally up to the cementoenamel junction. Tooth 84 had a mesial restoration. Tooth 46 was partially erupted

6.3.4.2 Step-by-Step Guide to Fabrication

Step 1: Abutment Tooth Prepared

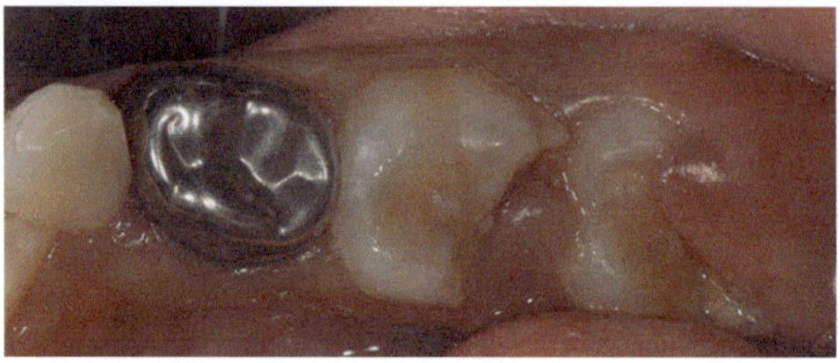

Abutment tooth 84 was prepared to receive a preformed metal crown

> **Clinical Notes**
> Due to the anatomy of the primary first molar, metal bands are not as stable as preformed metal crowns. Hence when the primary first molar is the abutment tooth, as in a reverse crown and loop or a distal shoe space maintainer, we prefer placing a preformed metal crown on the abutment tooth.

Step 2: Extraction

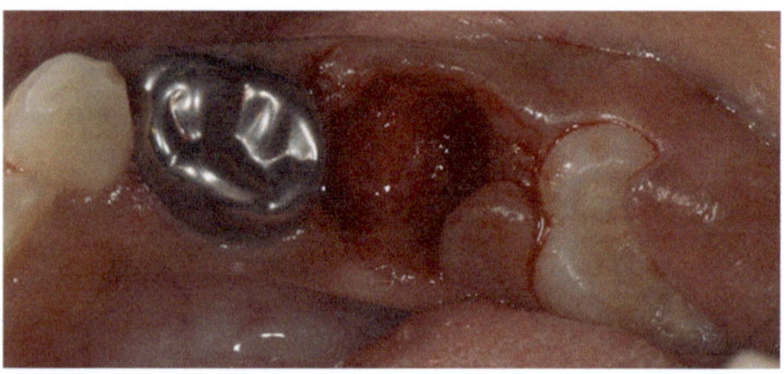

Tooth 85 was extracted

Step 3: Impression

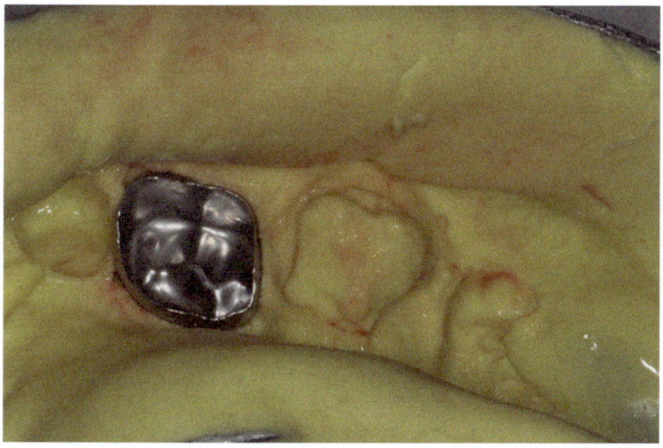

A sectional impression was recorded in alginate and the preformed metal crown transferred accurately into the impression

Clinical Notes

Impression is taken with the crown positioned on the abutment tooth. The impression should include the abutment tooth, site of extraction, and the tooth posterior to the extracted tooth, i.e., the partially erupted permanent first molar. The preformed metal crown is then transferred to the impression.

Step 4: Working Model

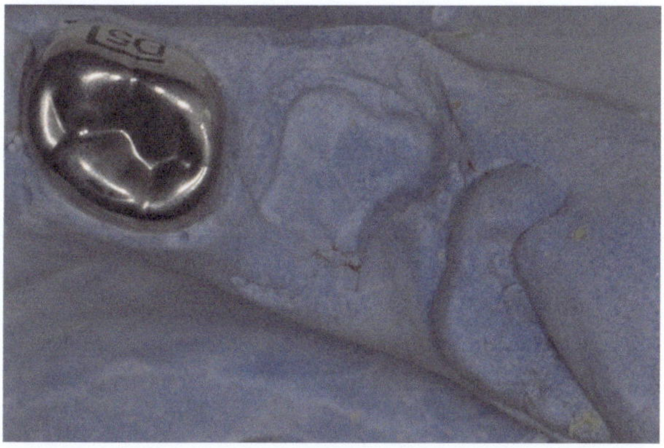

The working model ready for fabrication of the reverse crown and loop space maintainer

Step 5: Reverse Crown and Loop Fabricated

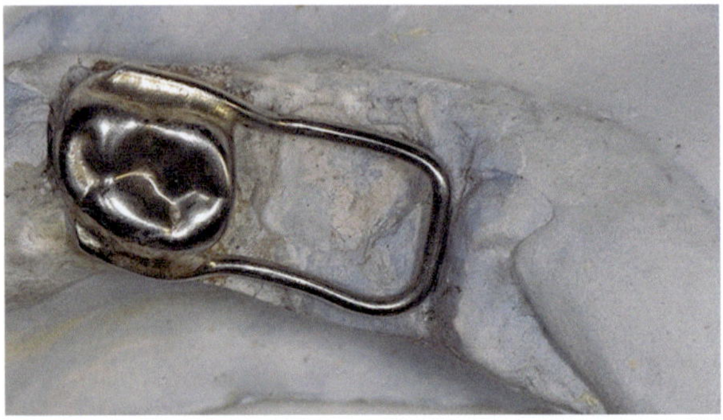

The loop should run parallel to the edentulous ridge and rest on the mesial surface of the erupting first permanent molar

Step 6: Space Maintainer Cemented

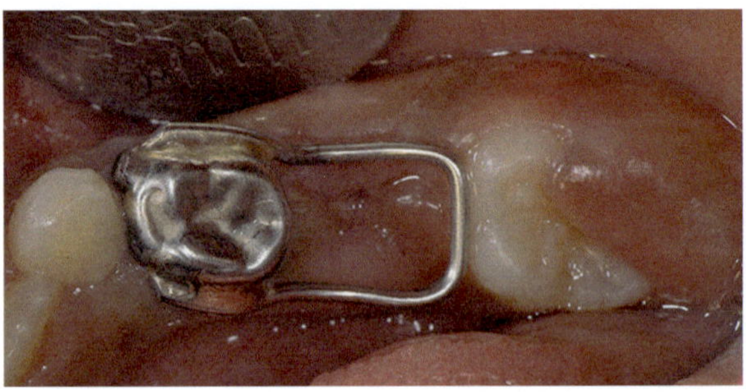

The space maintainer cemented using glass ionomer luting cement

Clinical Notes

The reverse crown and loop space maintainer should rest passively on the mesial surface of the erupting first permanent molar thereby preventing its migration mesially during and after eruption and the resultant space loss.

6.3.4.3 Long-Term Follow-Up

Six-Month Follow-Up

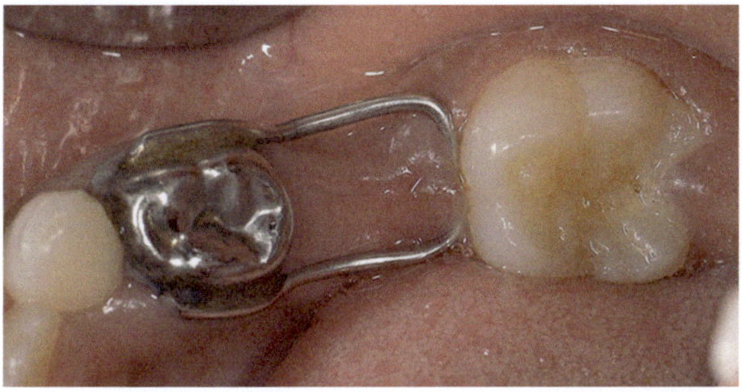

Follow-up shows the erupting first permanent molar guided by the space maintainer with no mesial migration

One-Year Follow-Up

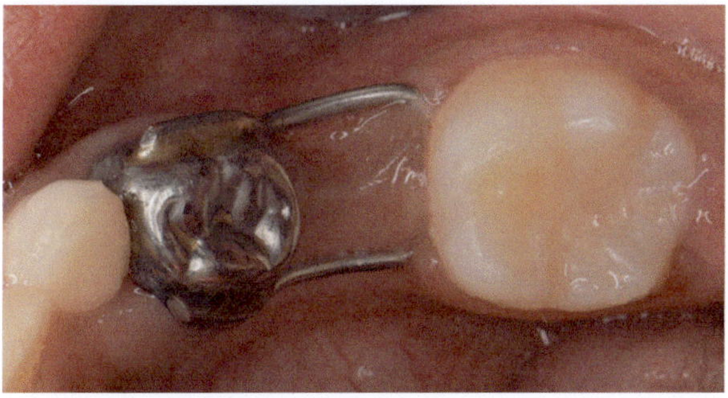

The 6-year molar has erupted in position

Clinical Notes
The loop can be cut off and a band and loop space maintainer placed with the first permanent molar as abutment, to prevent tipping of the first permanent molar following complete eruption.

6.3.5 Case Study 2: Prefabricated Reverse Crown and Loop Space Maintainer

6.3.5.1 Case Selection

Why Was This Case Selected for a Reverse Crown and Loop Space Maintainer?

- A 5-year-old child presented with severe pain in tooth 55. The child had repeated episodes of spontaneous pain in tooth 55.
- Tooth 55 had a non-restorable deep carious lesion. Carious lesions were noted in teeth 53 and 54.
- Tooth 16 was partially erupted.

Preoperative Occlusal View

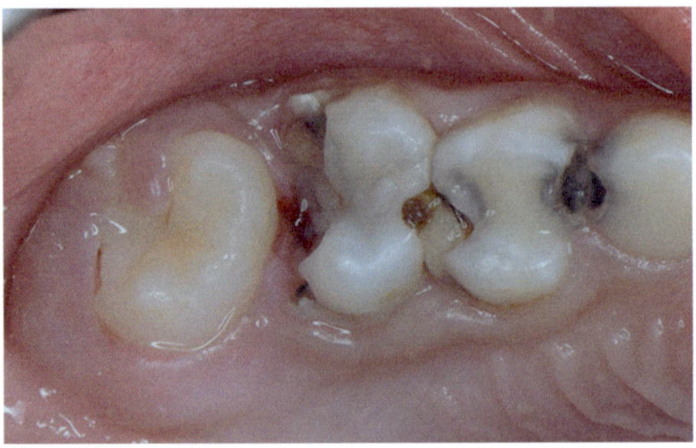

Carious lesions in 53, 54, and 55. Tooth 55 was non-restorable requiring extraction, 16 was partially erupted

Preoperative Radiograph

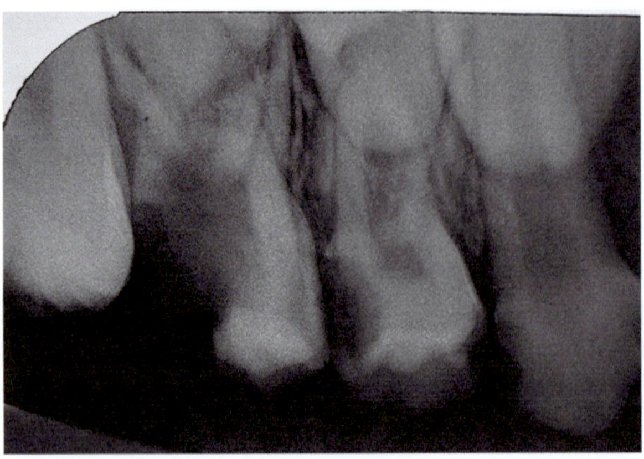

Tooth 55 showed a deep carious lesion involving the pulp and extending subgingivally. Tooth 54 had a deep carious lesion distally. Tooth 16 had erupted partially

Reverse Crown and Loop Space Maintainer Cemented

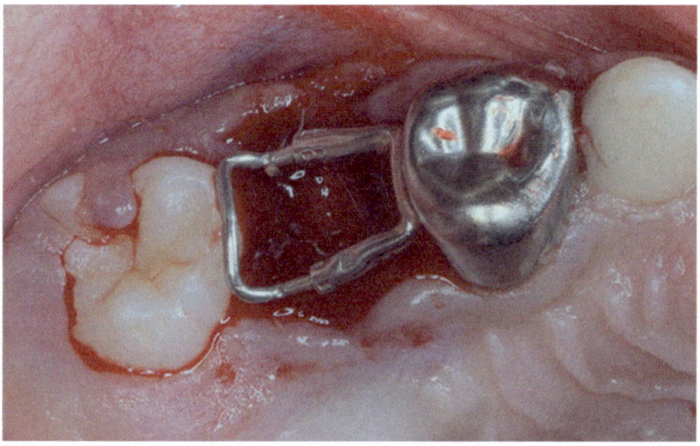

Tooth 55 was extracted. A prefabricated reverse crown and loop space maintainer (Denovo Dental, CA, USA) was adjusted and cemented on abutment tooth 54. Since abutment tooth 54 had a deep distal carious lesion, the preformed metal crown placed on tooth 54 worked on the principle of placing a Hall Crown (Chap. 1)

Five-Day Follow-Up Image

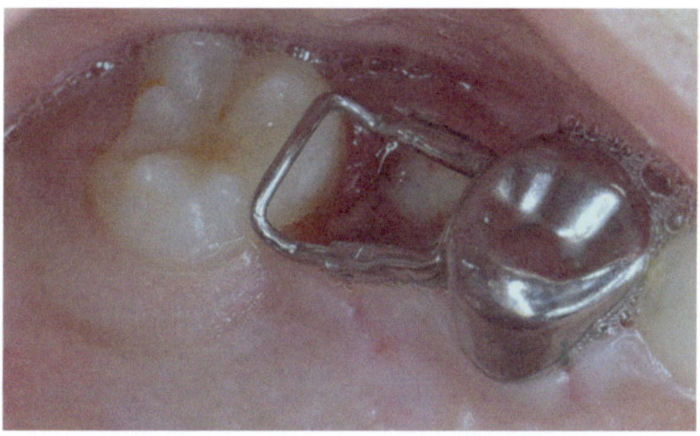

The loop of the space maintainer rests on the mesial wall of erupting tooth 16 preventing mesial migration and loss of arch length when tooth 16 is erupting

Clinical Notes

The space maintainer subsequently holds space until tooth 15 erupts but may require to be replaced by a band and loop space maintainer with tooth 16 as abutment if tipping of tooth 16 is noted. Hence regular follow-ups are a must. In the present case, the family was migrating to another country and needed urgent care for the present condition. They were advised on the need for regular monitoring and follow-up care.

6.4 Distal Shoe Space Maintainer

6.4.1 Introduction

The distal shoe space maintainer prevents severe space and arch length loss caused by the premature extraction of the second primary molar before the eruption of the first permanent molar. Also called “the intra-alveolar space maintainer,” it guides the unerupted first permanent molar into occlusion in the event that the second primary molar has to be extracted prematurely. It is a cantilevered space maintainer with the first primary molar acting as an abutment. The abutment tooth receives a preformed metal crown (PMC), and the loop travels in the reverse direction over and beyond the second primary molar. It then bends gingivally distal to the second primary molar into the socket extending roughly a millimeter below and just before the marginal ridge of the unerupted first permanent molar.

6.4.2 Indications and Contraindications

- The distal shoe space maintainer is specifically indicated when the second primary molar is lost before the eruption of the first permanent molar [2]. It is indicated in both maxillary and mandibular arches.
- It is contraindicated in medically compromised children especially in cardiac conditions that require antibiotic prophylaxis prior to dental treatment [12]. This is due to the intra-alveolar extension and the incomplete epithelization at the histological level that occurs following appliance placement [2].
- The other contraindications are multiple missing teeth leading to inadequate abutments [12].

6.4.3 Rationale

When the second primary molar is prematurely lost, the permanent first molar drifts mesially within the alveolar bone resulting in loss of arch length and the likely impaction of the second premolar [2]. The distal shoe space maintainer is most effective in this situation. Though considered an invasive appliance by some, since the intra-alveolar distal extension is placed in the extraction site at the time of extraction, it is extremely comfortable for the child patient and goes unnoticed by them. Though a removable space maintainer is considered an alternative to a distal shoe, it is inadequate because it cannot accurately guide the erupting first permanent molar like the distal shoe can. Removable appliances also have compliance issues. Since anchorage on the convergent first primary molar brings into question issues of stability, we always place a full coronal coverage metal crown on the abutment tooth. Following the full eruption of the first permanent molar, the intra-alveolar extension can be trimmed, and the appliance can continue to maintain space as a reverse crown and loop or be replaced with a conventional band and loop.

6.4.4 Case Study 1: Custom-Made Distal Shoe Space Maintainer

6.4.4.1 Case Selection

Why Was This Case Selected for a Distal Shoe Space Maintainer?

- A four and a half-year-old child presented with severe pain in relation to tooth 85. Deep carious lesion involving the pulp was noted in tooth 85. There was very poor remaining clinical crown structure.
- Tooth 84 had a distal proximal lesion but could serve as an abutment once restored.
- Radiograph showed a deep carious lesion in tooth 85 extending to the bifurcation area. Interradicular radiolucency was noted. Tooth 84 had a distal carious lesion.

Case Selection: Preoperative Occlusal View

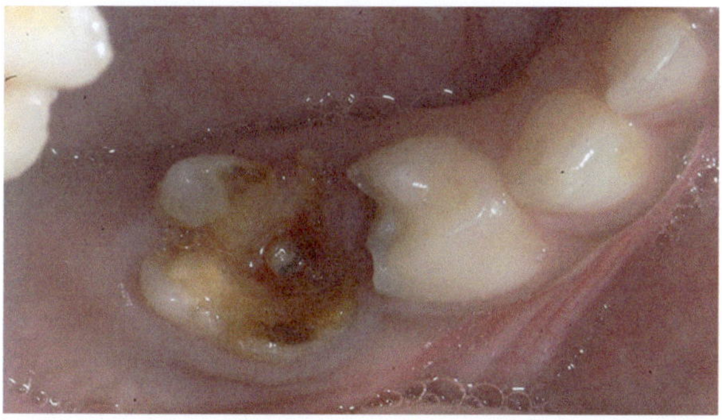

Tooth 85 had an extensive deep carious lesion with a visible pulp exposure. There was very little crown structure remaining and the tooth was not restorable. Tooth 84 had a distal proximal lesion

Case Selection: Preoperative Radiograph

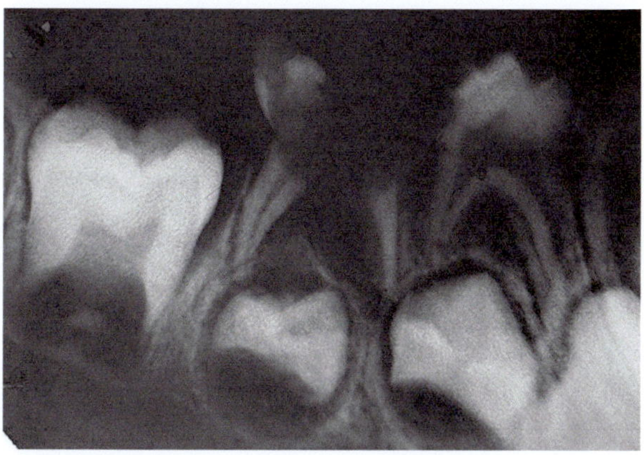

On the radiograph tooth 85 showed a large carious lesion extending to the bifurcation area. An interradicular radiolucency was noted. Tooth 84 had a moderately deep distal proximal lesion. Tooth 46 was as yet unerupted

6.4.4.2 Step-by-Step Guide to Fabrication

Step 1: Distal Shoe Fabricated on Working Model

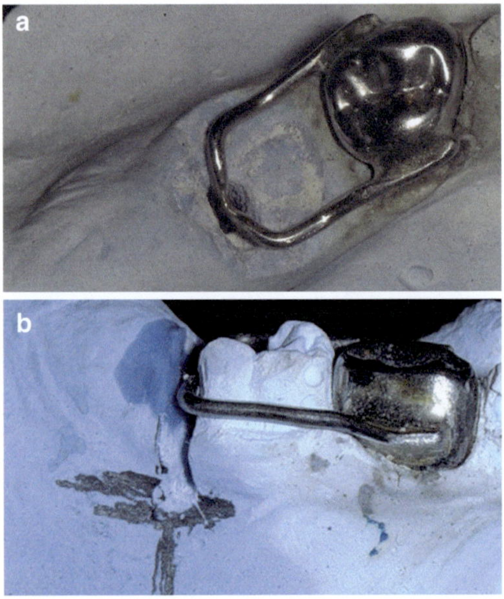

(**a**) The distal shoe space maintainer was fabricated on the working model with the crown on abutment tooth 84. (**b**) A vertical slot can be made in the cast along the distal surface of the second deciduous molar to accommodate the intra-alveolar extension of the distal shoe space maintainer (working model of another patient presented here)

Clinical Notes

The working model is made similarly as for all custom-made space maintainers. A preformed metal crown is placed on the abutment tooth 84 and a sectional impression is recorded in alginate. The preformed metal crown is transferred accurately into the impression, and a working model is made in stone.

Step 2: Fabricated Distal Shoe Space Maintainer

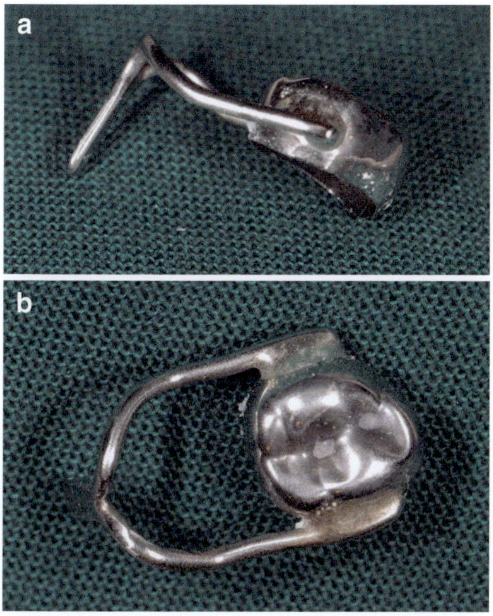

(**a**) The loop is similar to the loop of the band and loop appliance except for a narrow vertical U bend in the middle of the distal aspect of the wire. (**b**) This vertical extension serves as a guide for the eruption of the first permanent molar

Step 3: Extraction and Placement of Space Maintainer

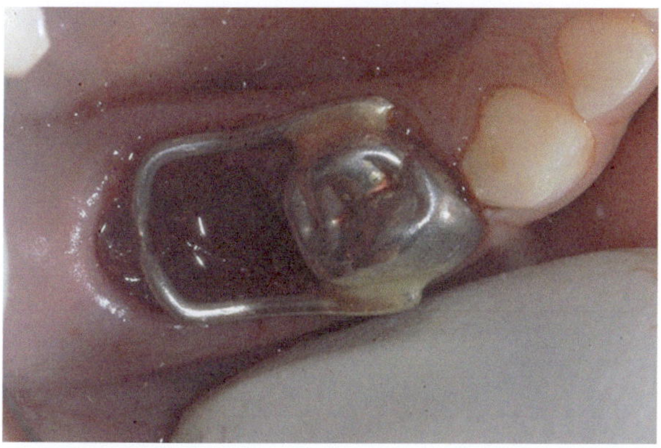

Tooth 85 was extracted; the fabricated distal shoe is tried intraorally and cemented

Clinical Notes

A periapical radiograph is recorded before cementation to check the extensions of the intra-alveolar portion in relation to the unerupted first permanent molar. Adjustments in the mesiodistal plane are made to ensure correct angulation before cementation.

Step 4: Radiograph Post Cementation

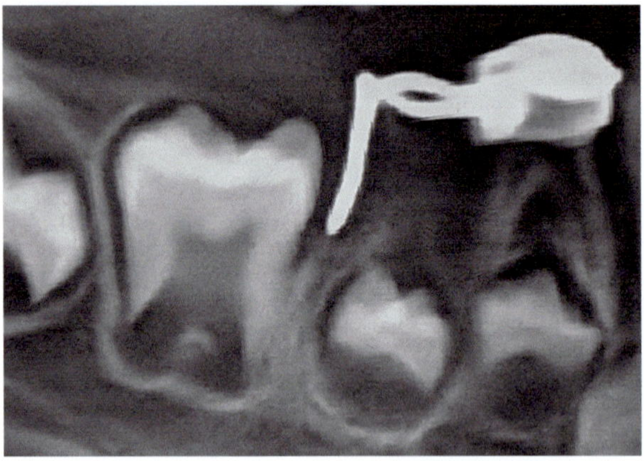

The vertical extension should be slightly short of the first permanent molar and should extend slightly beyond the mesial marginal ridge of the first permanent molar. A section of the orthopantomogram taken postoperatively is shown here

Follow-Up at 1 Week

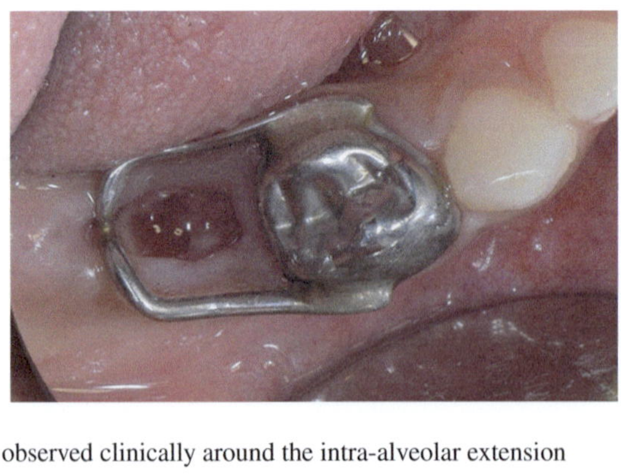

Good healing was observed clinically around the intra-alveolar extension

6.4.4.3 Long-Term Follow-Up

Eighteen-Month Follow-Up

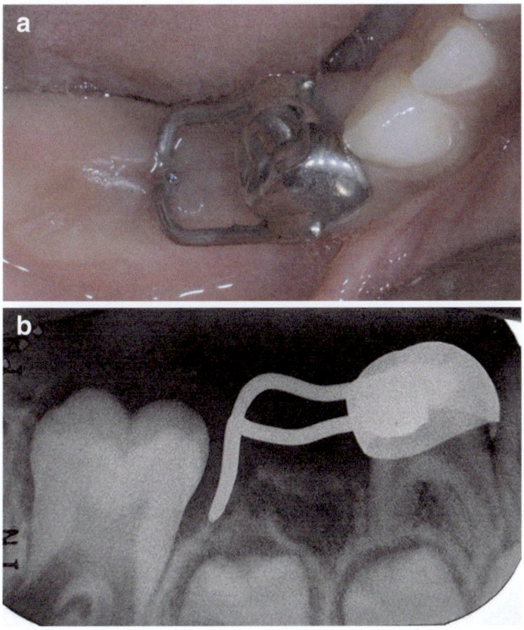

(**a**) Follow-up at 18 months showed healthy soft tissue and the bulge of the first permanent molar distal to the horizontal extension of the space maintainer. (**b**) Radiograph at 18 months showed tooth 46 maturing and moving further occlusally

Two and a Half-Year Follow-Up

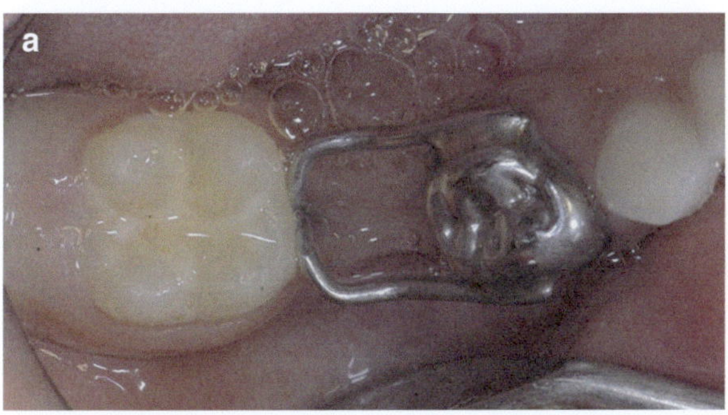

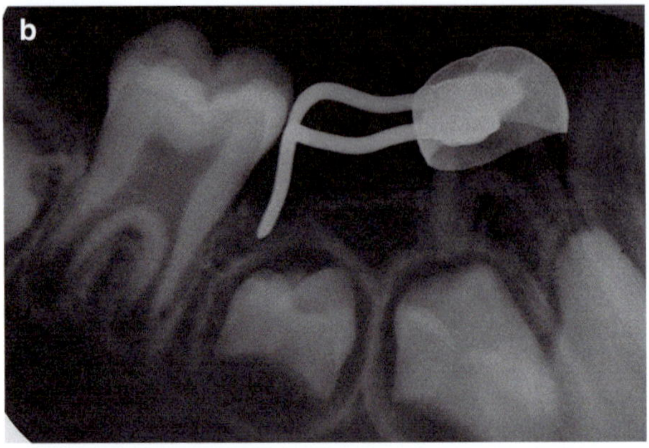

Two and a half-year follow-up images indicate that the first permanent molar had been guided successfully by the distal shoe space maintainer to erupt while maintaining critical arch length. The extension of the space maintainer was ready to be removed. (**a**) The first permanent molar had erupted completely guided by the distal shoe space maintainer. (**b**) Radiograph showed tooth 46 erupted fully at the same occlusal plane as tooth 84

Clinical Notes
Once the first permanent molar has completely erupted, the extension of the space maintainer is removed. In custom-made space maintainers, it is easier to remove both horizontal and vertical extensions.

Step 5: Distal Shoe Extension Removed

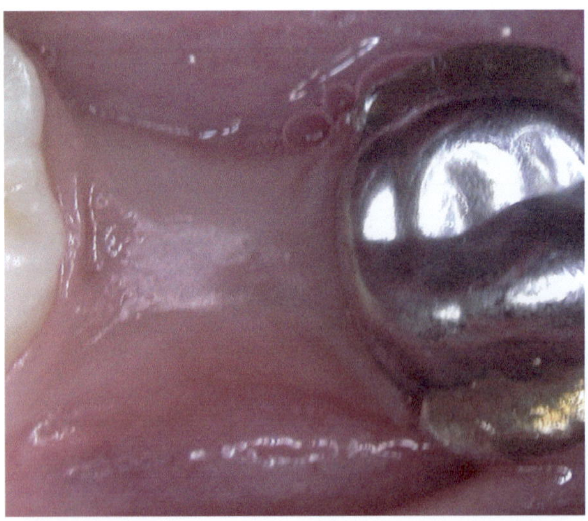

The distal shoe extension was cut off from the crown and removed. Note the epithelialized opening on the gingiva, mesial to the first permanent molar

Clinical Notes

The horizontal extension is cut off from the crown, and the distal shoe extension removed. Since the gingiva around the vertical extension is epithelialized, no local anesthesia is required when the extension is removed. The space mesial to the erupted first permanent molar is now maintained with a band and loop space maintainer.

Step 6: Band and Loop Space Maintainer Cemented

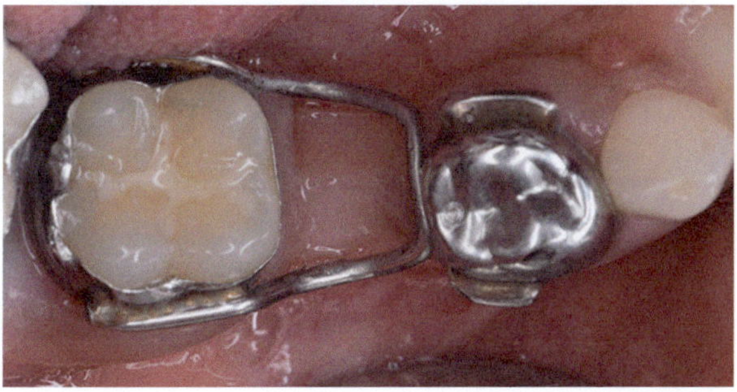

A band and loop space maintainer was cemented with tooth 46 as the abutment to hold space until the eruption of tooth 45

Four-Year Follow-Up Radiograph

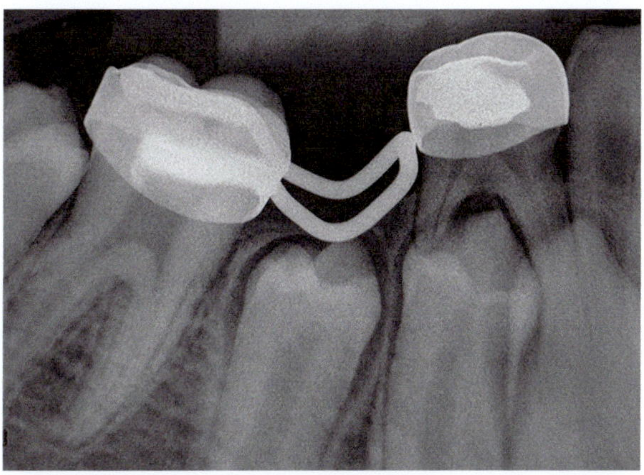

Band and loop space maintainer holding space for the erupting second premolar

Six-Year Follow-Up

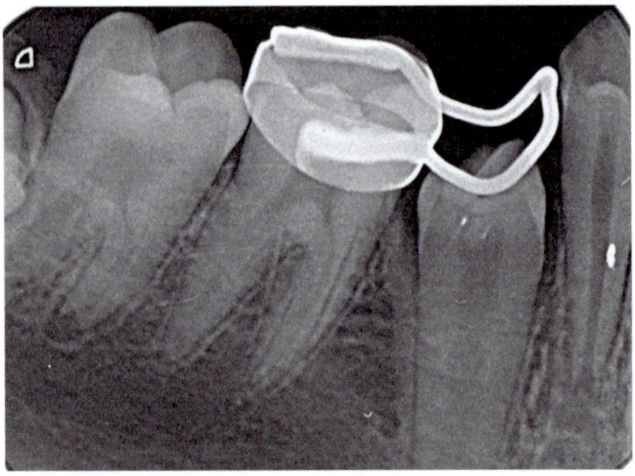

Band and loop space maintainer ready to be removed. Critical arch length has been maintained successfully

6.4.5 Case Study 2: Prefabricated Distal Shoe Space Maintainer

6.4.5.1 Case Selection

Why Was This Case Selected for a Distal Shoe Space Maintainer?

- A 5-year-old child presented with severe pain in relation to tooth 75. The tooth was indicated for extraction.
- Tooth 36 was unerupted and tooth 74 could serve as an abutment once restored.

Preoperative Occlusal View

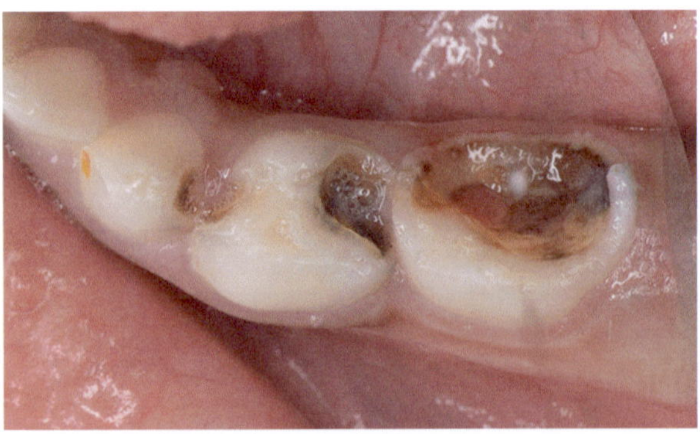

Tooth 75 presented with a deep carious lesion involving the pulp with very poor coronal tooth structure. A pulp polyp was visible at the base of the carious lesion. A deep carious lesion was evident in tooth 74. Tooth 36 was unerupted

Preoperative Radiograph

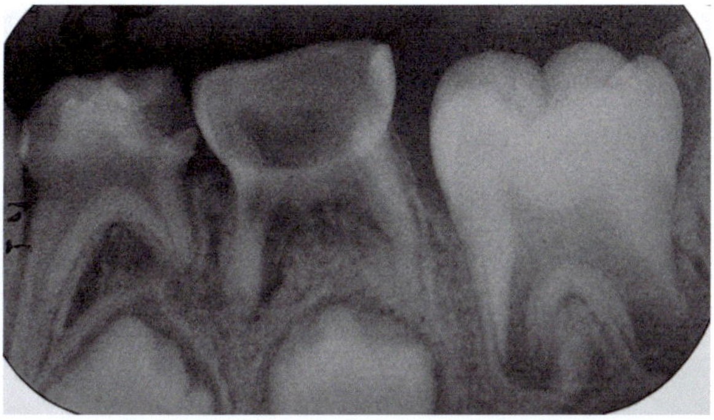

Note the deep carious lesion in tooth 75 involving the pulp with radiolucency extending to the interradicular area. Both mesial and distal roots showed severe root resorption. Tooth 74 showed a deep distal carious lesion with a thin layer of dentine separating the lesion from the pulp. Healthy radicular tissue was seen around tooth 74. Tooth 36 was unerupted

6.4.5.2 Step-by-Step Guide to Placement

Step 1: Selection of the Prefabricated Distal Shoe and Its Components

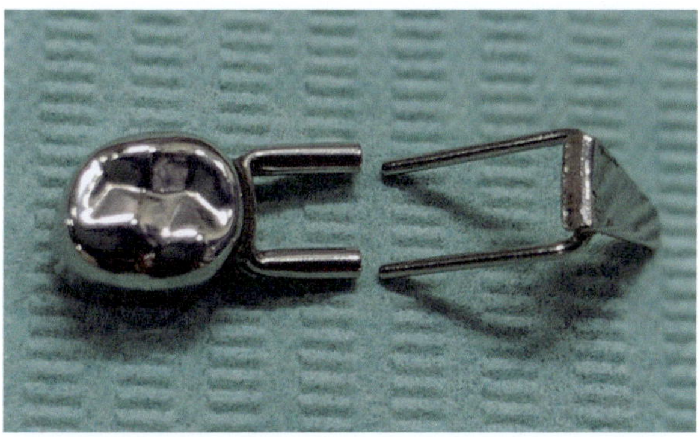

Note crown with the tubes attached, available in a variety of sizes and the distal shoe with the horizontal wires (Denovo Dental, CA, USA)

Clinical Notes

Following extraction of tooth 75, the crown with tubes is selected to seat on tooth 74 from a variety of sizes by trial and error. The horizontal wires of the distal shoe are trimmed to size and inserted into the tubes on the crown. Trimming of the horizontal wires to size is done by trial and error by placing the shoe in the tubes and seating the crown on tooth 74 so that the shoe is positioned perfectly along the mesial marginal ridge of tooth 36.

Step 2: Radiograph Before Cementing the Distal Shoe Space Maintainer

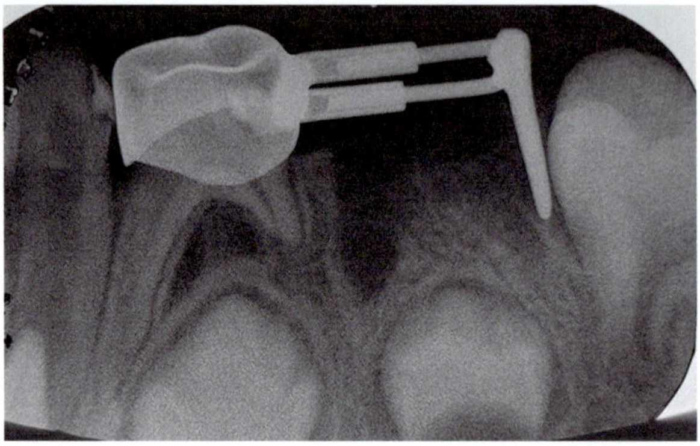

The distal shoe space maintainer was cemented on tooth 74 after radiographic confirmation of the correct position. The vertical subgingival component or shoe is located along the mesial marginal ridge of tooth 36 to guide its eruption

Clinical Notes

It was judged that tooth 74 would respond well to selective removal of carious tissue and sealing in with a crown (Chap. 2).

Step 3: Prefabricated Distal Shoe Space Maintainer Cemented

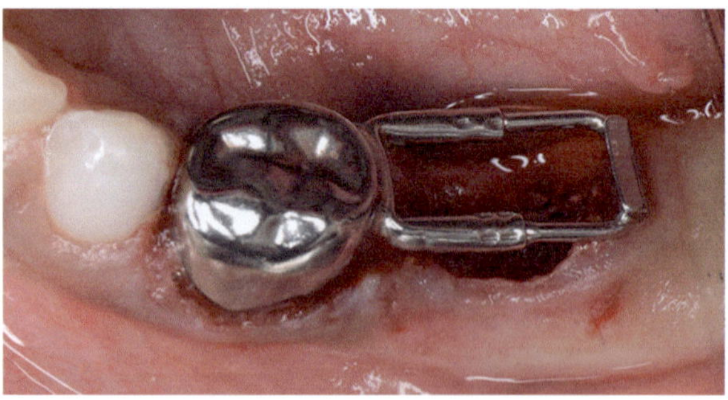

Prefabricated distal shoe space maintainer cemented after radiographic verification of position [12]

Healing at 1 Week

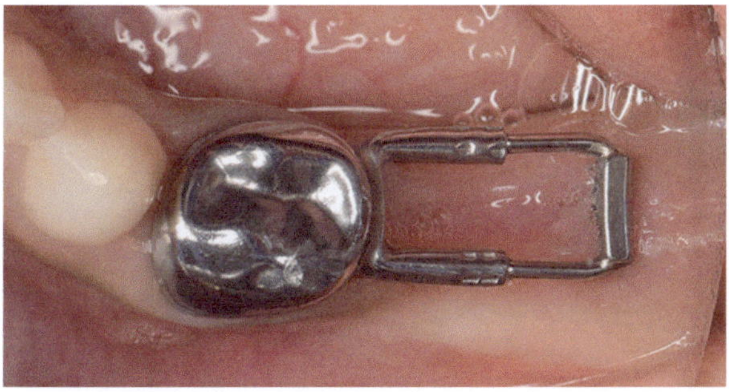

Soft tissue healing at 1-week follow-up showed a positive tissue response to the intra-alveolar extension

One and a Half-Year Follow-Up

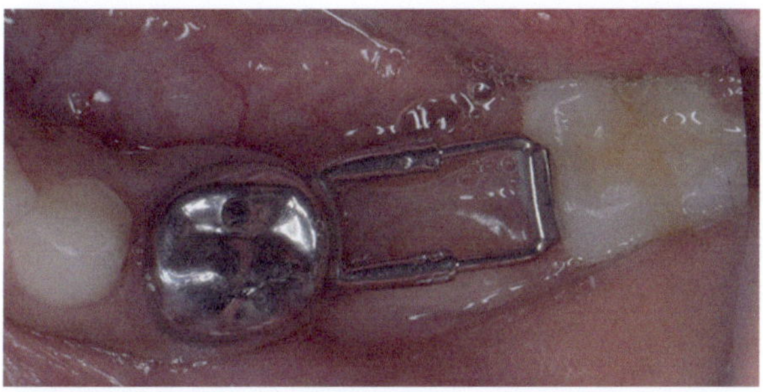

Note tooth 36 erupting in position guided by the distal shoe space maintainer. Thus critical arch length has been maintained. The intra-alveolar extension can be removed, and the space maintainer can continue to function as a reverse crown and loop. A band and loop space maintainer can be cemented following complete eruption of tooth 36

6.5 Conclusion

It should be the aim of every clinician treating children to care for the primary dentition through to natural exfoliation. However severe early childhood caries can cause irreparable damage to primary teeth making extraction the most ideal choice of treatment for some primary teeth. When teeth require to be extracted prematurely, maintaining the space created by the tooth loss is critical to prevent complex future orthodontic treatment requiring extraction of premolars. Accurate case selection, choice of appliance, and regular follow-ups help space maintainers fulfil their role in maintaining natural arch length in the growing child.

References

1. Bhujel N, Duggal MS, Saini P, Day PF. The effect of premature extraction of primary teeth on the subsequent need for orthodontic treatment. Eur Arch Paediatr Dent. 2016;17(6):423–34.
2. Christensen JR, Fields HW Jr. Space maintenance in the primary dentition. In: Casamassimo P, Fields H, Mctigue D, Nowak A, editors. Pediatric dentistry: infancy through adolescence. 5th ed. St. Louis, MO: Elsevier; 2013. p. 379–84.
3. Christensen JR, Henry W, Fields HW. Treatment planning and management of orthodontic problems. In: Casamassimo P, Fields H, Mctigue D, Nowak A, editors. Pediatric dentistry: infancy through adolescence. 5th ed. St. Louis, MO: Elsevier; 2013. p. 526–7.
4. Laing E, Ashley P, Naini FB, Gill DS. Space maintenance. Int J Paediatr Dent. 2009;19(3):155–62. https://doi.org/10.1111/j.1365-263X.2008.009514.
5. TunisonW F-MC, Elbadrawy H, Nassar U, El-Bialy T. Dental arch space changes following premature loss of primary first molars: a systematic review. Pediatr Dent. 2008;30:297–302.
6. Lin YTJ, Lin YT. Long-term space changes after premature loss of a primary maxillary first molar. J Dent Sci. 2017;12:44–8.
7. Kumari P, Kumari R. Loss of space and changes in the dental arch after premature loss of the lower primary molar: a longitudinal study. J Indian Soc Pedod Prev Dent. 2006;24:90–6.
8. Durward CS. Space maintenance in the primary and mixed dentition. Ann R Australas Coll Dent Surg. 2000;15:203–5.
9. Fields HW, Proffit WR. Moderate non skeletal problems in preadolescent children: preventive and interceptive treatment in family practice. In: Proffit WR, Fields HW, Sarver DM, editors. Contemporary orthodontics. 5th ed. St. Louis, MO: Mosby; 2013. p. 429–33.
10. Randall RC. Preformed metal crowns for primary and permanent molar teeth: review of the literature. Pediatr Dent. 2002;24(5):489–500.
11. Ekstrand KR, Christiansen J, Christiansen ME. Time and duration of eruption of first and second permanent molars: a longitudinal investigation. Community Dent Oral Epidemiol. 2003;31(5):344–50.
12. Brill WA. The distal shoe space maintainer chairside fabrication and clinical performance. Pediatr Dent. 2002;24(6):561–5.

Resin and Glass Ionomer-Based Pit and Fissure Sealants

7

7.1 Overview

Michael Buonocore in 1955 revolutionized dentistry through his innovative research on enamel surface preparations with weak acids. From here sprang the idea of adhesive dentistry opening the possibility that susceptible pits and fissures can be bonded and sealed with organic materials thereby preventing the caries process. Pit and fissure sealants have evolved a great deal since then in terms of materials and clinical technique. Resin-based sealants are the most commonly accepted pit and fissure sealant materials [1]. In both children and adolescents, resin-based sealants are effective for preventing carious lesions when the occlusal surfaces of permanent molars are treated with them [2]. But they still continue to be an underused mode of prevention [3]. Issues with isolation, lack of confidence in the sealant's bonding ability, and the concern of sealing over incipient carious lesions are reasons attributed to their low usage [4]. Glass ionomer sealants have proven useful in partially erupted molars [3] and where the use of the technique-sensitive resin-based sealants is challenged by age or disabilities. This chapter provides detailed step-by-step clinical guidance to the successful placement of a resin-based sealant. The clinical use of glass ionomer sealants is also elucidated.

7.2 Introduction

The morphology of pit and fissures provides an environment where bacteria and plaque are sheltered and harbored. The thin enamel in the pit and fissure region also accelerates the demineralization process. Oral hygiene maintenance remaining a challenge due to the age of the child and the long eruptive period of the permanent molars [5] further adds to the risk factors. Fluoride being less effective on occlusal as compared to proximal surfaces increases the need for specific preventive measures

M. S. Kher, A. Rao, *Contemporary Treatment Techniques in Pediatric Dentistry*,
https://doi.org/10.1007/978-3-030-11860-0_7

for the occlusal surface. First commercially introduced in 1971 [4], pit and fissure sealants are materials that are micromechanically bonded to the pits and fissures on the occlusal surfaces thus shielding them. The protective layer formed removes access of cariogenic bacteria to their nutrient sources [6].

7.3 Indications and Contraindications

Resin-based pit and fissure sealants are useful in both primary and permanent teeth. They are indicated in [7]:

- Non-carious posterior teeth with deep retentive fissures
- Self-cleansing pits and fissures in children determined to be high risk for dental caries
- Posterior teeth with incipient, stained, or noncavitated lesions

They are contraindicated in:

- Teeth with radiographic or clinical evidence of proximal lesions
- Teeth where isolation is questionable
- Partially erupted teeth

However, teeth that are partially erupted or where isolation is questionable can be sealed with glass ionomer sealants [3].

7.4 Rationale

Resin-based sealants are retained by micro-mechanical retention [6]. The etched enamel leads to an irregular surface into which the sealant material flows and forms resin tags. The polymerized resin covering the pits and fissures then acts like a physical barrier against plaque accumulation thereby preventing the formation of occlusal carious lesions [4]. In partially erupted teeth, the inability to maintain a dry field compromises the stability of the hydrophobic resin-based sealant. Glass ionomer cement with its fluoride release and ease of use is advantageous as a sealant in these teeth [3]. It is also invaluable as a sealant in children where the ability to cooperate is compromised.

7.5 Case Study: Resin-Based Sealants

7.5.1 Case Selection

7.5.1.1 Why Was This Case Selected for a Resin-Based Pit and Fissure Sealant?

- Tooth 36 was non-carious, but with deep retentive fissures.
- The child was determined to be at a high risk for dental caries.
- The child was cooperative and considered a good candidate for the technique-sensitive resin sealant procedure.

Case Selection: Preoperative Occlusal View

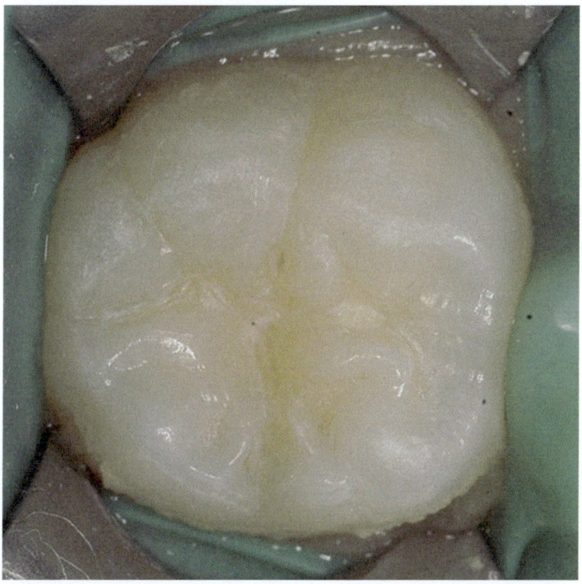

Tooth 36 to be sealed was isolated under dental dam. Note the tortuous anatomy of the grooves. On air-drying, the grooves appeared clean, and no staining or discoloration was visible

Clinical Notes

Though isolation can be achieved with cotton rolls and a high vacuum suction, even minimal exposure to saliva affects sealant retention [8]; hence, pit and fissure sealants are best applied under rubber dam isolation [3]. In the absence of rubber dam isolation, four-handed dentistry is advised to improve isolation and retention outcomes [3].

7.5.2 Step-by-Step Guide

Step 1: Tooth Cleaned with Pumice and Brush

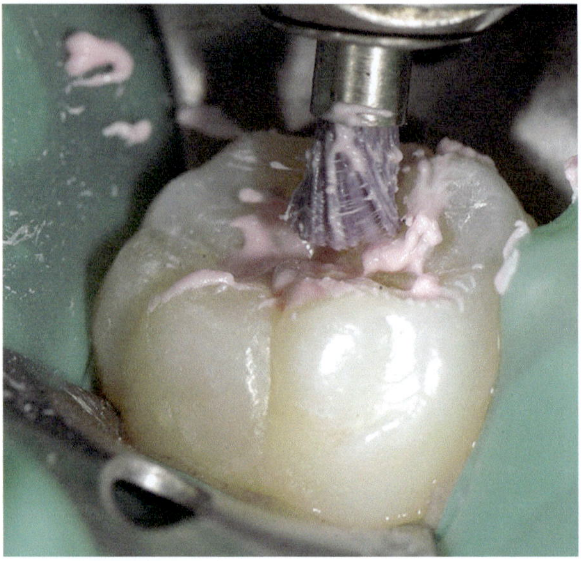

The grooves were cleaned with pumice paste and a bristle brush

Clinical Notes

The resin-based sealant can potentially penetrate deep into pits and fissures when free of debris. Following cleaning, the tooth is thoroughly rinsed with water, and a fine explorer should trace the fissures to remove any remnant of the pumice paste [9].

Evidence comparing surface cleaning methods suggests that sealant retention was similar when teeth were cleaned with a prophylaxis brush on a handpiece and running an explorer in the groove along with an air-water spray [10]. Supervised toothbrushing prior to sealant placement was found to be equally effective [11]. Hence, providing a well-cleaned surface, no matter what the technique, will offer optimal retention [3].

Step 2: Tooth Ready to Be Sealed

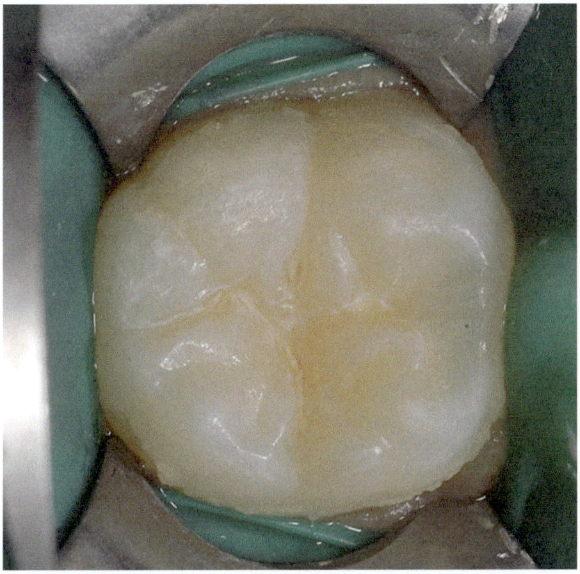

The tooth was air-dried. Note the clean, debris-free occlusal surface and the fissures ready to be sealed

Clinical Notes

Mechanical preparation of the tooth with a bur prior to sealant placement is not recommended because it is invasive [3]. Sealing stained fissures and fissures with incipient caries will not cause progress of the lesion [3]. The rationale is that a properly placed sealant will reduce bacterial counts and arrest the carious process underneath [12, 13] (Chap. 1).

Step 3: Acid Etching the Occlusal Surface

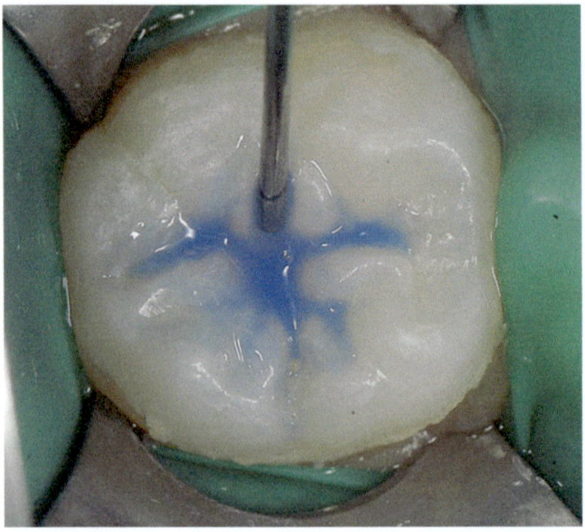

The etchant (35% phosphoric acid) was placed on the grooves and approximately 2 mm beyond the expected margins of the sealant

Clinical Notes

An etching time of 15 s is optimum on a tooth surface that has been cleaned and dried optimally [3].

Step 4: Tooth Dried

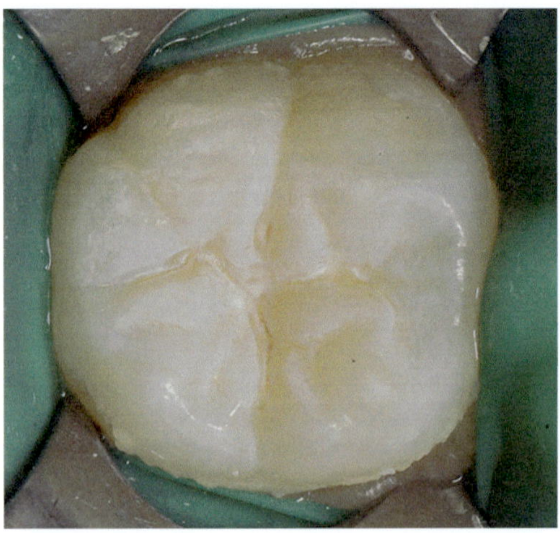

Note the chalky, frosted appearance following air-drying

Clinical Notes
The etchant is rinsed off the tooth for about 20 s, ensuring that no traces of the etchant are left on the tooth. The tooth is air-dried until a frosted appearance is visible. A well-dried tooth is critical because of the hydrophobic nature of the resin.

Step 5: Application of an Intermediate Bonding Agent

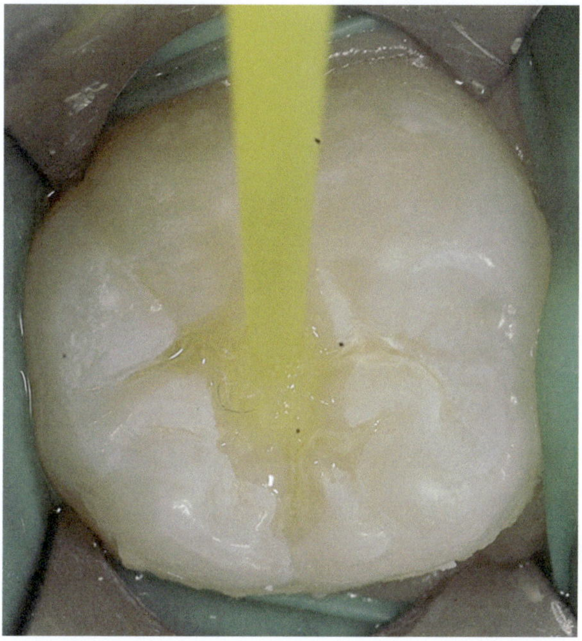

Bonding agent (etch and rinse adhesive) was scrubbed into the air-dried grooves

Clinical Notes
This step is optional. The idea is to counter the hydrophobic nature of the resin with the hydrophilic nature of the bonding agent in the presence of minute moisture contamination [4]. Though some studies have shown increased sealant-tooth bond strength with the use of an intermediate bonding agent [14], others have highlighted that this step is unnecessary in the absence of moisture contamination considering the increased chairside time and the reduced cost-effectiveness [9, 15].

Step 6: Bonding Agent Blow Dried

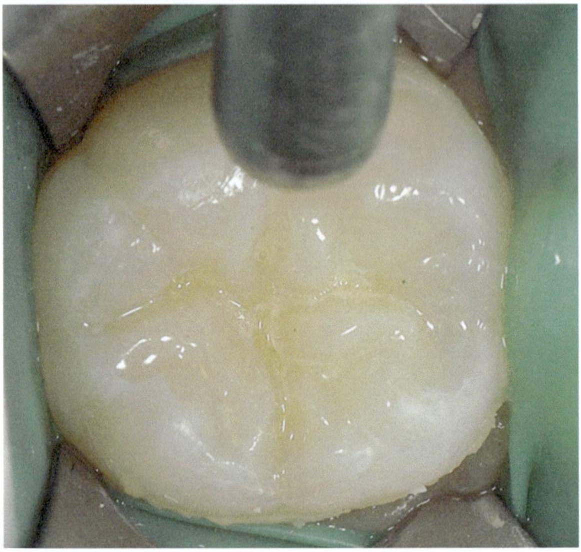

The bonding agent was gently blow dried after application

> **Clinical Notes**
> Note that the bonding agent is not photo-activated at this stage.

Step 7: Sealant Placement

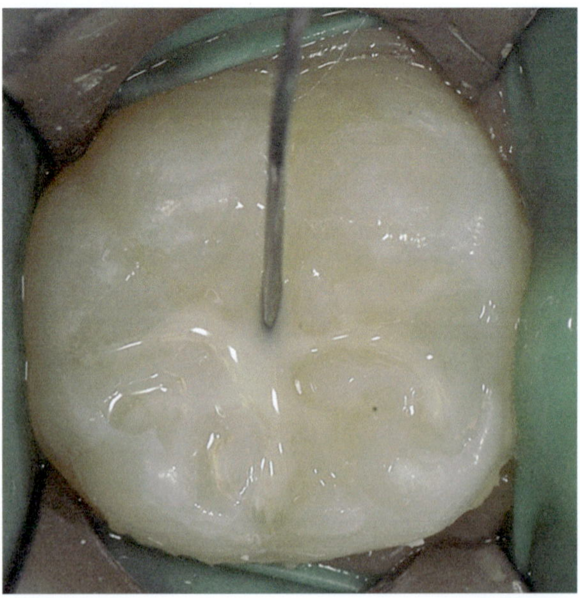

The resin sealant was placed taking care to avoid air bubbles and overfilling of the fissures

Clinical Notes

The sealant along with the bonding agent is light cured reducing one clinical step. Evidence shows that curing the bonding agent and sealant together does not affect bond strength [16].

Step 8: Adjusting Occlusion

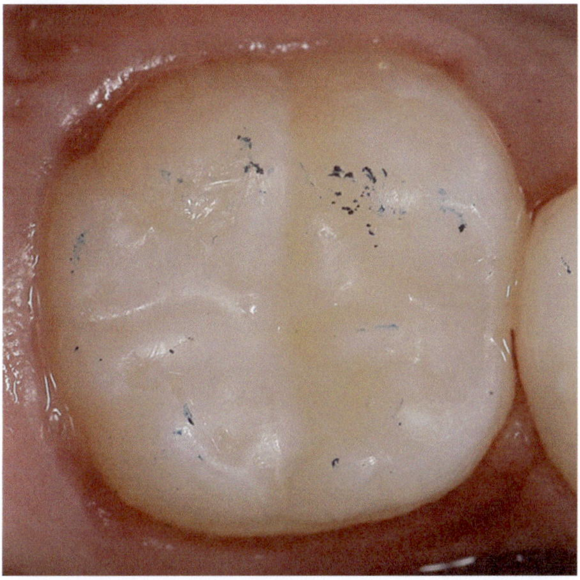

Overfilled areas were detected with articulating strips and any high points finished and polished

Clinical Notes

Cured sealant should be examined for areas of bubble entrapment and deficient areas. Material can be reapplied directly to these areas. Retention is tested by gently trying to dislodge the sealant with an explorer. The process of sealant application with all the steps has to be repeated for debonded areas.

Sealed Tooth After Finishing and Polishing

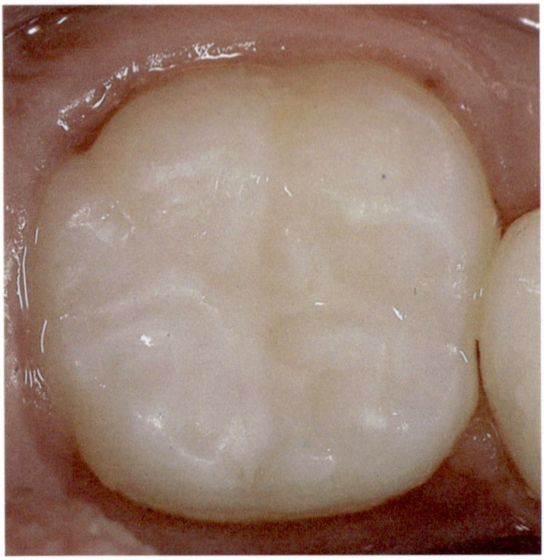

Note the well-sealed tooth with no deficient areas or air bubbles

> **Clinical Notes**
> Sealants have to be evaluated carefully for loss of retention during recall visits and reapplied where necessary accordingly [3].

7.5.3 Long-Term Follow-Up

Three-Year Follow-Up

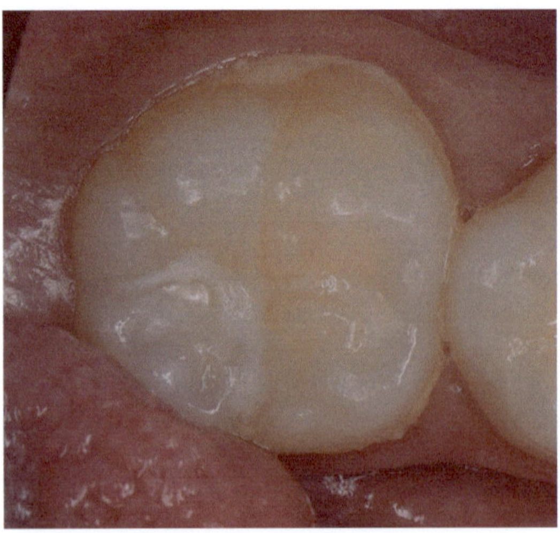

Note the intact sealant at the end of 3 years

7.6 What to Look for at Sealant Recalls?

Partial loss of sealant can leave the fissure caries susceptible. Clinicians must be aware that areas of sealant loss have a potential for stagnation of oral fluids and seepage under the retained sealant thus initiating a carious lesion [3]. Areas of sealant loss will have a greater propensity for plaque accumulation. Hence, timely recall and reapplication are advised.

Twelve-Year Follow-Up of Teeth That Received Resin-Based Sealants

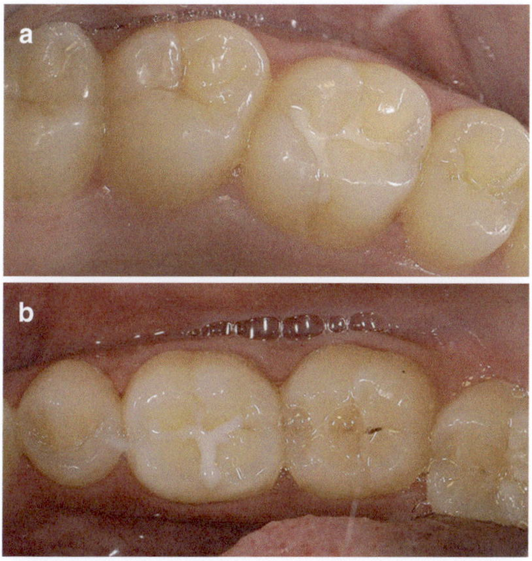

(**a**) Note the intact sealant in tooth 16. (**b**) Sealant intact in tooth 46. Note the tooth 47 shows a discolored groove and requires to be sealed

Eight-Year Follow-Up of Teeth That Received Resin-Based Sealants

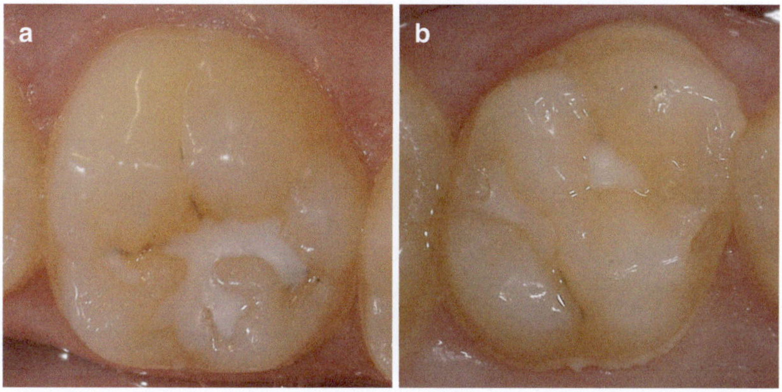

Teeth show wear and loss of sealant in part at 8-year follow-ups. (**a**) Partial loss of sealant seen on the mesial groove of tooth 36. (**b**) Wear and loss of sealant partially on the distobuccal groove of tooth 16

7.7 Glass Ionomer Sealant in a Partially Erupted Molar

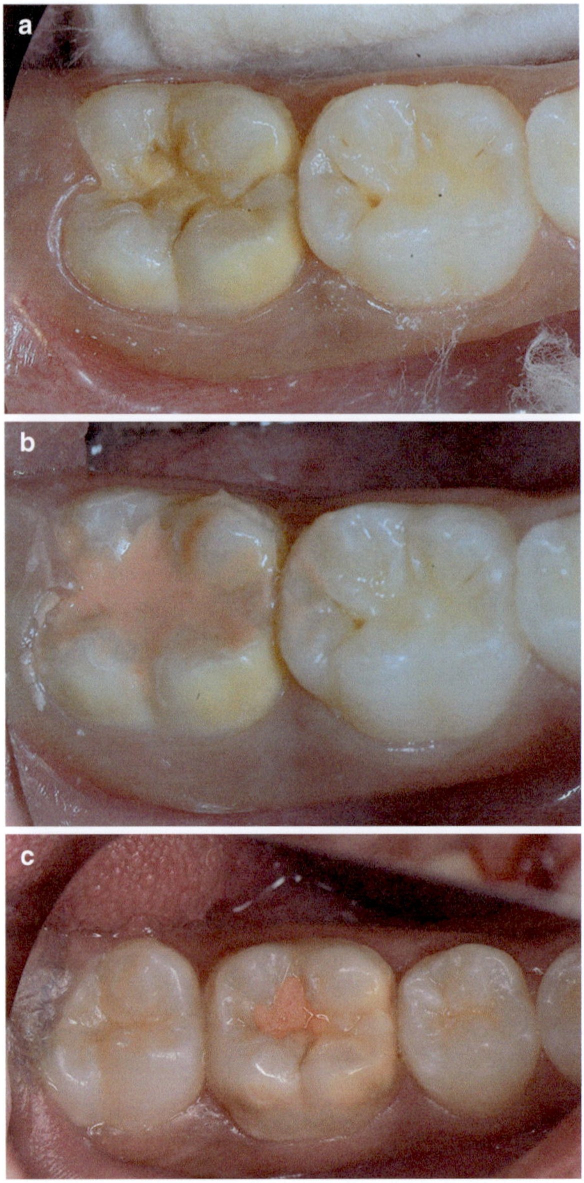

Application of glass ionomer sealant—GC Fuji VII (Triage) (GC Corporation, Tokyo, Japan)—on tooth 46 that presented with molar incisor hypomineralization and was not fully erupted. (**a**) Preoperative view of tooth 46. Note the hypomineralized occlusal surface and the possibility of plaque stagnation. The retromolar pad covered the distal marginal ridge. (**b**) Fuji 7 (Triage) applied on tooth 46. (**c**) Four-year follow-up showing the glass ionomer intact in the central occlusal area and grooves. There is peripheral wear. No carious lesion or enamel breakdown is seen. Tooth 45 has erupted and tooth 47 has erupted partially

Clinical Notes

When molars are partially erupted, moisture control is hampered. A sealant using glass ionomer releases fluoride, chemically bonds to the tooth surface, is less technique sensitive, and is best suited in these teeth [3].

7.8 Conclusion

There is little room for doubt that pit and fissure sealants are a primary method of preventing occlusal caries. The technique being demanding, diligent study and application of the clinical steps will ensure success of resin-based sealants. Glass ionomer sealants work best in partially erupted molars and when cooperation is challenged by age or disabilities. Recent literature [17] suggests a greater role for high-viscosity glass ionomer (HVGI) sealants.

References

1. Forss H, Saarni UM, Seppä L. Comparison of glass-ionomer and resin-based fissure sealants: a 2-year clinical trial. Community Dent Oral Epidemiol. 1994;22(1):21–4.
2. Ahovuo-Saloranta A, Forss H, Walsh T, Nordblad A, Mäkelä M, Worthington HV. Pit and fissure sealants for preventing dental decay in permanent teeth. Cochrane Database Syst Rev. 2017;(7):CD001830. https://doi.org/10.1002/14651858.CD001830.pub5.
3. Simonsen RJ, Neal RC. A review of the clinical application and performance of pit and fissure sealants. Aust Dent J. 2011;56(1 Suppl):45–58.
4. Wells MH. Pit and fissure sealants: scientific and clinical rationale. In: Casamassimo P, Fields H, Mctigue D, Nowak A, editors. Pediatric dentistry: infancy through adolescence. 5th ed. St. Louis, MO: Elsevier; 2013. p. 467–89.
5. Ekstrand KR, Christiansen J, Christiansen ME. Time and duration of eruption of first and second permanent molars: a longitudinal investigation. Community Dent Oral Epidemiol. 2003;31(5):344–50.
6. Simonsen RJ. Pit and fissure sealants. In: Clinical applications of the acid etch technique. 1st ed. Chicago, IL: Quintessence Publishing; 1978. p. 19–42.
7. Hicks J, Flaitz CM. Pit and fissure sealants and conservative adhesive restorations: scientific and clinical rationale. In: Pinkham JR, Casamassimo P, Fields HW, et al., editors. Pediatric dentistry: infancy through adolescence. 4th ed. St. Louis, MO: Elsevier; 2005.
8. Barroso JM, Torres CP, Lessa FC, Pécora JD, Palma-Dibb RG, Borsatto MC. Shear bond strength of pit-and-fissure sealants to saliva-contaminated and noncontaminated enamel. J Dent Child (Chic). 2005;72(3):95–9.
9. Khare M, Suprabha BS, Shenoy R, Rao A. Evaluation of pit-and-fissure sealants placed with four different bonding protocols: a randomized clinical trial. Int J Paediatr Dent. 2017;27(6):444–53. https://doi.org/10.1111/ipd.12281.
10. Muller-Bolla M, Lupi-Pégerier L, Tardieu C, Velly AM, Antomarchi C. Retention of resin-based pit and fissure sealants: a systematic review. Community Dent Oral Epidemiol. 2006;34:321–36.
11. Gray KS, Griffin SO, Malvitz DM, Gooch BF. A comparison of the effects of toothbrushing and handpiece prophylaxis on retention of sealants. J Am Dent Assoc. 2009;140:38–46.
12. Oong EM, Griffin SO, Kohn W, Gooch BF, Caufield P. The effect of dental sealants on bacteria levels in caries lesions: a review of the evidence. J Am Dent Assoc. 2008;139:271–8.

13. Griffin SO, Oong E, Kohn W, Vidakovic B, Gooch BF, CDC Dental Sealant Systematic Review Work Group, Bader J, Clarkson J, Fontana MR, Meyer DM, Rozier RG, Weintraub JA, Zero DT. The effectiveness of sealants in managing caries lesions. J Dent Res. 2008;87(2):169–74.
14. Asselin ME, Sitbon Y, Fortin D, Abelardo L, Rompre PH. Bond strength of a sealant to permanent enamel: evaluation of 3 application protocols. Pediatr Dent. 2009;31(4):323–8.
15. Marks D, Owens BM, Johnson WW. Effect of adhesive agent and fissure morphology on the in vitro microleakage and penetrability of pit and fissure sealants. Quintessence Int. 2009;40(9):763–72.
16. Torres CP, Balbo P, Gomes-Silva JM, Ramos RP, Palma-Dibb RG, Borsatto MC. Effect of individual or simultaneous curing on sealant bond strength. J Dent Child (Chic). 2005;72(1):31–5.
17. Mickenautsch S, Yengopal V. Caries-preventive effect of high-viscosity glass ionomer and resin-based fissure sealants on permanent teeth: a systematic review of clinical trials. PLoS One. 2016;11(1):e0146512. https://doi.org/10.1371/journal.pone.0146512.

Strategies for Pulp Therapy in Immature Permanent Teeth

8

8.1 Overview

When a permanent tooth first erupts into the oral cavity, the tooth root is immature, and the apex is open. The root supported by a vital pulp continues to mature after eruption. Apical closure occurs 3–4 years post clinical eruption. However, a pulpal episode from a carious exposure or a traumatic injury may result in the premature loss of a functioning pulp in the tooth, arresting root growth.

When root formation is arrested in an immature permanent tooth, it can have many unfavorable consequences, the most relevant being thin dentinal walls easily susceptible to root fracture [1]. Hence, continued root formation to apical closure and root maturation is critically important for the long life span of the tooth. A tooth can be pulpally involved either due to a traumatic injury as in a complicated crown fracture or due to a pulpal carious invasion. In order to maintain continued root growth, the treatment options in a pulpally involved immature permanent tooth come broadly under two categories. In vital teeth, the aim is to maintain tooth vitality and thus continued root growth through procedures called "apexogenesis" [2]. These most commonly include partial pulpotomy and cervical pulpotomy. In nonvital teeth, continued root growth is achieved through a relatively new procedure called "regenerative endodontic procedure." The following section deals with all the three procedures step by step along with their indications, contraindications, and rationale.

M. S. Kher, A. Rao, *Contemporary Treatment Techniques in Pediatric Dentistry*,
https://doi.org/10.1007/978-3-030-11860-0_8

8.2 Apexogenesis

8.2.1 Partial Pulpotomy for Traumatic Exposures (Cvek Pulpotomy)

8.2.1.1 Introduction

The term pulpotomy traditionally involved complete removal of the coronal pulp leaving intact healthy radicular pulp tissue. A medicament or a wound dressing to help promote healing then covered the site of amputation. A conservative form of pulpotomy involving removal of pulp tissue only to a depth clinically judged inflamed or degenerated is called as partial pulpotomy [1]. In a traumatically involved complicated crown fracture, a partial pulpotomy done removing only 2–3 mm of inflamed superficial pulp tissue beneath an exposure to reach healthy pulp tissue is called Cvek pulpotomy [3].

8.2.1.2 Indications and Contraindications

Cvek pulpotomy is indicated in [3]:

- Traumatically exposed vital immature permanent teeth.
- A delay of less than 9 days between incidence of trauma and treatment rendered is considered a safe period. The individual merits of the case will decide the depth of pulpal resection and a clinical call should be based on the presenting clinical scenario.
- Traumatic exposures where the size of the pulp exposure is less than 4 mm.
- A mature permanent tooth with a complicated crown fracture where a simple restoration like a direct composite buildup will suffice as the final restoration. If a more complex final restoration like a post and core is planned, then Cvek pulpotomy is contraindicated in such cases.
- In a mature permanent tooth, the presence of a concomitant luxation injury may affect the prognosis of Cvek pulpotomy, and hence it is contraindicated in such teeth.

8.2.1.3 Rationale

Cvek pulpotomy has an extremely good prognosis to the extent of 94–96% [4]. The reasons attributed for this high success rate are

- The flat fractured surface in a complicated crown fracture enables salivary cleansing thus preventing accumulation of contaminated debris. This leads to a hyperplastic/proliferative reaction keeping the inflammation superficial [3].

- Removal of superficial inflamed pulp enables placement of the medicament on non-inflamed pulp tissue [4].
- Preservation of the coronal pulp, which is rich in cells, facilitates healing [3].
- The depth in the prepared pulp cavity retains the medicament (mineral trioxide aggregate (MTA)/Biodentine or any calcium silicate-based cement), which provides a bacteria-tight seal. This aids healing of the pulp tissue [4].
- The pulp capping material sets hard enabling it to form a base for the final restoration to be placed. This further enhances the seal against bacteria [4].

8.2.1.4 Case Study 1: Cvek Pulpotomy

Case Selection

Why Was This Case Selected for a Partial Pulpotomy?

- An 8-year-old child presented 30 h after trauma with a complicated crown fracture in tooth 21.
- A pinpoint exposure was seen at the fracture site.
- There was no subluxation or luxation injury on the tooth.
- Radiograph showed immature root development in tooth 21 and an open apex.

Case Selection: Preoperative View of Tooth 21

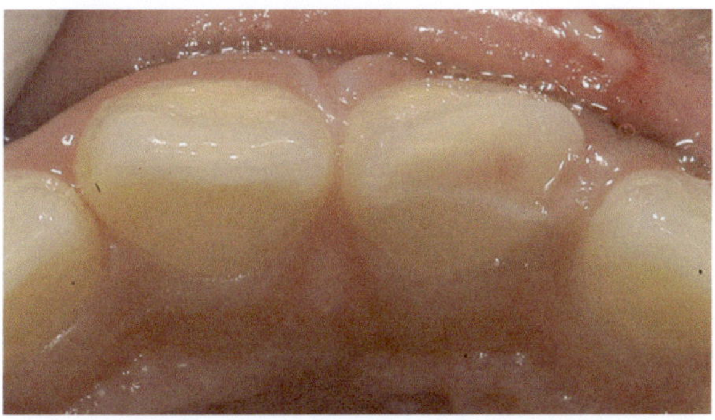

Child presented with a complicated crown fracture in tooth 21 and laceration of the upper lip. Note the pinpoint exposure site in tooth 21

Case Selection: Preoperative Radiograph

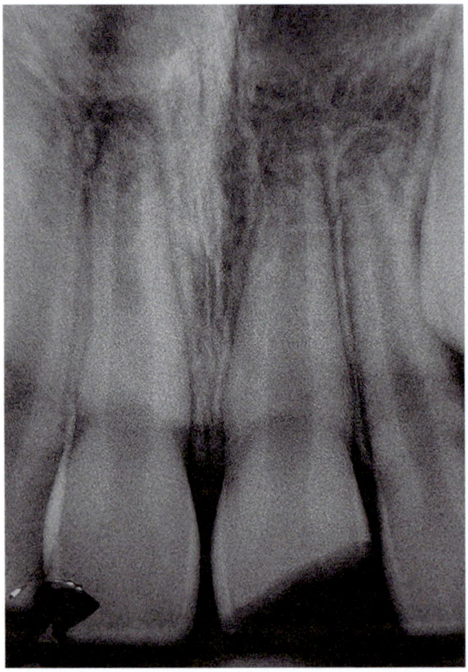

Complicated crown fracture in tooth 21. Note the immature root and open apex

Step-by-Step Guide

Step 1: Tooth Isolated

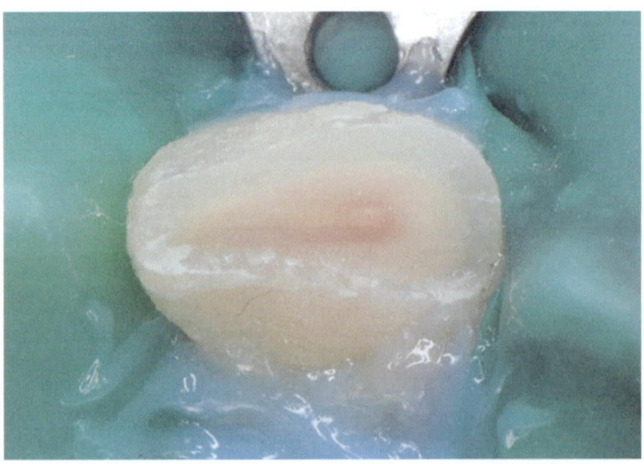

Local anesthesia was administered, and tooth 21 was isolated under rubber dam and the exposure site clearly visualized

Step 2: Deroofing to Gain Access

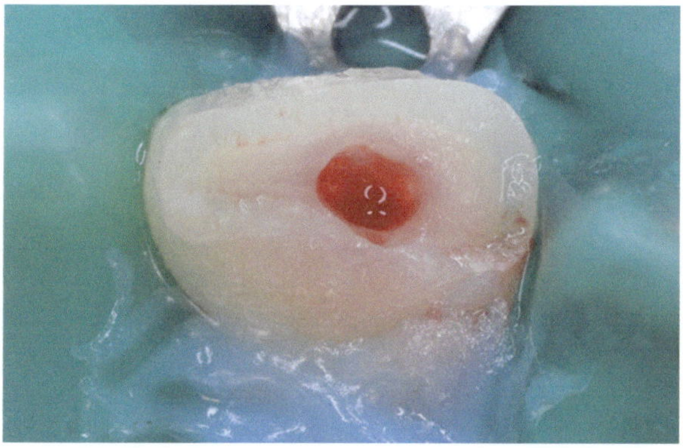

In order to remove the pulp judged to be inflamed, the pulp tissue at the site of exposure was deroofed with a sterile diamond bur mounted on a high-speed handpiece

Step 3: Partial Pulp Amputation

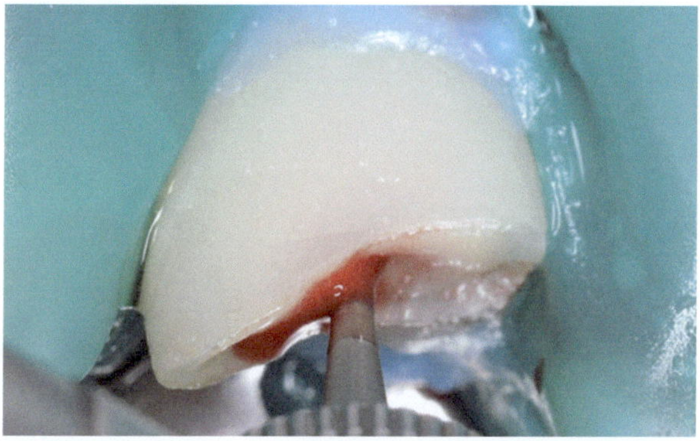

Pulp tissue was resected to a depth of 1–2 mm into the pulp cavity with a sterile carbide bur mounted on a slow speed handpiece under copious saline irrigation

Clinical Notes

The extent of the pulp cavity depth is dictated by the amount of hemorrhage. Excessive hemorrhage indicates pulpal inflammation in which case the depth of amputation is increased until moderate hemorrhage is encountered [4].

Step 4: Irrigation

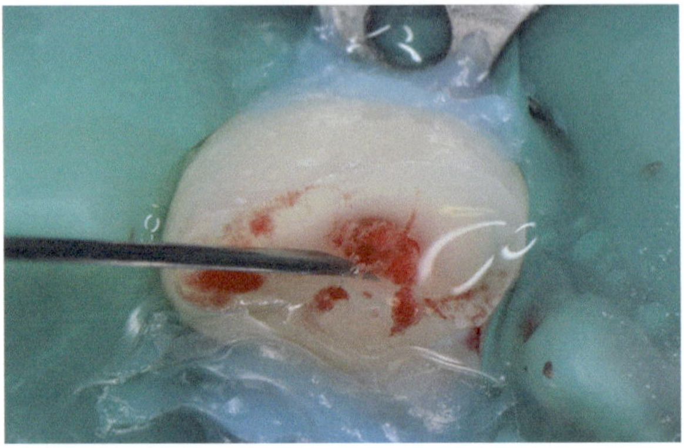

The cavity was gently rinsed with sodium hypochlorite [5] and saline

Clinical Notes
Placing the pulp medicament on a healthy non-inflamed pulp is critical to the success of vital pulp therapy. Sodium hypochlorite irrigation will provide the best antimicrobial wash in addition to hemorrhage control, removing debris and superficial dentin chips [4].

Step 5: Moist Cotton Pellet

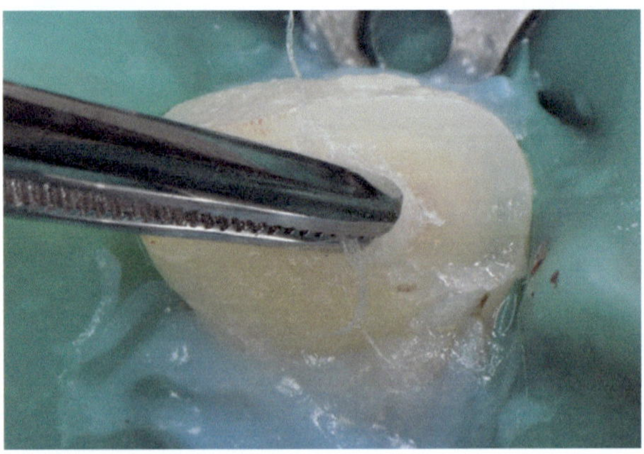

Once hemorrhage was controlled, the cavity was dried with sterile moist cotton pellets

Clinical Notes
The prognosis will be negatively influenced if a blood clot develops and care is taken to avoid formation of a blood clot [6].

Step 6: Hemorrhage Control

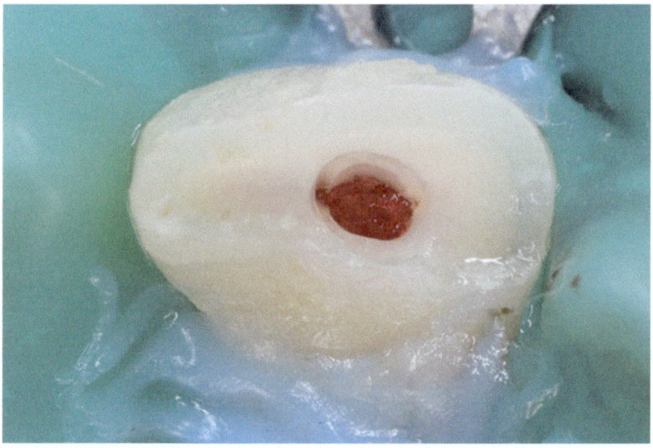

Note that hemostasis was obtained, and healthy pulp tissue was seen in the pulp cavity

Clinical Notes
The pulp cavity will also serve to retain the pulp medicament and the restorative material thus ensuring a bacteria-tight coronal seal [4].

Step 7: Placement of Pulp Medicament

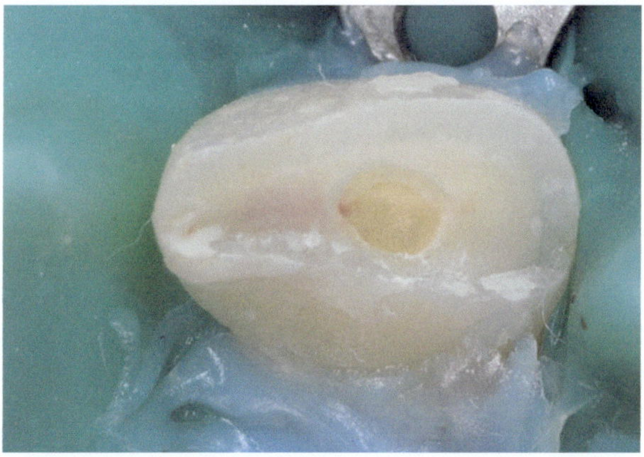

Calcium silicate-based cement—Biodentine (Septodont, Saint-Maur-des-Fosses, France)—was mixed and gently placed into the pulp cavity over the pulp tissue for a bacteria-tight seal

Clinical Notes

A bacterial tight seal of the pulp is a very critical factor for success. Calcium silicate- based cements are suitable pulp medicaments because of their excellent sealing capability and greater ability to stimulate reparative dentine. The medicament should be at least 1.5 mm thick and should completely cover the exposure site and the dentin surrounding it [2]. We prefer using Biodentine among the calcium silicate-based cements for anterior teeth because of its lesser staining potential and faster setting time [7, 8].

Step 8: Coronal Seal

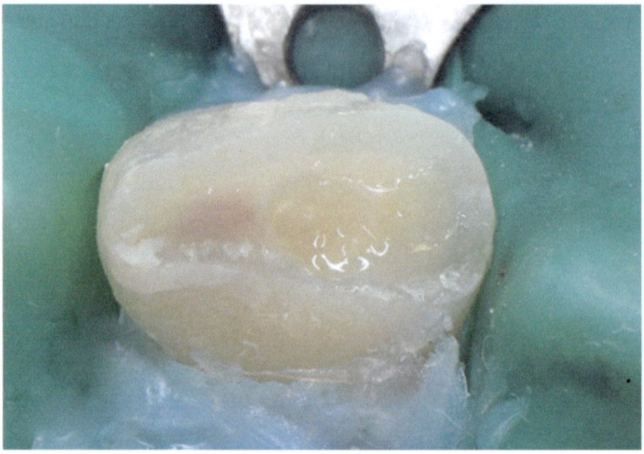

Resin-modified glass ionomer restorative cement was placed over the Biodentine to reinforce a bacteria-tight seal [2]. Note the restorative material placed lower than the fracture surface to facilitate reattachment of the fractured fragment post pulp therapy

Clinical Notes

When calcium silicate-based cements are used as pulp medicaments, it is advisable to etch the cavity and apply bonding agent on the walls of the pulp cavity after placing RMGI cement (see "Sect. 8.2.2.4, Step 6: Coronal Seal" and "Sect. 8.3.4.2, Step 12: Second Appointment (PS): Coronal Seal"). This will minimize discoloration of the tooth in the aesthetic zone [9]. The adhesive applied on the dentinal walls occludes the dentinal tubules reducing the chances of discoloration. Tooth discoloration caused by Bioactive Endodontic Cements (BEC) can be treated by internal bleaching [10].

Step 9: Crown Fragment Reattached

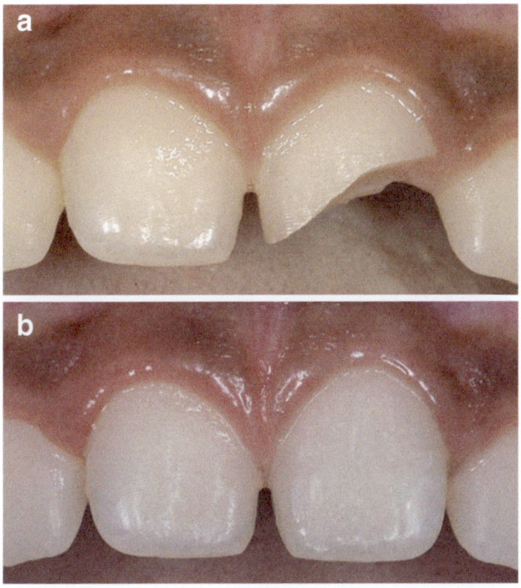

(**a**) Tooth 21, 1 week following Cvek pulpotomy. (**b**) Postoperative labial view of tooth 21 following crown fragment reattachment. Note the superior aesthetics of this minimally invasive procedure

Step 10: Postoperative Radiograph

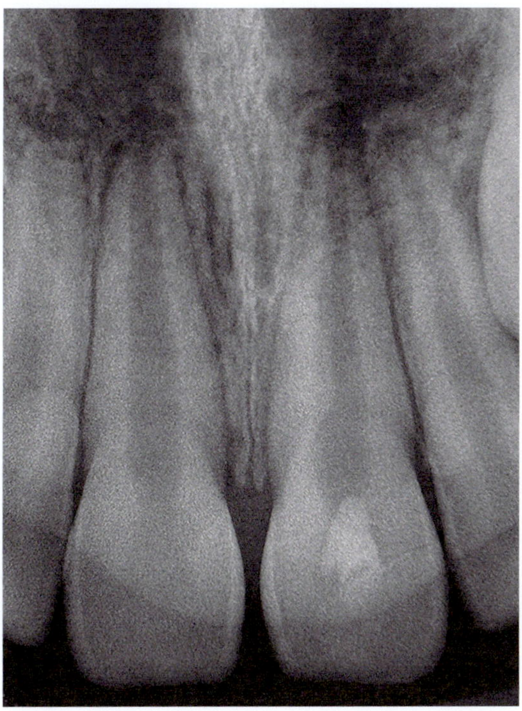

Note tooth 21 following Cvek partial pulpotomy and fragment reattachment

Long-Term Follow-Up

Two-Year Follow-Up Radiograph

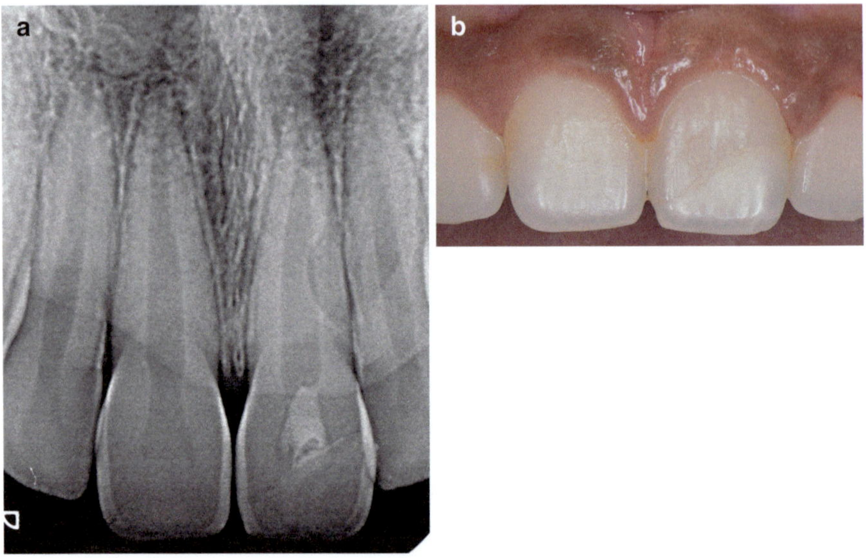

On a 2-year follow-up. (**a**) Note further root maturation and apical closure in tooth 21 indicating success of the Cvek pulpotomy procedure; the intact reattached fragment is also clearly visible. (**b**) Labial view at 2 years shows success of the reattached fragment and this minimally invasive restorative procedure

Clinical Notes

Cvek pulpotomy allows vitality testing in the follow-up visits because of the remaining coronal pulp tissue. A vital pulp, absence of pain or swelling, continued root growth, absence of internal resorption, calcifications, and periapical radiolucency indicate a successful outcome [2].

8.2.1.5 Case Study 2: Cvek Pulpotomy with a Long-Term Follow-Up

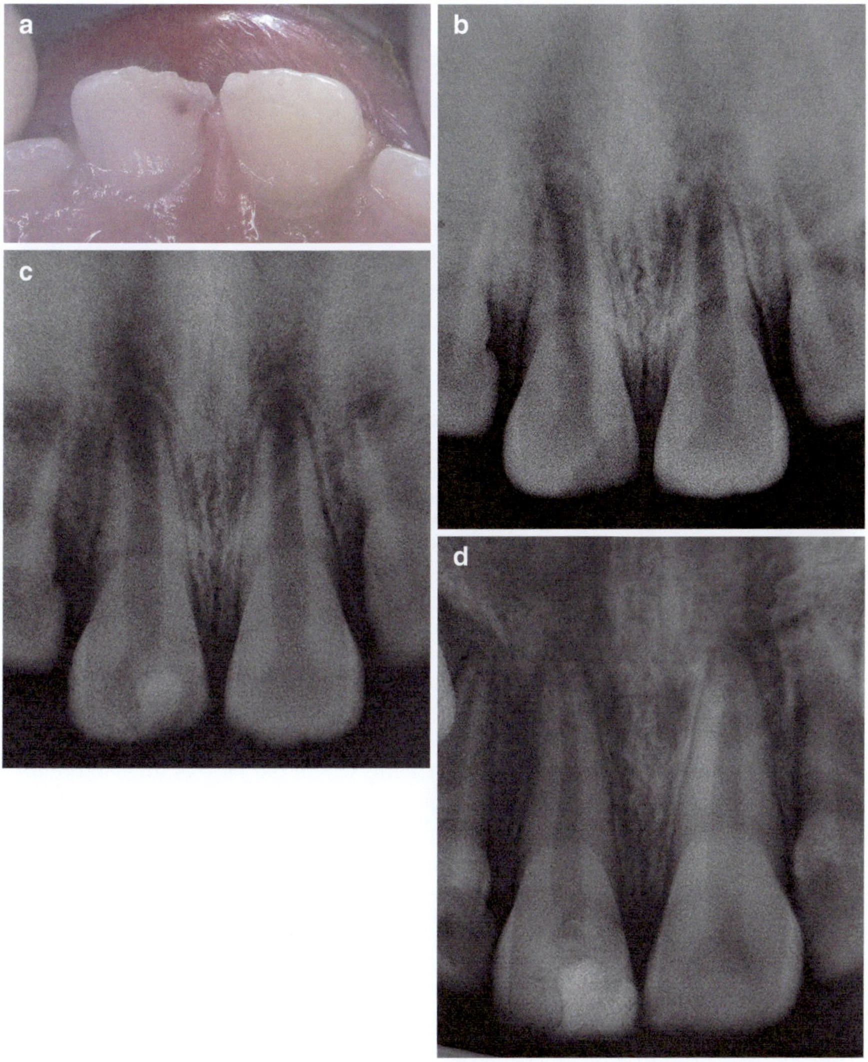

(**a**) Tooth 11 presented with a complicated crown fracture 40 h after trauma; note the exposed pulp. (**b**) Preoperative radiograph of tooth 11 with crown fracture, immature root, and open apex. (**c**) Postoperative radiograph following partial pulpotomy. (**d**) Four-year follow-up radiograph of tooth 11 showing root maturation and apical closure

8.2.2 Full Pulpotomy in Immature Permanent Teeth

8.2.2.1 Introduction

Pulpotomy is the removal of part of the pulp tissue displaying inflammatory or degenerative changes followed by placement of a medicament to preserve the vitality of the remaining underlying tissue [1]. This definition can imply either a partial pulpotomy or a full pulpotomy. A full pulpotomy is the removal of the entire coronal portion of the pulp to the level of the root orifices [4]. A full pulpotomy has traditionally been a classic pulp therapy protocol in primary teeth exhibiting carious or mechanical exposures [2]. In an immature permanent tooth involved pulpally, it is performed as a treatment to encourage continued physiologic root growth or apexogenesis.

8.2.2.2 Indications and Contraindications

A full pulpotomy in an immature permanent tooth is indicated in:

- Teeth where the clinical judgment of the extent of coronal pulp inflammation becomes challenging [4]. Clinically, it may be seen as continued hemorrhage from the pulp. In such a scenario, to avoid placing the medicament on inflamed pulp, a full pulpotomy is preferred.
- In teeth where the size of the pulp exposure in a complicated crown fracture is more than 4 mm or the child reports more than 9 days post trauma, a partial pulpotomy is contraindicated [3], and a full pulpotomy is indicated. However, the clinician is advised to select the treatment modality depending on the individual merits of each case.
- In symptomatic teeth with a history of pain, where the pulp is involved due to carious or traumatic exposures, the depth of pulp inflammation will be difficult to predict, and a full pulpotomy is indicated [11]. It should be noted that in such cases, sometimes a deeper pulp resection into the root canals might be required to obtain hemorrhage control [1].

8.2.2.3 Rationale

The success of vital pulp therapy lies in the removal of all the inflamed pulp tissue, eliminating bacteria from the dentine-pulp complex with a bacteria-tight seal and ensuring placement of a medicament on the remaining non-inflamed pulp [4]. This creates an environment where apexogenesis can successfully occur. Full pulpotomy involves the removal of all coronal pulp tissue to obtain hemorrhage control and the placement of calcium silicate-based cements over non-inflamed tissue. Calcium silicate based cements provide a bacterium tight seal through predictable dentin bridge formation and preservation of the remaining pulpal health [2]. It also sets hard allowing it to function as a base for the overlying restoration, which further reinforces the coronal seal [4].

8.2.2.4 Case Study 1: Full Pulpotomy in a Tooth with Traumatic Exposure

Case Selection

Why Was This Case Selected for a Full Pulpotomy?

- A 9-year-old child presented 2 weeks after trauma with a complicated crown fracture in tooth 21.
- A large linear area of pulp exposure (>4 mm) was seen at the site of fracture.
- Patient reported that a dressing on the exposed pulp had been placed by a previous dentist that dislodged the next day.
- Radiograph showed immature root development in tooth 21 with a complicated crown fracture and an open apex.

Case Selection: Incisal View of Fractured 21

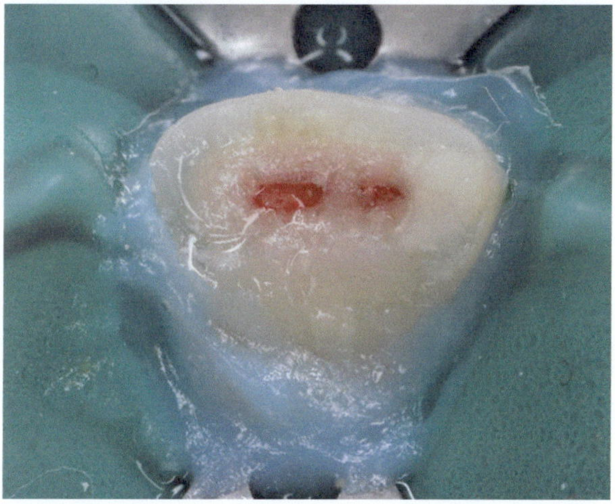

Note the large linear exposure site

Clinical Notes

Interval between the traumatic episode and the initiation of therapy was more than 2 weeks. It was likely that the pulp tissue was bacterially contaminated and that pulpal inflammation had progressed deep into the coronal pulp. Hence, a full pulpotomy was planned.

Case Selection: Preoperative Radiograph

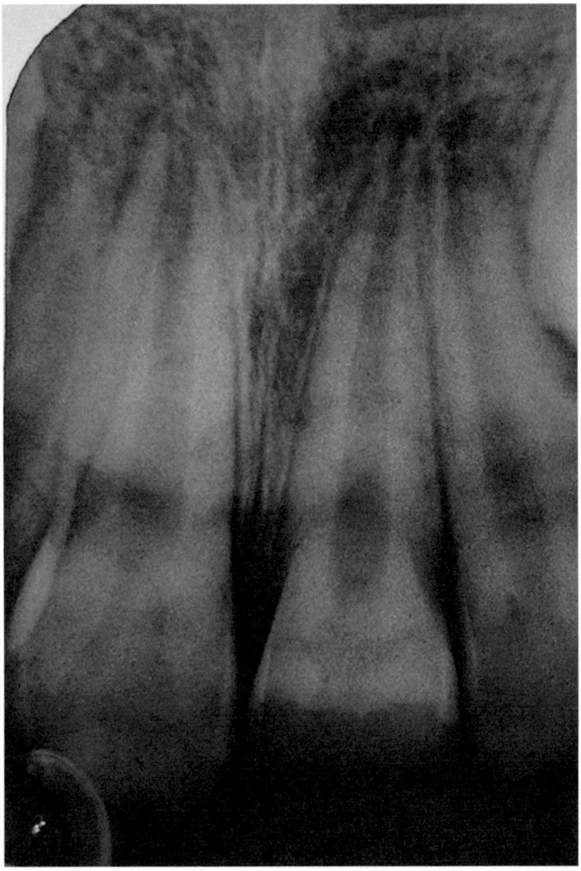

Tooth 21 presented with a complicated crown fracture. Note the immature root and open apex in tooth 21

Step-by-Step Guide

Step 1: Access Cavity Preparation

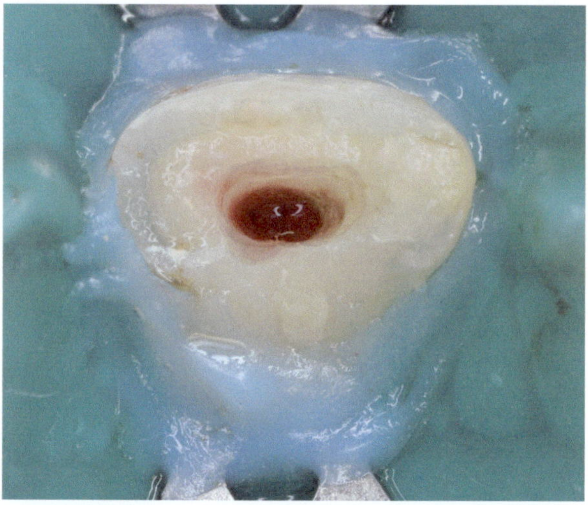

Local anesthesia was administered and rubber dam applied. A straight-line access without undercuts in the access cavity preparation was made. The coronal pulp tissue was amputated to the cervical or the orifice level

Clinical Notes
The pulp chamber is irrigated with 2.5% sodium hypochlorite [11].

Step 2: Hemorrhage Control

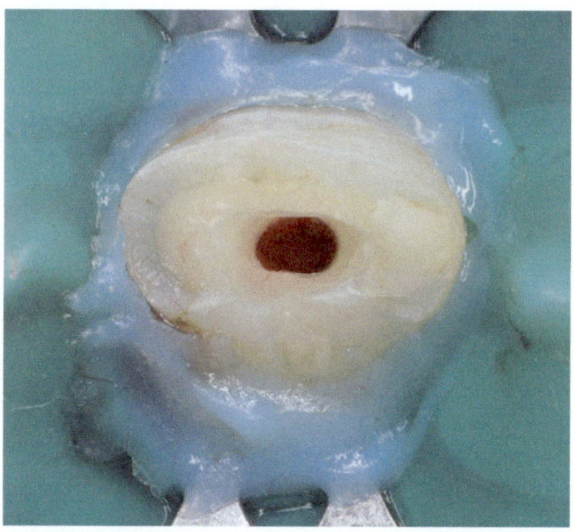

Note that the bleeding is controlled

Clinical Notes

The sodium hypochlorite solution may be left on the exposed pulp tissue to obtain hemorrhage control. This is followed by moderate pressure from a moist cotton pellet. Continued bleeding indicates deeper levels of the pulpal inflammation warranting a deeper level of pulp resection.

Step 3: Placement of Mineral Trioxide Aggregate (MTA)

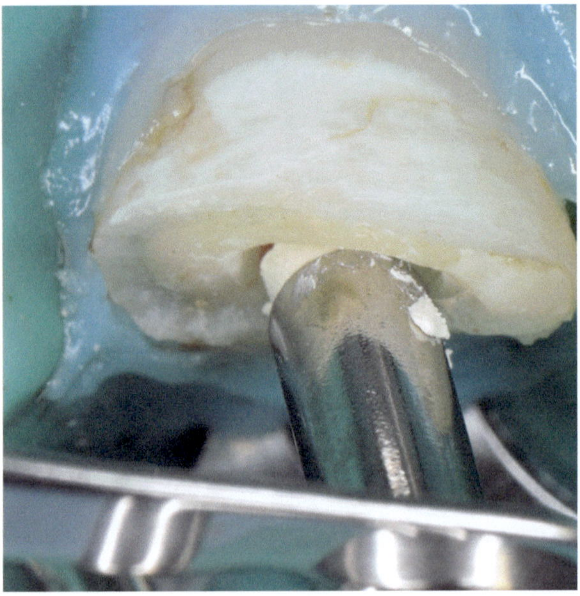

MTA was placed over the pulp stump (NuSmile NeoMTA, NuSmile Ltd, Houston, TX, USA)

Clinical Notes

While MTA shows highly successful results as a biomaterial for pulpotomy, evidence so far does not prove that any one bioactive endodontic cement (BEC) is superior to the other [12].

Step 4: MTA Condensed

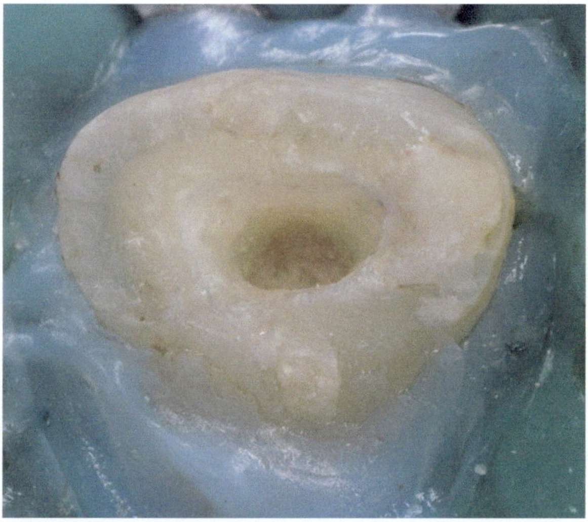

MTA is seen here placed over the pulp stump

> **Clinical Notes**
> A moist cotton pellet is used to gently condense the MTA. We now prefer using Biodentine among the calcium silicate-based cements for anterior teeth because of its lesser staining potential [7, 8].

Step 5: RMGI Cement Application

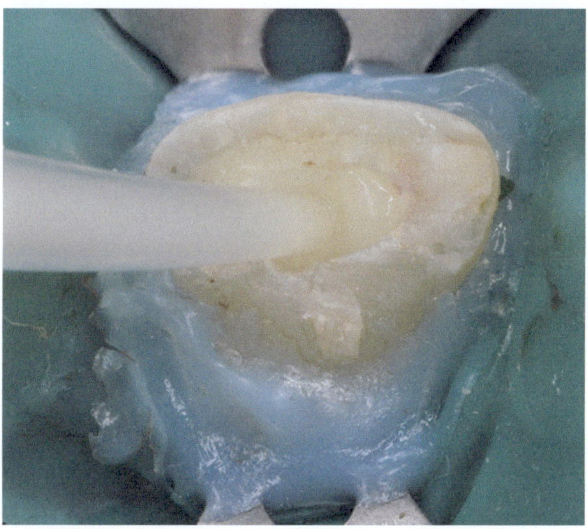

A layer of resin-modified glass ionomer cement (Fuji II LC, GC Corporation, Tokyo, Japan) was placed over the MTA

Clinical Notes

A bacteria-tight seal is a very critical factor for success of vital pulp therapy. A well sealing pulpal dressing and subsequent restoration with an adhesive material ensure this. MTA has a prolonged setting time, and placing a temporary dressing over MTA to allow it to set would risk compromising the seal [13]. Resin-modified glass ionomer (RMGI) restorative cement placed immediately after placing MTA protects it and allows MTA to set underneath permitting the final restoration to be placed in the same sitting without any compromise of the seal [13]

Step 6: Coronal Seal

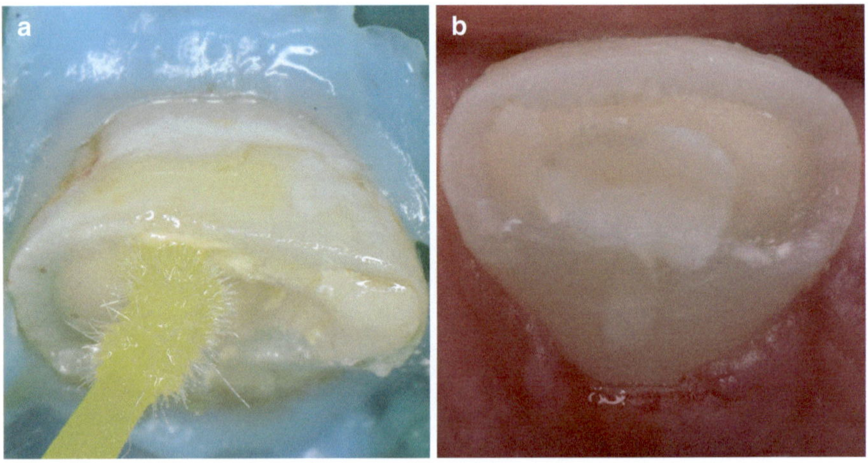

(**a**) Bonding agent applied on the walls of the access cavity after etching. (**b**) Composite resin was placed for a tight coronal seal

Clinical Notes

The walls of the access cavity are etched, and bonding agent is applied following the placement of a layer of RMGI cement over the MTA; also see "Sect. 8.3.4.2, Step 12: Second Appointment (PS): Coronal Seal." This will minimize staining caused by MTA [9, 10].

Step 7: Postoperative Radiograph

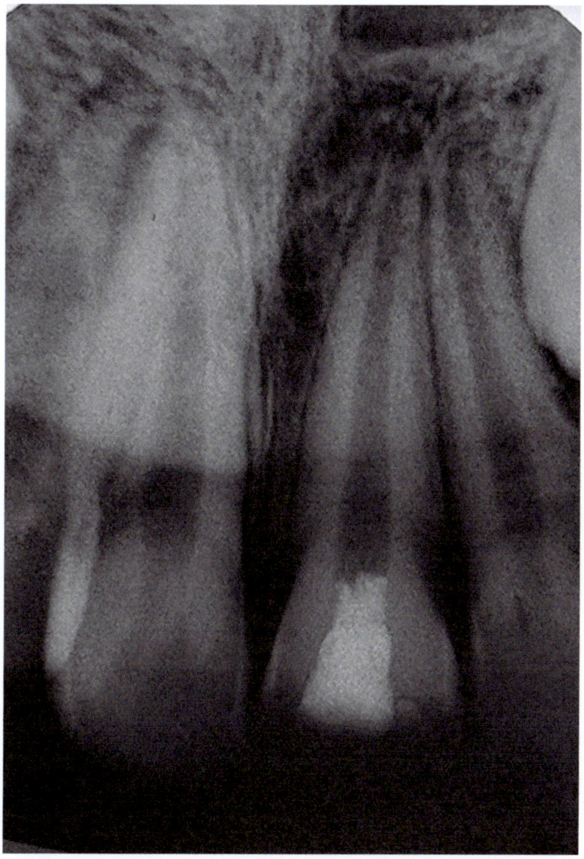

A radiograph was taken immediately following cervical pulpotomy

Clinical Notes

Owing to the loss of the coronal pulp, sensitivity testing is not possible in case of a full pulpotomy. Hence, a radiographic follow-up to access signs of apical periodontitis and to monitor root maturation is important. This is done at 6 months and yearly thereafter.

Long-Term Follow-Up

Two-Year Follow-Up Radiograph

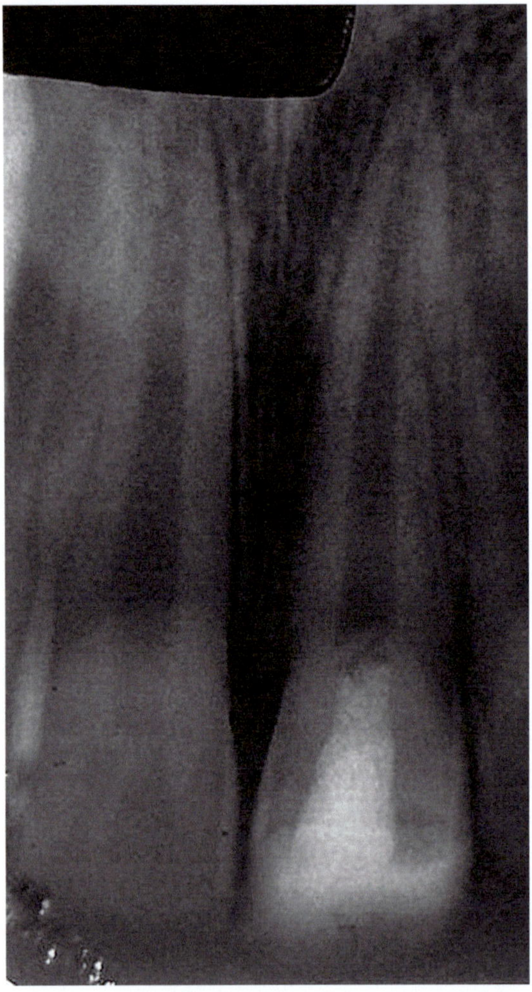

At the end of 2 years, note the calcific barrier formation and continued root maturation proving the presence of vital pulp tissue

Clinical Notes

Reentry is not required unless the tooth gets symptomatic [1]. Regular radiographic screening is advised to detect possible sequelae such as pulp necrosis.

Long-Term Follow-Up of a Full Pulpotomy in a tooth with Traumatic Exposure: Case 2

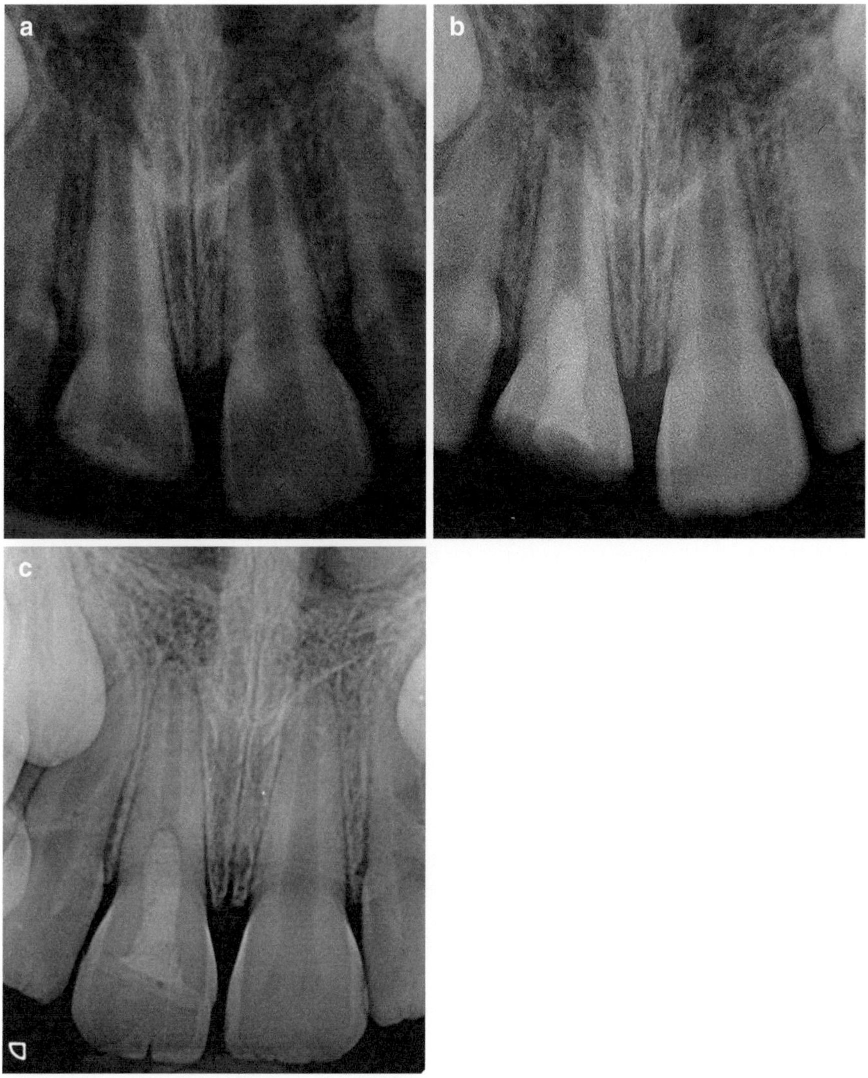

(**a**) Tooth 11 with a complicated crown fracture and a pulp exposed for 2 months. Child was referred after the dentist placed a glass ionomer dressing 1 month post trauma. (**b**) A deeper level of pulp resection was carried out because of continued bleeding despite pulp amputation up to the level of the cementoenamel junction. (**c**) One-year follow-up demonstrating root maturation and apical closure. Note the tooth fragment that was reattached successfully

8.2.2.5 Case Study 2: Full Pulpotomy in a Carious Immature Permanent Molar

Case Selection

Why Was This Case Selected for a Full Pulpotomy?

- A 7-year-old child presented with a deep carious lesion in tooth 46.
- The tooth had a history of two episodes of spontaneous night-time pain. The child was not chewing food on the right side. There was no history of an extraoral swelling.
- The tooth was tender to percussion. No intraoral abscess or draining sinus was visible.
- Radiograph showed a deep carious lesion exposing the pulp. The roots of tooth 46 were immature with open apices.

Case Selection: Preoperative Occlusal View

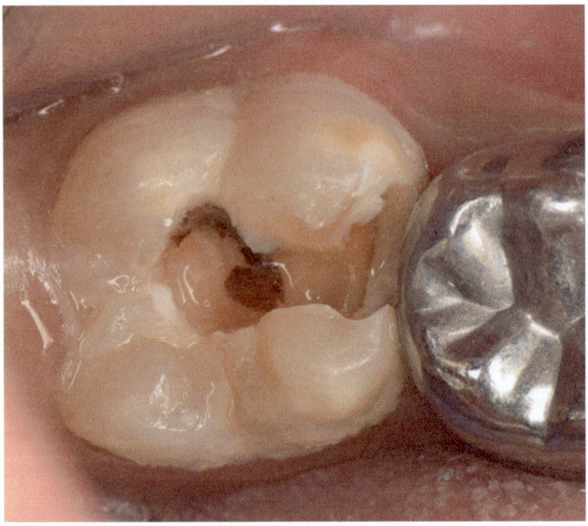

Tooth 46 showed a deep carious lesion. The soft tissue around the tooth appeared normal

Case Selection: Preoperative Radiograph

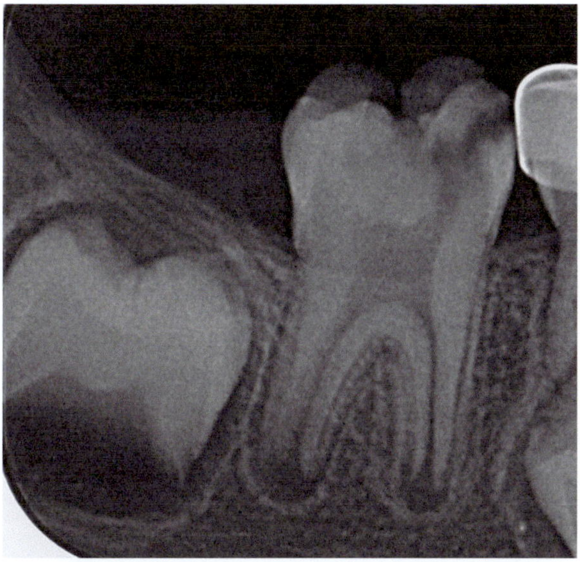

Note the immature open apices in tooth 36. There were no signs of furcal or periapical pathosis

Step-by-Step Guide

Step 1: Tooth Isolated

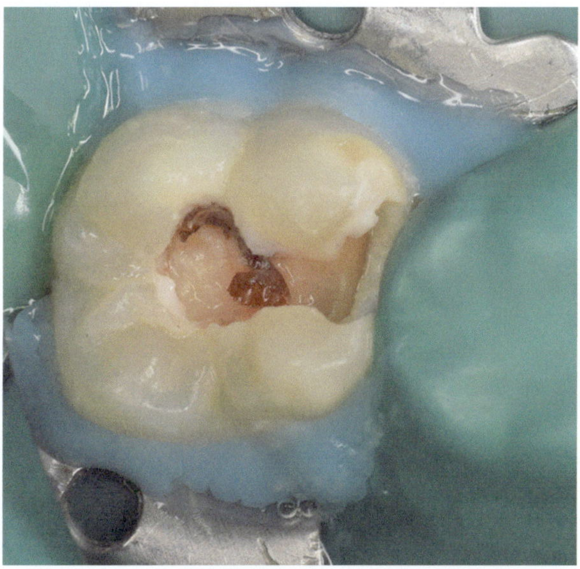

Local anesthesia was administered, and tooth 46 was isolated and clearly visualized

Clinical Notes

The tooth may have a history of severe spontaneous pain consistent with a diagnosis of irreversible pulpitis. There should however not be any signs of non-vitality like the presence of a swelling, sinus tract, or pathologic mobility.

Step 2: Complete Unroofing

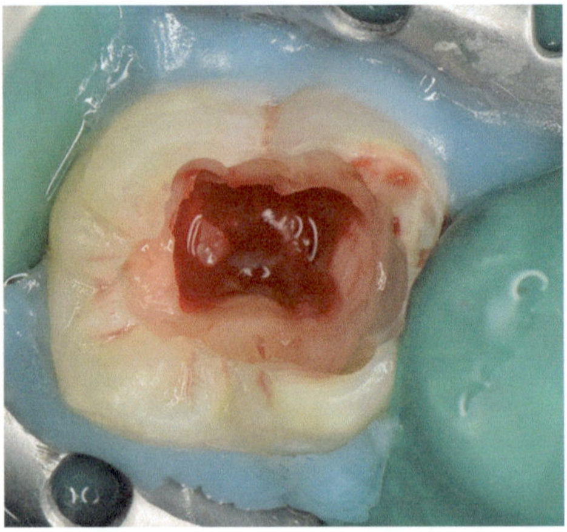

The pulp chamber was unroofed with a water-cooled high-speed sterile bur removing all undercuts after complete removal of carious tissue

Step 3: Hemostasis Obtained at the Radicular Orifices

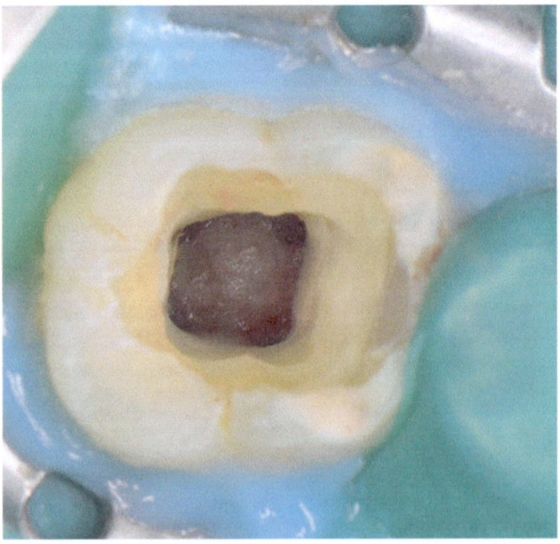

Note hemostasis obtained in all four canal orifices

Clinical Notes

Coronal pulp amputation is performed with a sterile round bur mounted on a slow speed handpiece under copious saline irrigation. Managing the health of the remaining pulp tissue is achieved by controlling bleeding by bathing the chamber with 2.5% sodium hypochlorite. The exposed pulp tissue can be allowed to soak in sodium hypochlorite for up to 10 min [11]. A fresh solution can be used every 3–4 min [1]. A saline-soaked blot dried cotton pellet is applied under gentle pressure to achieve hemostasis. If required, deeper pulp resection into the canals can be undertaken until bleeding is controlled.

Step 4: MTA Placed

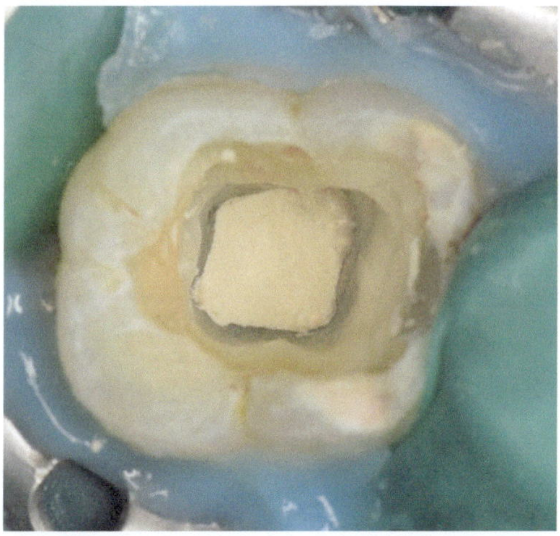

Mineral trioxide aggregate (Angelus MTA Angelus, Londrina, PR, Brazil) 2 mm thick [11] was placed over the pulp stumps and condensed

Step 5: Coronal Seal

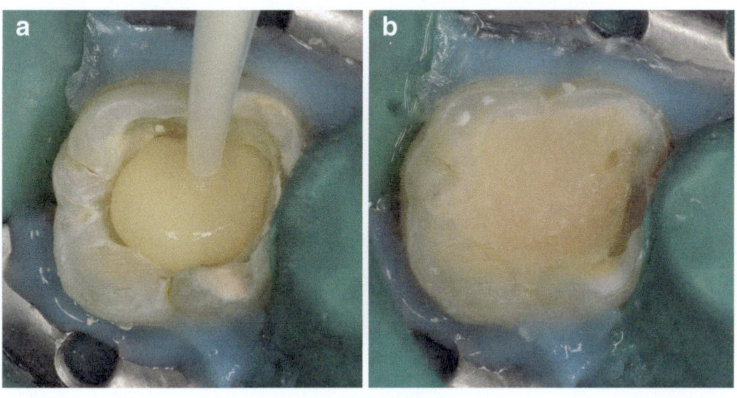

(**a**, **b**) Resin-modified glass ionomer restorative cement was used as a core buildup material over the MTA [13]

Step 6: Preformed Metal Crown

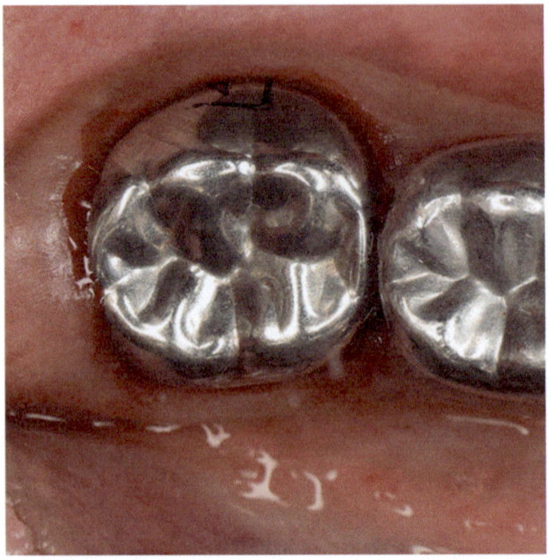

A preformed metal crown was placed for a stable long-term coronal seal

Clinical Notes
The tooth preparation being minimally invasive for a steel crown, they are an excellent treatment choice following pulp therapy in young permanent teeth (Chap. 4).

Step 7: Postoperative Radiograph

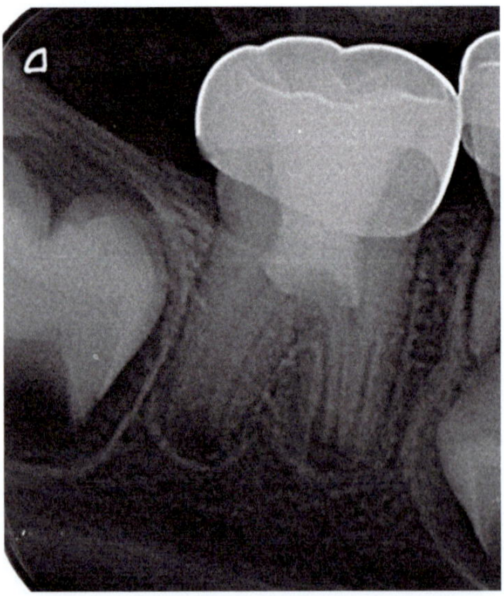

Pulpotomy in tooth 36 followed by full coronal coverage with a preformed metal crown

Clinical Notes
Owing to the loss of the coronal pulp, sensitivity testing is not possible in case of a full pulpotomy. Hence, a radiographic follow-up to access signs of apical periodontitis and to monitor root maturation is important.

Six-Month Follow-Up Radiograph

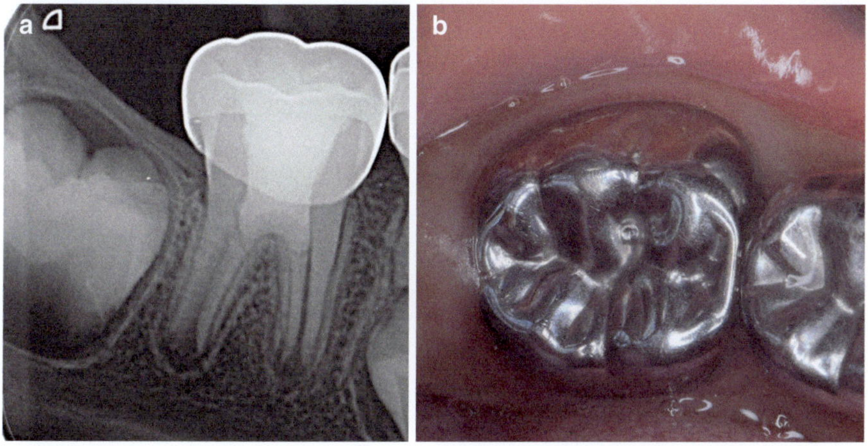

Six-month follow-up. (**a**) Periapical radiograph showing root maturation as compared to the post-operative radiograph. (**b**) Occlusal view of tooth 46 at 6 months showing excellent soft tissue response and a stable crown

Long-Term Follow-Up of a Full Pulpotomy in a Carious Molar - Case 2

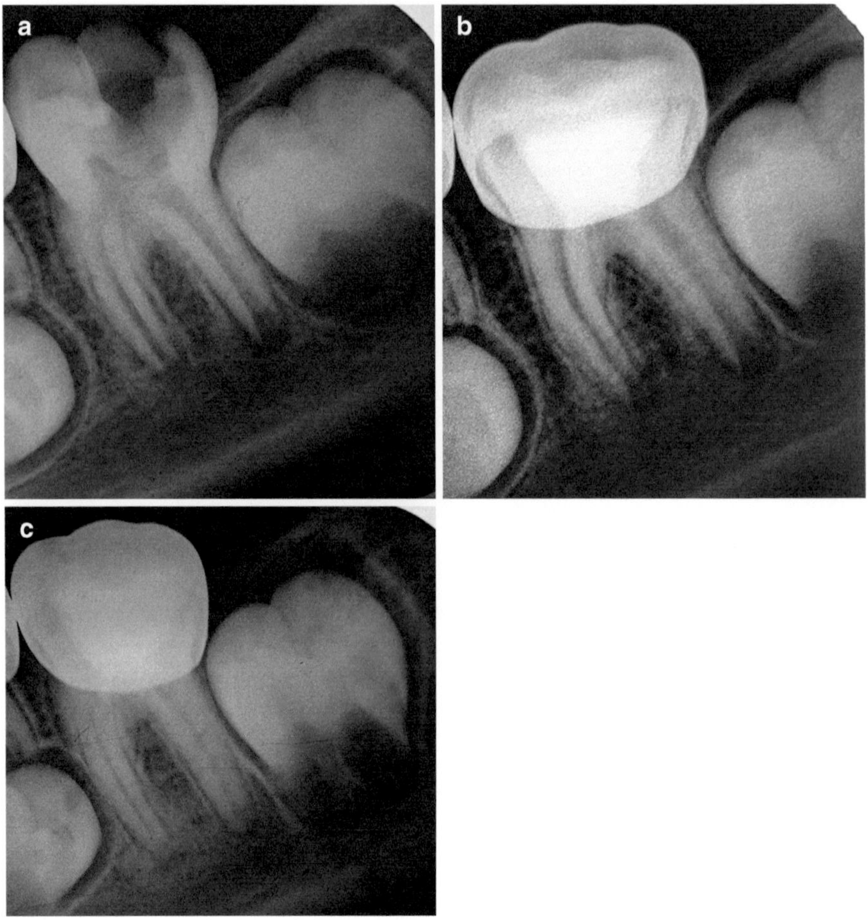

(**a**) Tooth 36 with a deep carious lesion extending to the pulp. The roots were immature. (**b**) Postoperative radiograph shows pulpotomy performed and a preformed metal crown cemented in tooth 36. (**c**) At the end of 30 months, note the root maturation and apical closure in tooth 36 following successful apexogenesis

8.3 Regenerative Endodontic Procedures

8.3.1 Introduction

A young permanent tooth with an incompletely formed root is dependent on the continued vascular supply of the pulp for its root development and completion. In the case of such a tooth becoming non-vital due to trauma or a carious attack, the root development stays arrested. This scenario leaves the tooth with an unfavorable crown root ratio and weak dentinal walls susceptible to fracture [1]. Traditionally, these teeth were treated with apexification using calcium hydroxide or mineral trioxide aggregate to induce an artificial barrier at the level to which root development was complete. But the lack of further root development leads to a high percentage of root or cervical crown fractures [14].

Regenerative endodontic procedures are defined as "biologically based procedures designed to replace damaged structures, including dentin and root structures, as well as cells of the pulp-dentin complex" [15]. In non-vital immature permanent teeth, present "regenerative endodontic procedures" (REPs) allow for resolution of infection and continued root development. Banchs and Trope in 2004 described a clinical protocol to promote root growth and apical closure in immature infected permanent teeth [16]. Popularly called "revascularization," the term maturogenesis has also been proposed for these procedures since they promote continued root development and maturation in necrosed immature permanent teeth [14]. The following is a step-by-step depiction of this procedure.

8.3.2 Indications and Contraindications

REPs are indicated in:

- Immature permanent teeth with a necrotic pulp [17]
- Necrotic immature teeth where the final restoration does not require a post/core [17]
- Necrotic immature teeth where the apical diameter of the root is more than 1 mm. Larger apical diameters promote predictable outcomes [14]
- The American Society of Anesthesiologist's ASA1 or ASA2 patients [17]

They are contraindicated in:

- Patients in whom a regular follow-up is not possible
- Parents, who do not consent to the possibility of crown discoloration, no response to treatment, or treatment failure resulting in pain/infection [17]

8.3.3 Rationale

Tissue engineering is the science that aims at regenerating cells, tissues, and organs so that normal function is reestablished. Stem cells, growth factors, and scaffolds are the three parameters required for its success. Stem cells are undifferentiated cells with the potential to differentiate into other cell types. Scaffolds ensure support for the cell differentiation. Growth factors are proteins that stimulate cell differentiation [18]. Current protocols for REPs integrate the principles of tissue engineering with a bacteria-free environment in an attempt to return vascularity and bring about root growth in non-vital immature permanent teeth. A bacteria-free root canal system and a bacteria-tight seal to prevent reinfection are important criteria that promote root growth in non-vital immature permanent teeth.

- REPs firstly disinfect the pulp space with medicaments [18].
- Following the removal of the medicament, irrigation with ethylenediaminetetraacetic acid (EDTA) releases growth factors from dentin. Studies have shown dentin to contain an abundance of bioactive molecules, which play an important role in the REP when released [18].
- Bleeding stimulated from the periapical area through the large apical opening bring along with them the stem cells most likely the " stem cells from apical papilla" (SCAP) which in the developing root are known to be present in the periapical region [19].
- The resulting blood clot acts like a scaffold that provides support for new cell formation and proliferation. The blood clot also possesses numerous growth factors [18].
- Further sealing the tooth with calcium silicate-based cements followed by a resin-modified glass ionomer cement prevents bacterial reinfection [18].
- Residual vital pulp cells, stem cells from the periodontal ligament, and Hertwig's epithelial root sheath (HERS) cells that have survived the onslaught of the bacterial infection could also contribute to the regenerative process under sterile and optimal conditions [14].

8.3.4 Case Study 1: Regenerative Endodontic Procedure

8.3.4.1 Case Selection

Why Was "Tooth 11" Selected for a Regenerative Endodontic Procedure?

- A 9-year-old child presented 3 months after trauma with a gingival parulis in relation to tooth 11.

- The child suffered trauma to teeth 11, 12, and 21 3 months before the current presentation. Tooth 21 was treated with a partial pulpotomy and crown fragment reattachment. Tooth 11 suffered extrusive luxation. Tooth 11 was repositioned, and a flexible splint was placed for 15 days. Follow-up was uneventful until the child presented after 3 months with signs of a non-vital pulp.
- Radiograph showed no periapical radiolucency but an immature root and an open apex with an apical diameter of close to 2 mm.

Case Selection: Preoperative Clinical View of Tooth 11

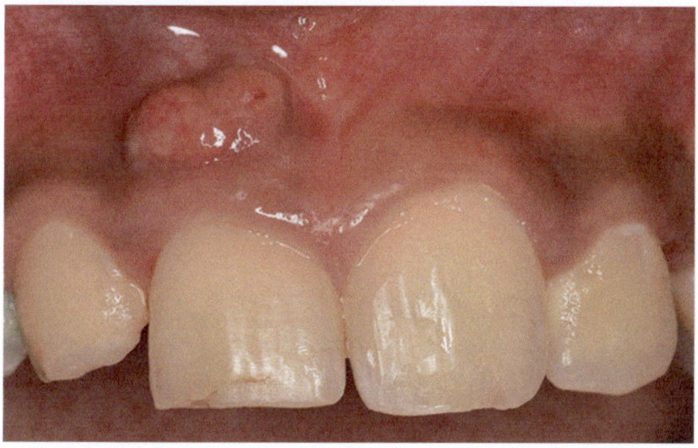

Note the parulis in relation to tooth 11

Clinical Notes

The parulis was observed 2 months after trauma. Tooth 11 had suffered extrusive luxation and was repositioned 12 h post trauma. The tooth was splinted with a flexible splint for 2 weeks. The parulis was observed on the follow-up visit after 2 months.

Case Selection: Preoperative Radiographic View of Tooth 11

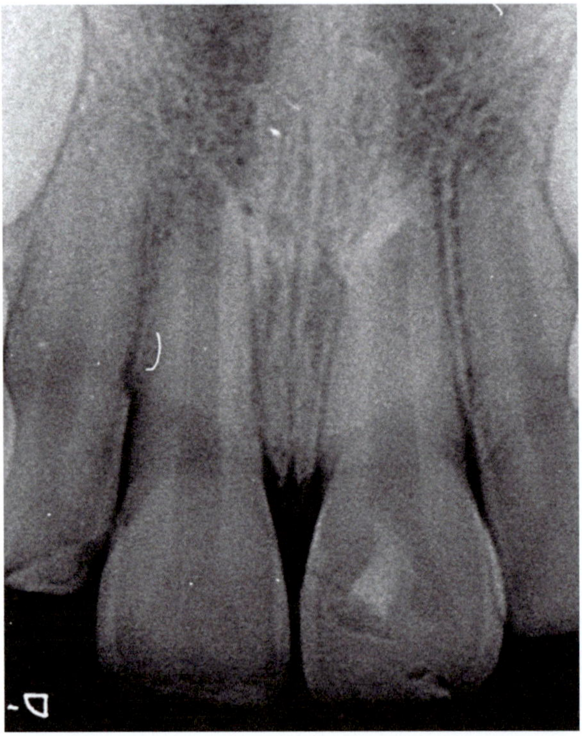

Tooth 11 showed an immature root and open apex with an apical diameter of close to 2 mm. Tooth 21 had been treated with a partial pulpotomy and fragment reattachment 3 months ago

Clinical Notes

Regenerative endodontic procedures are more predictable in teeth with an apical diameter of more than 1 mm [14].

8.3.4.2 Step-by-Step Guide

Step 1: First Appointment (Root Canal Disinfection (RCD)): Access Opening

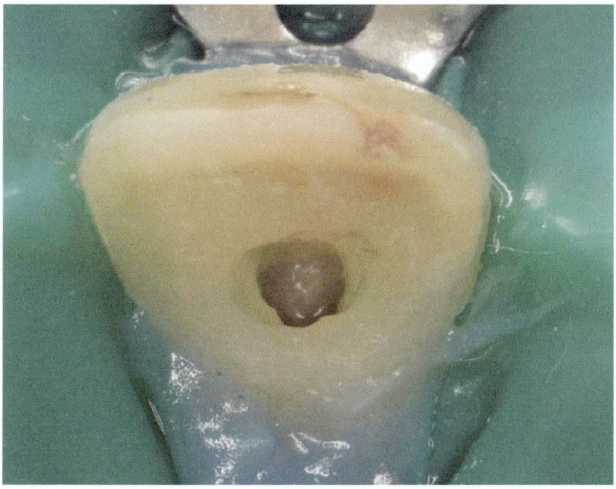

The tooth was isolated under rubber dam following administration of local anesthesia. Access cavity was opened to allow for purulent hemorrhagic discharge

Step 2: First Appointment (RCD): Working Length

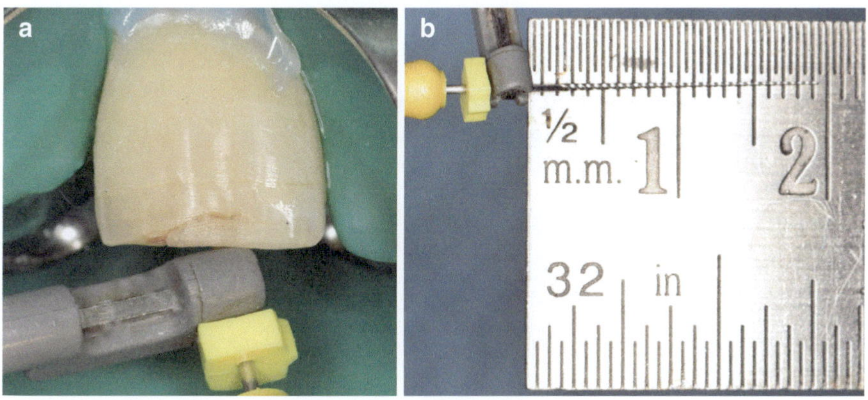

(**a**) The working length was measured with an electronic apex locator. (**b**) The measurement—19.5 mm—was noted. The same was confirmed with a diagnostic radiograph

Clinical Notes

This step is important in order to position the needle accurately during irrigation [14] and position the endodontic file accurately while inducing periapical bleeding in the second appointment.

Step 3: First Appointment (RCD): Irrigation

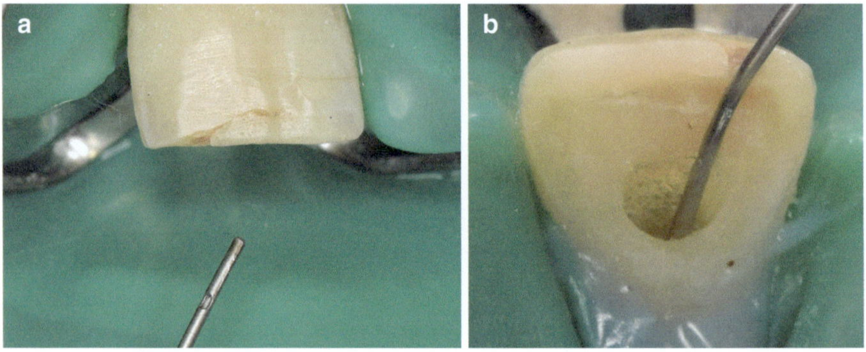

(**a**) Side-vent needle with closed ends was used for irrigation. (**b**) The tooth was irrigated for 5 min with 20 mL of 1.5% NaOCl [17] using a stopwatch

Clinical Notes

Copious and gentle irrigation is recommended with the needle kept 1 mm short of the working length. This is to reduce cytotoxicity to the apical stem cells. Side-vent needles are recommended since they reduce any chances of extrusion of the irrigating solution through the open apex into the periapical area. Irrigation with low concentration NaOCl is followed by irrigation with 20 mL of EDTA for 5 min [17].

Step 4: First Appointment (RCD): Dry Canal

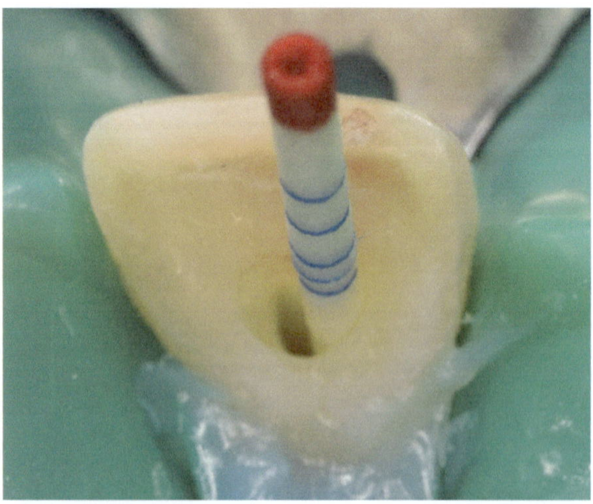

The canal was dried well with paper points

Step 5: First Appointment (RCD): Medicament Inserted

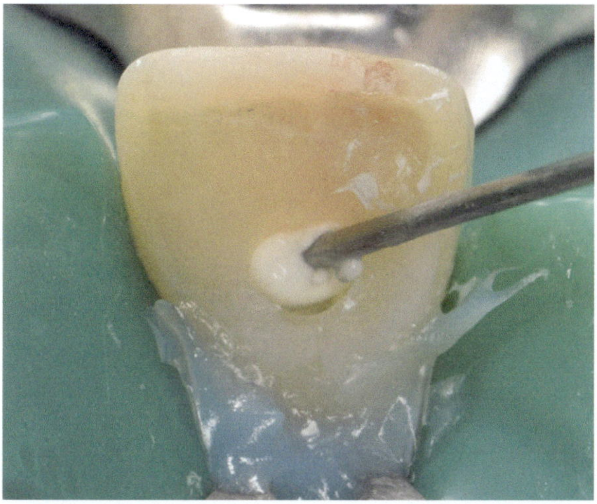

Calcium hydroxide paste was delivered into the root canal with a syringe system

> **Clinical Notes**
> Alternately, a low concentration triple antibiotic paste (1:1:1 ciprofloxacin/metronidazole/minocycline to a final concentration of 1–5 mg/mL) placed well below the CEJ can be used as an intracanal medicament. The pulp chamber sealed with a dentine bonding agent will minimize staining caused by minocycline. A double mix paste omitting minocycline can also be used, or minocycline can be substituted with amoxicillin, clindamycin, or cefaclor [17].

Step 6: First Appointment (RCD): Coronal Seal

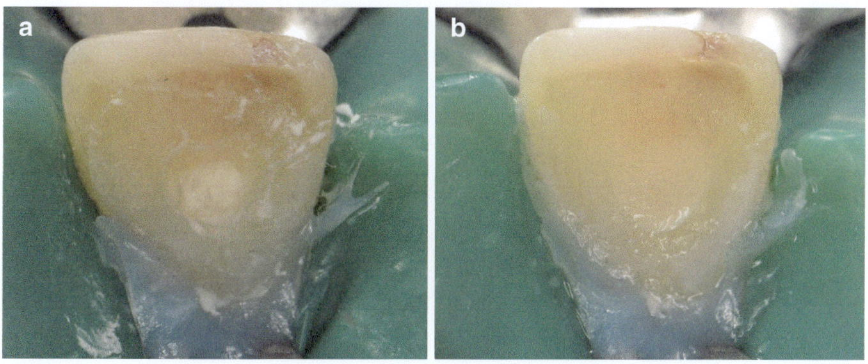

(**a**) The paste was condensed with a cotton pellet. (**b**) RMGI restorative cement seal of 3–4 mm was placed

Clinical Notes
A depth of 3–4 mm of the temporary restorative material will ensure the essential stable coronal seal [17].

Labial View: End of First Appointment

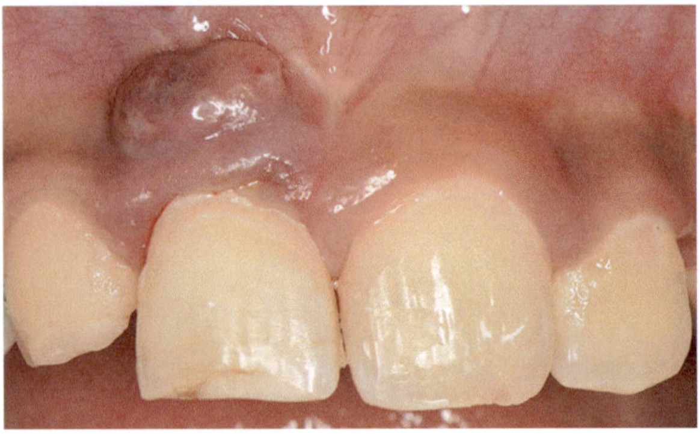

Note the parulis looking hemorrhagic and slightly collapsed at the end of appointment

Radiograph: End of First Appointment

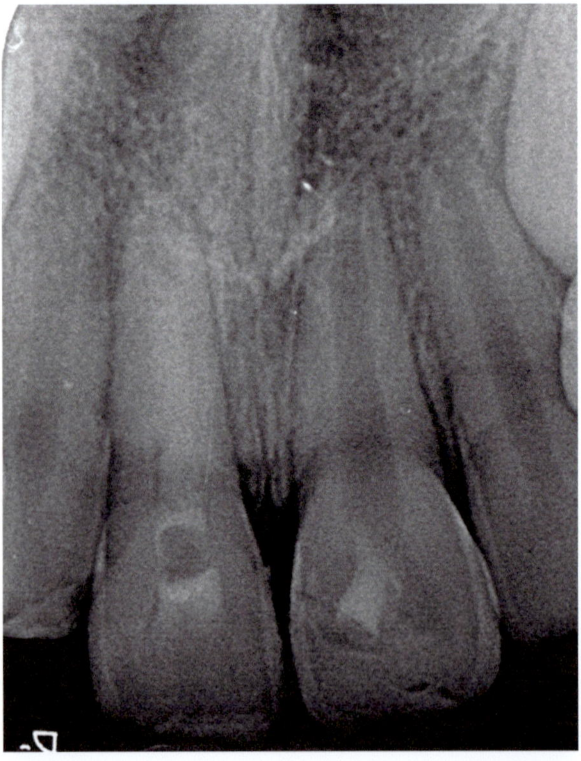

A postoperative IOPA was recorded at the end of appointment one. The next appointment was scheduled after 1–4 weeks [17]

Labial View: Start of Second Appointment

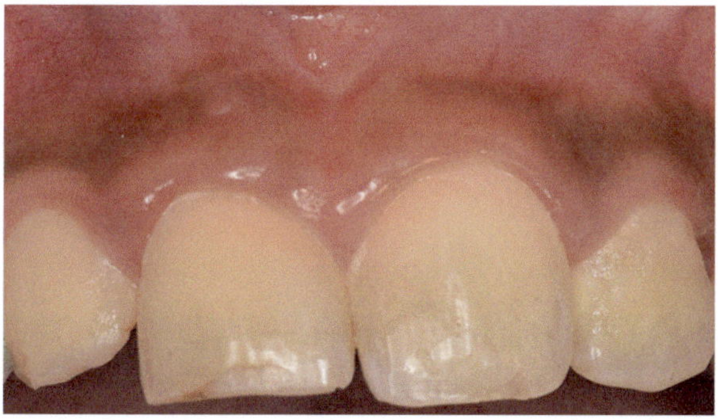

At the end of 2 weeks, before the start of the second appointment, note that the soft tissue appeared well healed

> **Clinical Notes**
> At the start of the second appointment, the tooth should show a resolution of all signs of infection such as purulent discharge, pain, abscess, or a sinus tract. Failing this, the disinfection time is increased. In cases of persistent infection, an alternate antimicrobial can be used and the disinfection process repeated [17].

Step 7: Second Appointment (Providing a Scaffold (PS)): Irrigation

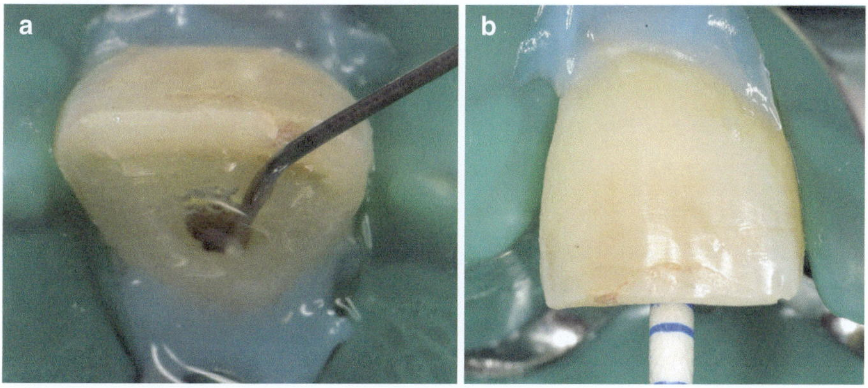

(**a**) Tooth was anesthetized using a local anesthetic without vasoconstrictor and isolated under dental dam. The canal was irrigated using 20 mL of 17% EDTA, gently and copiously [17]. (**b**) The canal was dried with paper points

Clinical Notes
EDTA being a chelating agent decalcifies the wall of the root dentin and exposes the collagen fibers. The decalcified dentin releases growth factors, which attract and stimulate the differentiation of new cells. The collagen aids in adhesion of the new cells onto the dentin [20].

Step 8: Second Appointment (PS): Inducing Bleeding

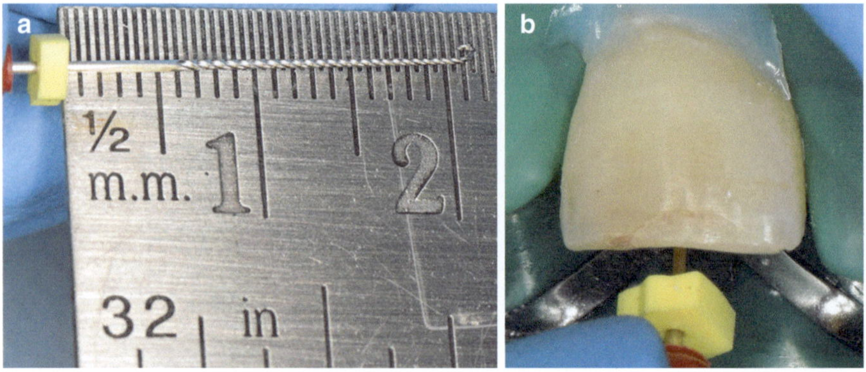

(**a**) A K-file was pre-curved and marked to 2 mm past the apical foramen. (**b**) To induce bleeding, a K-file was inserted into the canal to 2 mm beyond the apical foramen, the file is rotated, and the canal is over-instrumented [17]

Clinical Notes
The blood filled in the canal forms a stable blood clot that acts as a scaffold, which provides a framework for the stem cells and vasculature [14].

Blood-Filled Canal

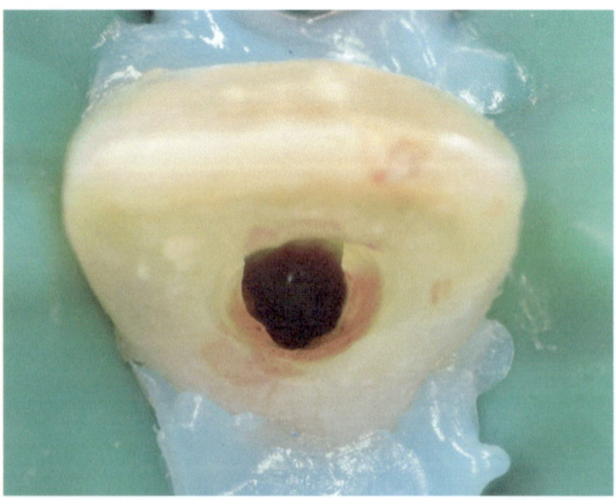

Note the entire canal was filled with blood to the level of the cementoenamel junction. The blood was allowed to clot 3 mm short of the cementoenamel junction

Clinical Notes
Placing a sterile soaked cotton pellet in the orifice ensures that the blood clot forms below the CEJ at a depth that allows placement of a restorative material. A stable blood clot is usually established in 15 min [14]. Platelet-rich plasma (PRP), platelet-rich fibrin (PRF), or autologous fibrin matrix (AFM) can be used as an alternative or when bleeding is difficult to induce [18].

Step 9: Second Appointment (PS): Collagen Matrix Placed

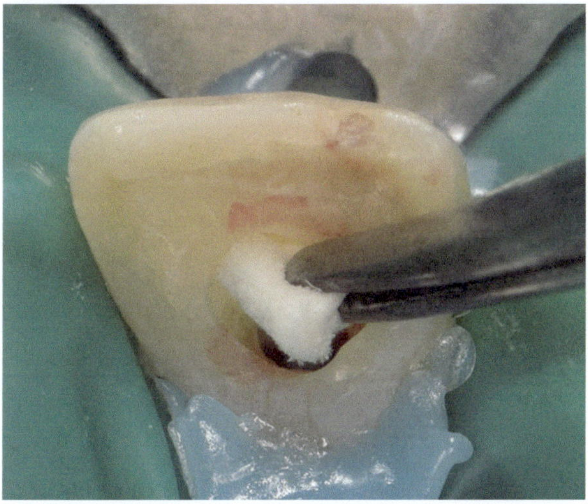

Resorbable collagen matrix was placed over the blood clot

Clinical Notes
A resorbable matrix placed over the blood clot stabilizes the clot and forms a more secure surface for the placement of a calcium silicate-based material like mineral trioxide aggregate or Biodentine [17].

Stable Blood Clot

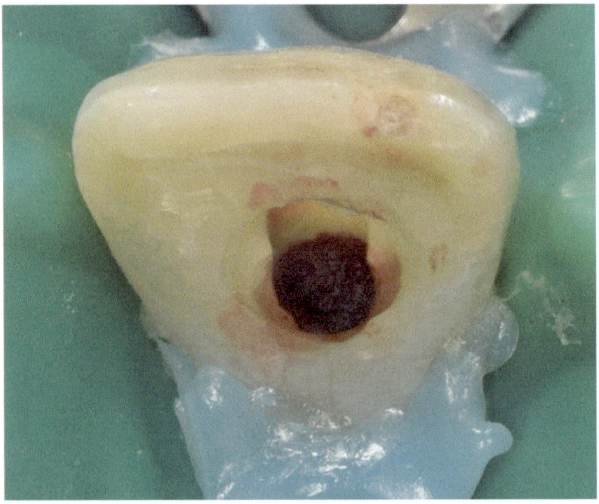

Note the stable blood clot seen below CEJ. The collagen matrix soaked in the blood clot stabilizes it

Clinical Notes

The collagen matrix soaked blood clot can be gently touched with the butt end of a large sterile paper point to confirm its stability [17].

Step 10: Second Appointment (PS): Biodentine Plug

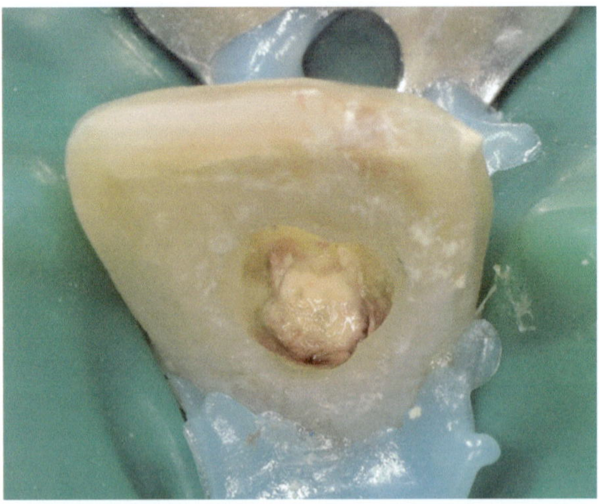

A 3 mm layer of Biodentine (Septodont, Saint-Maur-des-Fosses, France) was placed as a capping material over the stable blood clot up to the level of the cementoenamel junction

Clinical Notes

The calcium silicate-based material should be placed carefully on the clot so that the blood clot is not disturbed and the material does not get pushed further into the canal. New tissue regeneration does not happen in the area of the canal where the calcium silicate-based cement is placed predisposing that area to potential fracture. Hence, the capping material should be limited to around 3 mm below the CEJ [14].

Step 11: Second Appointment (PS): Resin-Modified Glass Ionomer

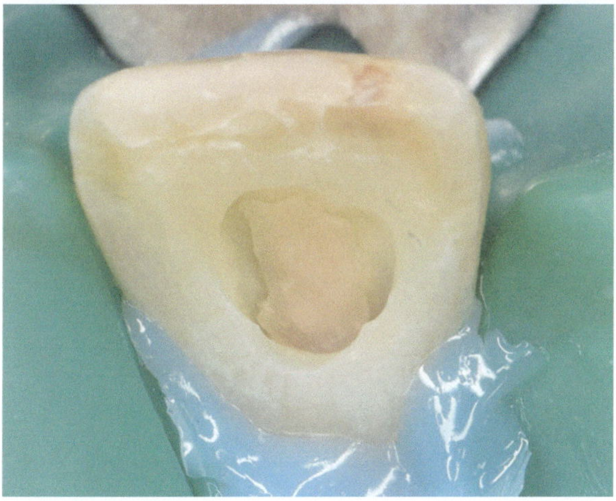

A thin layer of RMGI restorative cement was placed over the Biodentine and photo-activated

Step 12: Second Appointment (PS): Coronal Seal

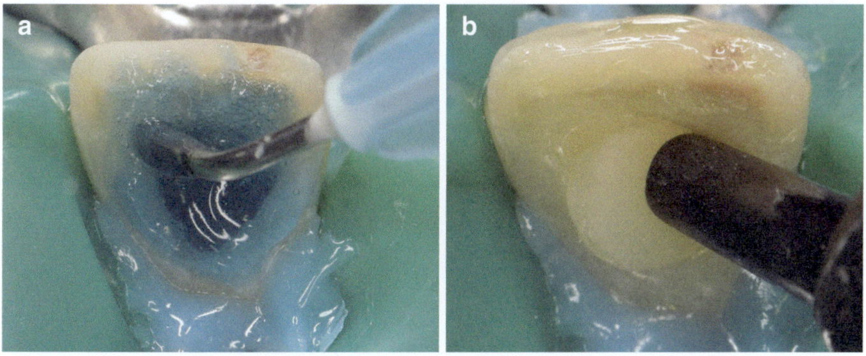

(**a**) Access cavity was etched and bonding agent applied to reduce any discoloration that the capping material may cause [9, 10]. (**b**) Composite resin placed for a stable coronal seal

Postoperative Radiograph

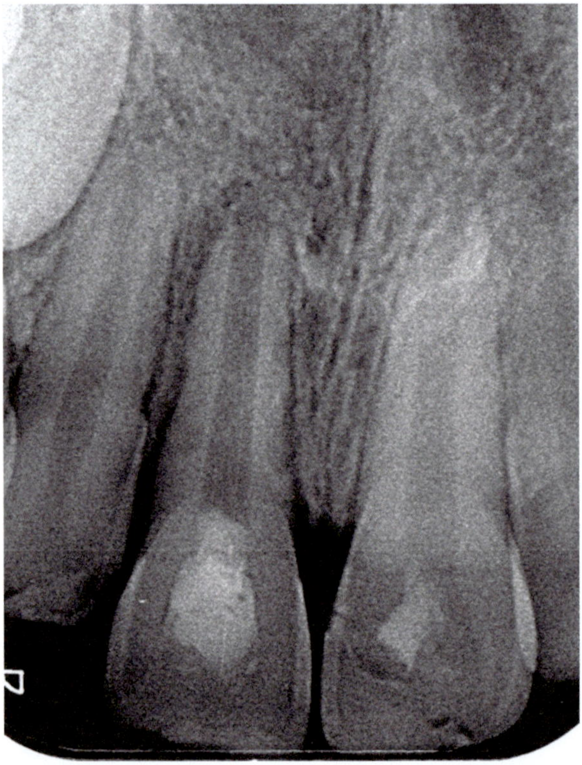

At the end of the second appointment, note the Biodentine plug at the level of the CEJ and the coronal seal in tooth 11. This radiograph was recorded for comparison with follow-up radiographs

Postoperative Clinical View

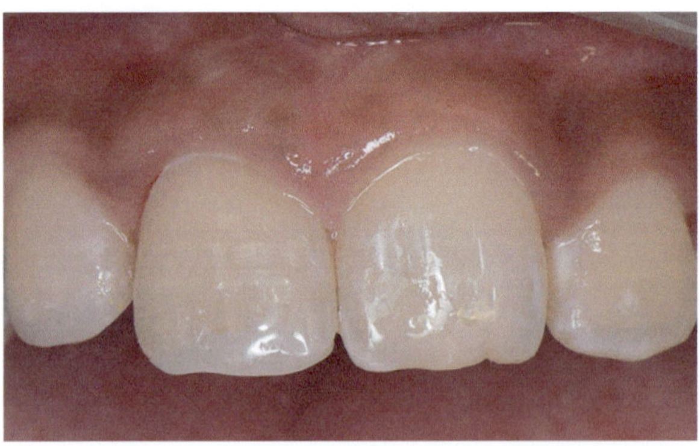

Labial view following aesthetic coronal restorations in teeth 11 and 21. Tooth fragment was reattached in tooth 21. Note the healthy soft tissue around tooth 11 indicating good healing and success in achieving the primary goals of the regenerative endodontic procedure

Six-Month Follow-Up Radiograph

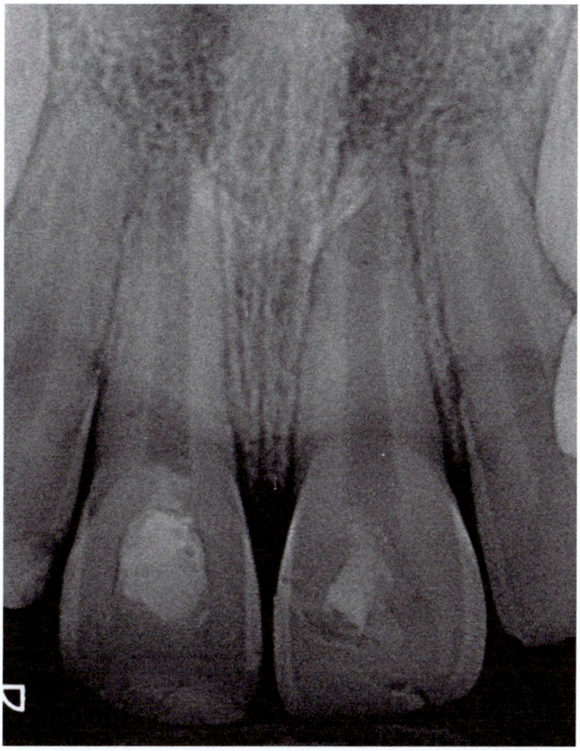

Radiograph at the end of 6 months shows that the primary indicators of success have been achieved. The secondary goals also seem to be achieved on careful examination of the radiograph at 6-month follow-up that shows increased root wall thickness and narrowing at the apex

Clinical Notes

The success of a regenerative endodontic procedure is measured through its primary, secondary, and tertiary goals achieved [17].

Primary Goal: Resolution of clinical signs and symptoms and evidence of bone healing.

Secondary Goal: Increased root wall thickness usually seen in 12–24 months posttreatment. This is ideally followed by an increase in root length.

Tertiary Goal: Positive response to vitality testing indicating a more organized pulp tissue.

However, even when a tooth is retained in the arch after REP without signs of continued root maturation, it is considered an acceptable outcome because the retained tooth allows alveolar bone growth that would facilitate future implant placement if required [19].

8.3.5 Case Study 2: Long-Term Follow-Up of a Regenerative Endodontic Procedure

Five-year follow-up of an 8-year-old child who presented with a parulis in relation to tooth 11, tenderness and mobility in tooth 11, and history of two episodes of extraoral swelling in relation to the same tooth. The child was treated in the year 2010.

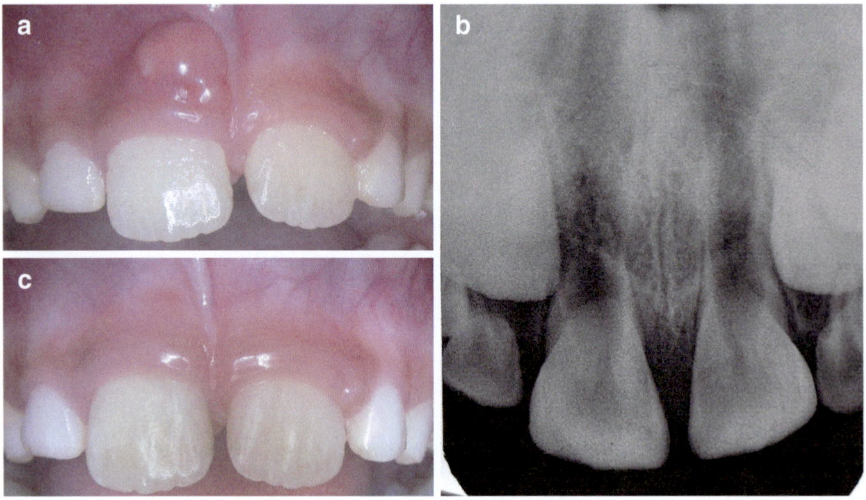

(**a**) Note the parulis in relation to newly erupted tooth 11. (**b**) Radiograph showed that tooth 11 was very immature with only one third root development. (**c**) Clinical view at the beginning of the second appointment showed well-healed gingiva. (**d**) Immediate follow-up radiograph at the end of the second appointment. Note the MTA placed just below the CEJ and the coronal seal. (**e**) One-year follow-up radiograph showed root growth that was lagging behind a little in comparison to tooth 21. (**f**) Five-year follow-up radiograph. Note that tooth 21 is fully mature. While the apical third of tooth 11 appears fully mature with apical closure, the middle third of the root shows lack of maturation and thin dentinal walls. However, there are no signs of apical pathology, and the radicular bone appears healthy. (**g**) Clinical image at the end of 5 years shows healthy gingiva and soft tissue. Tooth 11 appears slightly discolored which could be due to the use of minocycline in the antibiotic paste and the use of MTA as a capping agent

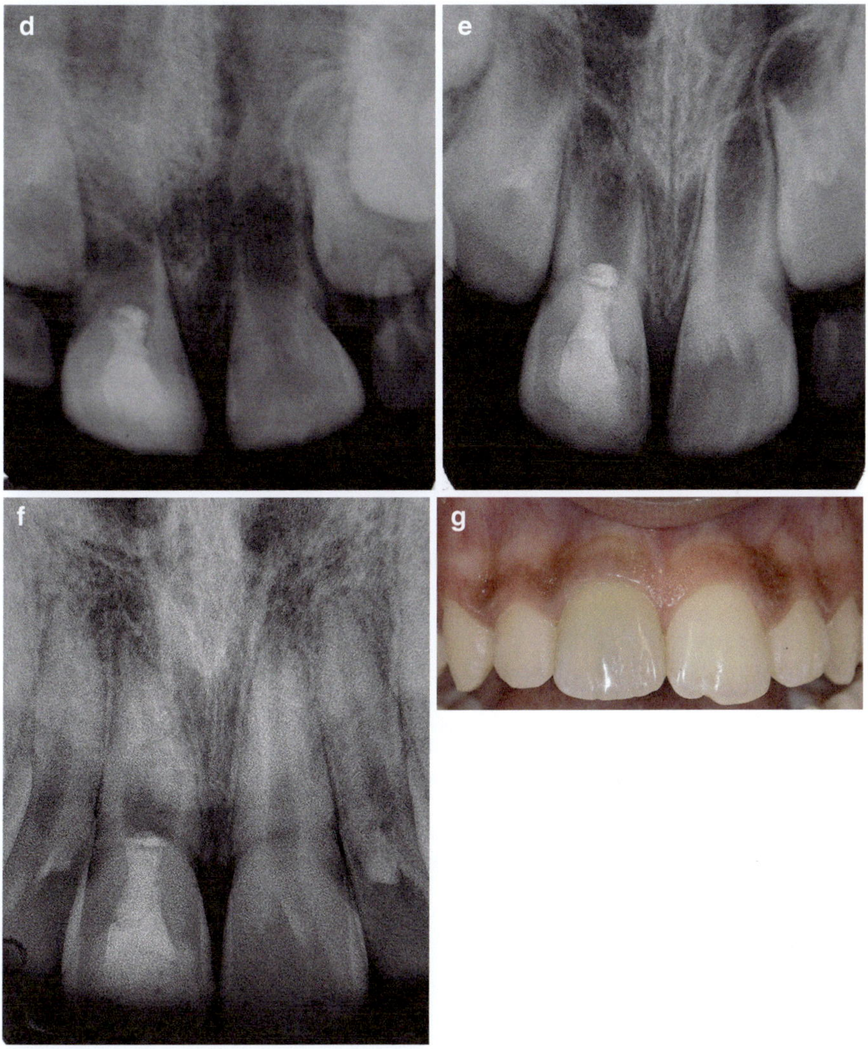

(continued)

Clinical Notes

While a weak and thin middle third of the root leaves the tooth susceptible to fracture, maintaining the tooth in the alveolar bone for as long as possible will allow alveolar bone growth and preserve healthy alveolar bone for successful implant placement in the anterior aesthetic zone in the future. The primary and secondary goals of the regenerative endodontic procedure have been successfully achieved.

8.4 Conclusion

The ideal goal of endodontic procedures in immature permanent teeth is to promote complete root growth to apical closure. Vital pulp therapy aims to remove diseased pulp tissue and preserve healthy pulp tissue to give nature a chance to fulfil this important objective. In non-vital teeth, regenerative endodontic procedures now give us new hope to fulfil this objective. In addition, future research in REP aims to completely regenerate a vital pulp-dentin complex capable of sensory neuronal signaling of tissue damage and mounting an immune response.

References

1. Waterhouse PJ, Whitworth JM, Camp JH, Fuks AB. Pediatric endodontics. In: Hargreaves KM, Cohen S, editors. Cohen's pathways of the pulp. St. Louis, MO: Elsevier; 2011. p. 808–56.
2. Pulp therapy for primary and immature permanent teeth. Pediatr Dent. 2017;39(6):325–33.
3. Bimstein E, Rotstein I. Cvek pulpotomy - revisited. Dent Traumatol. 2016;32(6):438–42. https://doi.org/10.1111/edt.12297.
4. Sigurdsson A, Trope M, Chivian N. The role of endodontics after dental traumatic injuries. In: Hargreaves KM, Cohen S, editors. Cohen's pathways of the pulp. St. Louis, MO: Elsevier; 2011. p. 620–54.
5. Cox CF, Tarim B, Kopel H, Gürel G, Hafez A. Technique sensitivity: biological factors contributing to clinical success with various restorative materials. Adv Dent Res. 2001;15:85–90.
6. Cvek M. A clinical report on partial pulpotomy and capping with calcium hydroxide in permanent incisors with complicated crown fracture. J Endod. 1978;4(8):232–7.
7. Marconyak LJ Jr, Kirkpatrick TC, Roberts HW, Roberts MD, Aparicio A, Himel VT, Sabey KA. A comparison of coronal tooth discoloration elicited by various endodontic reparative materials. J Endod. 2016;42(3):470–3.
8. Możyńska J, Metlerski M, Lipski M, Nowicka A. Tooth discoloration induced by different calcium silicate-based cements: a systematic review of in vitro studies. J Endod. 2017;43(10):1593–601. https://doi.org/10.1016/j.joen.2017.04.002.
9. Akbari M, Rouhani A, Samiee S, Jafarzadeh H. Effect of dentin bonding agent on the prevention of tooth discoloration produced by mineral trioxide aggregate. Int J Dent. 2012;2012:563203. https://doi.org/10.1155/2012/563203.
10. Torabinejad M, Parirokh M, Dummer PMH. Mineral trioxide aggregate and other bioactive endodontic cements: an updated overview – Part II: other clinical applications and complications. Int Endod J. 2018;51:284–317.
11. Linsuwanont P, Wimonsutthikul K, Pothimoke U, Santiwong B. Treatment outcomes of mineral trioxide aggregate pulpotomy in vital permanent teeth with carious pulp exposure: the retrospective study. J Endod. 2017;43(2):225–30. https://doi.org/10.1016/j.joen.2016.10.027.
12. Parirokh M, Torabinejad M, Dummer PMH. Mineral trioxide aggregate and other bioactive endodontic cements: an updated overview – Part I: vital pulp therapy. Int Endod J. 2018;51:177–205.
13. Hilton TJ. Keys to clinical success with pulp capping: a review of the literature. Oper Dent. 2009;34(5):615–25.
14. Wigler R, Kaufman AY, Lin S, Steinbock N, Hazan-Molina H, Torneck CD. Revascularization: a treatment for permanent teeth with necrotic pulp and incomplete root development. J Endod. 2013;39(3):319–26. https://doi.org/10.1016/j.joen.2012.11.014.
15. Murray PE, Garcia-Godoy F, Hargreaves KM. Regenerative endodontics: a review of current status and a call for action. J Endod. 2007;33(4):377–90.

16. Banchs F, Trope M. Revascularization of immature permanent teeth with apical periodontitis: new treatment protocol? J Endod. 2004;30(4):196–200.
17. AAE. Clinical considerations for a regenerative procedure. In: Clinical resources. Regenerative endodontics. 4 January 2018. Chicago, IL: American association of Endodontists; 2018.. https://www.aae.org/specialty/wp-content/uploads/sites/2/2018/06/ConsiderationsForRegEndo_AsOfApril2018.pdf. Accessed 2 Oct 2018.
18. Sedgley CM, Cherkas P, Chogle SMA, Geisler TM, Hargreaves KM, Paranjpe AK, Yamagishi VT-K. Regenerative endodontics. In: Endodontics colleagues for excellence: American Association of Endodontists. Spring 2013. Chicago, IL: American association of Endodontists; 2013.. https://www.aae.org/specialty/wp-content/uploads/sites/2/2017/06/ecfespring2013.pdf. Accessed 1 Oct 2018.
19. Law AS. Considerations for regeneration procedures. Pediatr Dent. 2013;35(2):141–52.
20. Galler KM, D'Souza RN, Federlin M, Cavender AC, Hartgerink JD, Hecker S, Schmalz G. Dentin conditioning codetermines cell fate in regenerative endodontics. J Endod. 2011;37(11):1536–41. https://doi.org/10.1016/j.joen.2011.08.027.

MIX
Papier aus verantwortungsvollen Quellen
Paper from responsible sources
FSC® C105338

If you have any concerns about our products,
you can contact us on
ProductSafety@springernature.com

In case Publisher is established outside the EU,
the EU authorized representative is:
Springer Nature Customer Service Center GmbH
Europaplatz 3, 69115 Heidelberg, Germany

Printed by Libri Plureos GmbH
in Hamburg, Germany